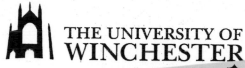

THE UNIVERSITY OF WINCHESTER

HEALTH CARE IN THE CITIES

HEALTH CARE IN BIG CITIES

Edited by LESLIE H.W. PAINE

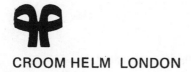

CROOM HELM LONDON

© 1978 International Hospital Federation
Croom Helm, 2-10 St John's Road, London SW11

British Library Cataloguing in Publication Data

Health care in big cities.
  1. Medical care. 2. Cities and towns
  I. Paine, Leslie Harold William
  362.1'09173'2   RA394

ISBN 0–85664–590–7

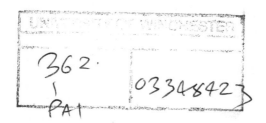

Printed in Great Britain by Biddles Ltd, Guildford, Surrey

CONTENTS

ACKNOWLEDGEMENTS

There are many people to whom debts of gratitude are owed for their help towards the preparation of this book.

First of all, to the Trustees of the City Parochial Foundation in London, whose grant enabled the project to get started.

Then to the individuals and organisations in each of the cities concerned, whose efforts represented a very considerable expenditure of time, skill and money from their own resources.

To Dr George Cust (Chief Medical Officer of the Health Education Council in London), who compiled the comparative statistical tables from the varied data supplied by each city.

And last but not least to Dr R.F. Bridgman (formerly Inspector-General of Social Affairs, Paris; and formerly Chief Medical Officer, Organisation of Medical Care, World Health Organisation, Geneva), who chaired all the 'big cities' sessions at the Tokyo Congress and who gave much help and advice during the course of the project.

The International Hospital Federation is deeply grateful to this wide circle of friends and helpers for their contributions in what it is hoped will be a continuing exchange of information and ideas between these and other cities.

ACKNOWLEDGEMENTS

FOREWORD

R.F. Bridgman

The structure and organisation of the health services in big cities with
more than a million inhabitants are dependent on many historical,
political and socio-economic factors which must be analysed to enable
us to control their future development. Perhaps we should remind
ourselves that, if the big city is not a really new phenomenon — Rome,
Peking and Constantinople were very big cities in the past — many big
cities of today have experienced very rapid growth since the beginning
of the century and the number of large urban centres throughout the
world will rise before the century ends. This phenomenon is even more
important in several of the developing countries and is creating
problems which these countries are ill prepared to solve. The reader will
notice that the term 'large urban centres' was used above instead of
the previous 'big cities'. This is because, in many countries, the
authorities are trying to limit the growth of the urbanised centre
constituted by the town proper as an administrative and geographic
entity. Sometimes this centre, which represents the historic nucleus,
is even becoming slowly depopulated, as we can see in Paris and several
large American cities. But the urban area around it, whether it has
developed rather chaotically in the form of unorganised suburban
sprawl, or whether it has been possible to structure it to some extent
in the recent form of satellite towns or conurbations, is in most cases
growing at a very rapid rate. Now the whole urbanised area is mostly
administered by a mosaic of local authorities, which means immediately
that some co-ordinating agency is necessary; and this is all the more
indispensable if the big city is the capital of a region with a total
population of considerably more than the two million generally
recognised as the optimum for regional administration. Thus the
regions with Tokyo, New York or Paris as their capital are approaching
or have even gone beyond ten million inhabitants.

In many countries, health service administration has always been
in the hands of the local authorities and private enterprise, both profit-
and non-profit-making. It is not surprising that the health services,
considered as systems which attempts are now being made to analyse,
are particularly complex, little known and poorly co-ordinated, made
up as they are of public and private curative institutions, preventive

medicine services, environmental health services and liberal professions represented by doctors, pharmacists, dentists, nurses and other members of the paramedical professions. The cost of these services has made it necessary to introduce various financing procedures, taking the form generally of social insurance, often distinct from the governmental authorities. There are also certain specific sectors such as the organisation of emergency care, psychiatric services, ambulatory care services, both preventive and curative, the rehabilitation of the physically handicapped, home care, care of the elderly, etc

● If we can now discover, thanks to the new methods of analysis at our disposal, the met demand for medical care — provided the private institutions co-operate — it is more difficult to measure potential demand and even harder to assess the medical care needs of the population. In the great conurbations with a very heterogeneous population from the points of view of demographic composition, standard of living and financial capabilities, needs vary considerably with the different socio-professional groups. Knowledge of these needs is still very fragmentary.

Among the most urgent problems facing the public authorities today is the distribution of the hospitals throughout the conurbation. For clear historical reasons, most of them were built in the old city centre and on its immediate periphery, which is completely built up today. It follows that there is now an excessive concentration of facilities in a restricted area which is nearly impenetrable to means of communication, contrasting with a shortage of facilities in the outer belt and in the satellite towns. This unevenness of distribution may be observed also in the medical staff, since most of the specialists, working at least partly in the hospitals, are concentrated in the heart of the towns. In addition, the fact that, in many cases, the preventive services are in the hands of the local authorities, the political tendencies and financial resources of which vary considerably, causes great inequalities in distribution and efficiency.

Let is imagine that we have complete knowledge of the met demand — by area, by age group, by sex, by socio-professional group, and that the planners can therefore work out a reasonably correct assessment of needs. Then the construction of a network of hospitals capable of meeting these needs has many prerequisites. The sites on which future hospitals will be built will have to be reserved long in advance, decisions will have to be taken on long-term spatial and financial planning, the necessary staff will have to be provided and trained and the over-all running costs will have to be estimated. In fact, many years have to pass between the initial decision to set up a large new hospital and its opening. The problem is further complicated, in big cities, by the fact that the health services make a contribution to medical education and research, and this makes co-ordination absolutely necessary inside the governmental authorities.

These considerations all come down to a recommendation for the strengthening of the research, planning and co-ordinating agencies, which can lead to a centralisation of authority. But one must know when to stop! And this must be before such a rigid authoritarianism has been imposed that it is impossible to adjust to the changes coming in all spheres and that local initiative, both public and private, is stifled.

We should, therefore, encourage the International Hospital Federation which, with the help of other organisations, has had the great merit of recognising the size of the problem and undertaking to study it at its twentieth congress. The volume and diversity of the preparatory documents and papers relating to many contemporary big cities have shown the complexity of the problem. Despite the accumulation of statistical data, often difficult to interpret and compare, we find that our knowledge of the situation is very poor and that we cannot fully control its future development. This book is only one stage in a long-term research programme. It is essential to pursue these studies on the basis of a clear plan in order to arrive at solutions that will be applicable and rational.

To persist either in improvising or in trying to adapt often outdated systems to the rapid changes being experienced by the great conurbations would lead to unmitigated failure. Without guiding principles based on a clear formulation of the problem, one would only be perpetuating a situation which is already fairly chaotic; and this would end in an unbearable financial burden and a squandering of resources in men and materials.

There is no doubt that in our century the health of urban populations has improved to the point where it is much better than that of their rural counterparts. But setting aside the positive activities of the environmental health services which have produced spectacular results in the field of communicable diseases, what are the respective contributions made by the curative services and by the improvement in living standards as seen in housing, nutrition, personal hygiene and general education? No one can answer this vital question at present. The health services are too extravagant in staff and money ever to hope to obtain the necessary resources to develop, even to survive, if they cannot provide proof of their efficiency.

We must therefore hope that the initial efforts of the International Hospital Federation, the results of which appear on the pages that follow, may be pursued and result in a methodology for the study and planning of health services in big cities.

INTRODUCTION

Miles Hardie

By the end of this century perhaps half the world's population will be
city-dwellers, and the number of cities with over a million population
will have increased to over 270, as compared with 75 in 1950. Few
people feel that the quality of city life is improving, and many fear
that standards of physical and mental health may fall rather than rise
as city populations expand or city centres decline.

In rural and urban areas alike, the improvement of health standards
depends upon many things beside the development of health services.
Housing, sanitation, nutrition, transport, education, wage levels and
pensions are just some of the factors that have a profound influence
upon the health of any population. Political, social and economic
change will often have far greater effect in improving health standards
than changes in the organisation and management of health services.
Increasing attention is being paid world-wide to problems of health
care in rural areas; in many cities, the problems of maintaining and
improving health standards and health services can also be acute.

It was against this background that late in 1974 the International
Hospital Federation (IHF) decided to initiate a project aimed at
promoting the exchange of information and ideas between policy-
makers, planners and managers in a number of big cities on
problems and progress in improving health standards and developing
more effective health and social services, particularly for the more
disadvantaged sections of the community. The over-all objectives of
the project were defined as being, first, to identify some of the main
problems influencing the improvement of health standards and the
development of health services in some of the big cities of the world;
second, to collect, collate and disseminate information about the
organisation of health care in these cities and about the good ideas and
practices that have been introduced, or are planned, to help overcome
some of the main problems; and third, through the medium of the
IHF congress in Tokyo in May 1977, and through other conferences
and workshops or projects, to promote the exchange of information
and ideas on this topic and to stimulate discussion and action to
improve health standards and health services.

The project was launched in November 1974 with the help of a grant from the City Parochial Foundation in London. It was agreed from the outset that the project should not be treated as a purely theoretical academic exercise, but rather as a review of problems and progress which it was hoped would be of practical help to those engaged in the planning and provision of health services and in the improvement of standards of health. It was also emphasised that the project was not intended or expected to provide complete definitive answers to the problems of big cities in a short space of time, but that it should be considered rather as a reconnaissance or exploration, an attempt to identify some of the problems that need further study, to illustrate some of the ways in which some cities have been able to mitigate or overcome some of the problems that beset them, and to find out whether there are lessons that cities can usefully learn from each other about the planning and management of their health services, despite obvious differences in economic, social and other factors.

The chapters of this book represent first of all the general descriptive papers that the participating cities prepared as background material for publication in the IHF quarterly journal *World Hospitals* prior to the Tokyo congress, together with the papers that were given at the congress itself on particular aspects of health services.

For the descriptive papers, each city was asked to provide a two-part statement, one part giving factual information about the existing health services of the city, covering demographic and other data, planning and organisation, finance, community participation and health-related agencies, and the other part giving some facts and opinions under three main headings: some of the main problems affecting the planning and provision of health services in the city; some of the good ideas in planning and provision in the city that other big cities might usefully study, adopt or adapt for themselves; some of the changes in planning and provision, and some of the studies or experiments, that might be discussed or implemented to help promote improvement in health standards and health services in the city. When submitting these papers, each city was asked to indicate which aspects of its health services it would like to suggest as possible choices for presentation and discussion at the congress, and it was from these suggestions that the final selection of topics was made for the congress programme.

Within the constraints of time, money and staff available, both for the IHF and for the participating cities, to develop the project, it was not practicable to have all the information received from each city reorganised and presented in identical format. Nor indeed was it considered desirable, at this exploratory stage of the project, to try to impose a rigid pattern of presentation upon each city, but rather to let each tell its own story in its own way, and then to use this basic information as a springboard for future collaborative study and action. And this in fact is what has been happening. Further initiatives are developing: a project concerned with the collection and dissemination of information on good ideas and practices in mental health in urban areas has started from a London base with support from two British foundations; a consortium of European cities is developing a project on health care planning in urban areas; a study on aspects of primary care in big cities is at a pilot stage, and different aspects of big city health services are in the programme of several IHF regional conferences and workshops.

There is no shortage of problems that need resolving, and the scope for study and action is enormous. There is also scope for publicising more widely what is going well in health care in big cities: too many good ideas are born to blush unseen, or at any rate to exist unheeded by all but a few. There is much that cities can learn by sharing their problems and their successes. The purpose of this book is therefore to inform, to explore and to stimulate: to spread information about present patterns of 'big city' health services; to encourage further exploration of problems and possible solutions in the development of these services; to stimulate a greater exchange of information and ideas within and between big cities. The IHF will be glad to hear from any readers interested in promoting further collaboration between cities with the aim of improving standards of health and health services.

PART ONE:
HEALTH SERVICES IN BIG CITIES

1 LONDON

Miles Hardie

A. THE PATTERN OF EXISTING SERVICES

Introduction

Health services for the 7.2 million people living in the 610 square miles of Greater London are provided as part of the country's National Health Service (NHS). The NHS was created by legislation in 1946 which aimed to promote 'the establishment in England and Wales of a comprehensive health service, designed to secure improvement in the physical and mental health of the people of England and Wales, and the prevention, diagnosis and treatment of illness'. Through this legislation, which came into force on 5 July 1948, the Minister of Health was made responsible to Parliament for seeing that health services of every kind were made available to everyone in the country.

Under the NHS, the essential freedoms have been safeguarded, for the public is free to use the service or not. The patient is free to choose his family doctor (usually termed general practitioner or GP) and to change to another if he wishes to do so. The doctor is free from interference in his clinical judgement, and may accept private patients while taking part in the service. The service is available free of charge at the time of use to all residents in London (and in the rest of Britain) according to their medical need, except that certain small charges are made for some items. For the patient, access to the medical services of the NHS in London and elsewhere in the country is through the GP with whom he has chosen to register. Except in the case of accident or emergency, access to hospital services may only be arranged through the GP, and not direct by the patient.

Organisation

From 1948 to 1974, the NHS was administered in three parts — the hospital and specialist services, the general practitioner services and the local authority services. Under the NHS Reorganisation Act of 1973 these services were unified. For England and Wales, there are now just over 100 regional and area health authorities in place of over 600 boards, committees and councils that had previously been responsible for them. For London and its environs, there are four metropolitan regional health authorities, within whose boundaries there are in Greater London itself 16 areas comprising 36 districts, as outlined in Figure 1.1. Within Greater London there are nearly 300 hospitals with a total of about 75,000 beds (i.e. almost 10 beds per 1,000 population): other basic statistics about health and health services in London are shown in Appendix A at the end of this chapter. The 1973 Act came into force on 1 April 1974 and provides for four levels of planning and administration: central strategic planning and monitoring by the Department of Health and Social Security; regional planning and general supervision of operation by regional health authorities (RHAs); area planning and operational control by area health authorities (AHAs); local day-to-day planning and running of the services in health districts by district management teams (DMTs). Figure 1.2 shows the relationships between these four levels. At each level there are various professional advisory committees, of which the Medical Advisory Committees are the most influential.

The Department of Health and Social Security (DHSS)

The DHSS has over-all responsibility for the planning and operation of London's health services within the NHS. The DHSS came into being on 1 November 1968 as an amalgamation of the Ministry of Health (first established in 1919) and the Ministry of Social Security. The section dealing with health has a staff of about 7,500 people, and is mainly a central supervisory department for the general organisation, planning and financing of the health and welfare services. The Secretary of State for Social Services is the head of the DHSS: this is a political appointment, as are those of the Minister of State and the Parliamentary Under-Secretary of State (Health) and the Parliamentary Under-Secretary of State (Social Security). The two senior permanent officials of the DHSS are the Permanent Secretary and the Chief Medical Officer: these are both members of the Civil Service, as are the rest of the staff of the DHSS. But none of the staff employed by regional and area authorities in the NHS are civil servants. Within the DHSS there are officers who have a particular responsibility for helping to co-ordinate health services in London, working in close collaboration with the regional and area authorities in London.

Regional Health Authorities (RHAs)

There are four metropolitan RHAs for the geographical area of London and its environs. These RHAs are responsible for a population totalling

Figure 1.1: The NHS Boundaries within the Greater London Area

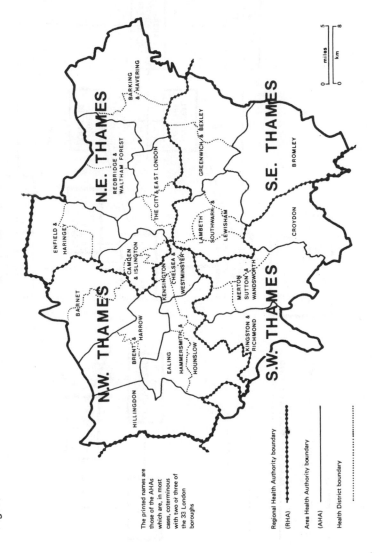

The printed names are those of the AHAs which are, in most cases, coterminous with two or three of the 33 London boroughs

N.E. THAMES

BARKING & HAVERING

REDBRIDGE & WALTHAM FOREST

THE CITY & EAST LONDON

GREENWICH & BEXLEY

S.E. THAMES

BROMLEY

ENFIELD & HARINGEY

LAMBETH

SOUTHWARK &

LEWISHAM

CROYDON

CAMDEN & ISLINGTON

KENSINGTON &

CHELSEA &

WESTMINSTER

BARNET

MERTON

SUTTON &

WANDSWORTH

N.W. THAMES

BRENT & HARROW

KINGSTON & RICHMOND

HILLINGDON

EALING

HAMMERSMITH &

HOUNSLOW

S.W. THAMES

miles 5
km 8
0
0

Regional Health Authority boundary

(RHA)

Area Health Authority boundary

(AHA)

Health District boundary

Figure 1.2: Relationship between the Four Levels of Metropolitan Regional Health Authorities

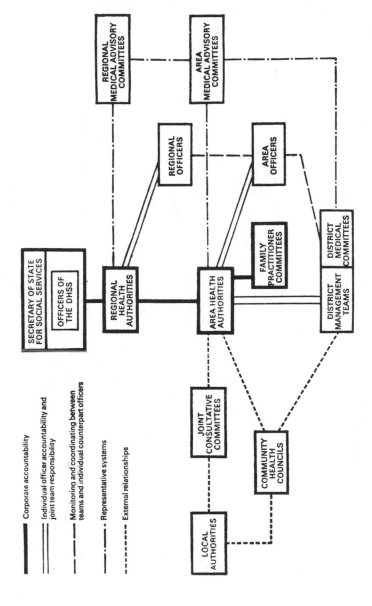

Figure 1.3: Structure of the Area Health Authority

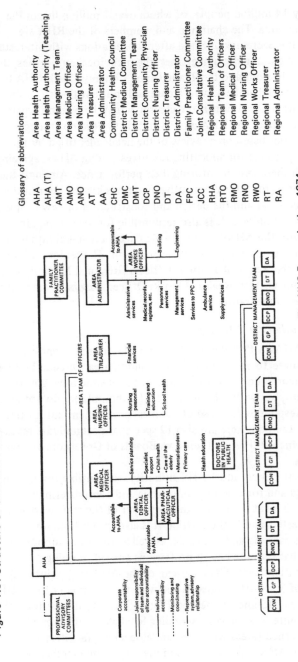

Glossary of abbreviations

AHA	Area Health Authority
AHA (T)	Area Health Authority (Teaching)
AMT	Area Management Team
AMO	Area Medical Officer
ANO	Area Nursing Officer
AT	Area Treasurer
AA	Area Administrator
CHC	Community Health Council
DMC	District Medical Committee
DMT	District Management Team
DCP	District Community Physician
DNO	District Nursing Officer
DT	District Treasurer
DA	District Administrator
FPC	Family Practitioner Committee
JCC	Joint Consultative Committee
RHA	Regional Health Authority
RTO	Regional Team of Officers
RMO	Regional Medical Officer
RNO	Regional Nursing Officer
RWO	Regional Works Officer
RT	Regional Treasurer
RA	Regional Administrator

Source: Reproduced from Office of Health Economics publication *The NHS Reorganisation*, 1974

approximately 14 million people, of whom over 7 million live in the Greater London area. The chairman and members of the RHA are appointed by the Secretary of State after consultations with interested organisations, including the universities, the main local authorities, the main health professions and the Trade Union Congress. Each RHA has between 15 and 20 members, who are unpaid (but entitled to travelling and other allowances), although the chairman may be paid on a part-time basis. The role of the RHA and its staff is to develop strategic plans and priorities based on a review of the needs identified by the AHAs. It is responsible for allocating resources among AHAs, agreeing area plans with them and monitoring their performance. Amongst the most important of the RHAs' executive functions are the distribution of medical manpower and the design and construction of new hospitals and other health buildings. It is also responsible for identifying, in consultation with the AHAs, services which need a regional rather than an area approach and arranges for their provision. The senior staff of the RHA form the Regional Team of Officers (Regional Medical Officer, Regional Nursing Officer, Regional Works Officer, Regional Treasurer and Regional Administrator).

Area Health Authorities (AHAs)

There are 23 AHAs within the boundaries of the four metropolitan RHAs and of these 16 cover the Greater London area. Outside London, the AHA boundaries coincide with those of the elected local government authorities, but within London the AHA boundaries do not in every case correspond with those of the local government authorities (boroughs). In London there are also 12 specialist postgraduate teaching hospitals which still retain their own Boards of Governors separate from any AHA.

The AHA is the operational NHS authority, responsible for assessing needs in its area and for planning, organising and administering area health services to meet them. It is the employer of the staff who work at area headquarters and in the district. It is also responsible for services such as catering and domestic, as well as for other supportive services which back up the health professions and, in so doing, contribute to patient care. The chairman of the AHA is appointed by the Secretary of State after consultation with the chairman of the RHA. There are between 15 and 25 members for each AHA, at least four of whom are appointed by the corresponding local authorities, one by the university concerned (areas with substantial teaching facilities are administered by AHAs (Teaching)) and the remaining members are appointed by the RHA after consultation with the main professions, the trade unions and other organisations. An AHA always includes doctors and at least one nurse or midwife, but otherwise the proportion of professional members is not prescribed. Members are unpaid (but entitled to travelling and other allowances) but the chairman may be paid on a part-time basis. Figure 1.3 shows the structure of the AHA. Associated with each AHA is a Family Practitioner Committee (FPC). The FPC consists of 30 members appointed by the AHA, with half the members nominated by the doctors in the area, and each FPC is responsible to the AHA for the administration of the general medical, dental, ophthalmic and pharmaceutical services for the area. The senior paid staff of the AHA form the Area Team of Officers (Area Medical Officer, Area Nursing Officer, Area Treasurer and Area Administrator).

Health Districts

There are 36 health districts within the 16 areas covering the Greater London area. These districts are responsible for the day-to-day running of the services. Each district contains a district general hospital (DGH) and in London 12 of the DGHs are also teaching hospitals for the undergraduate training of medical students. There is no statutory authority at district level, as there is at area or region, and responsibility for the day-to-day operation of the services at district level lies with the district management team (DMT) of about six senior paid staff (District Administrator, District Treasurer, District Nursing Officer, District Community Physician and members of the District Medical Committee). At district level there are also health care planning teams whose function is to determine health care needs of groups of patients (e.g. elderly, mentally ill, mentally handicapped children, etc.) or to look at particular problems (e.g. review of primary care services, reorganisation of out-patient department, etc.).

London Ambulance Service

Two important services organised on an all-London basis are the London Ambulance Service (LAS) and the Emergency Bed Service (EBS). The LAS looks after the eight million people who live in Greater London or who visit or come to work in the capital each day. The present service had its beginning in 1965 when the nine services in the area were amalgamated into a single unit, responsible for conveying some three million patients a year to and from 400 different hospitals and clinics. Since April 1974 the South West Thames Regional Health Authority has taken over administrative responsibility

for the LAS with its 1,000 vehicles based at 78 stations with some
2,500 operational and control staff. The work of the LAS falls into
two categories – the emergency service, which deals with around 1,500
calls a day, and the non-urgent service which undertakes some 9,000
journeys a day conveying patients to and from treatment at hospital
or clinic. The cost of the LAS is covered by the NHS, so that no direct
charges are made to any patient using the service.

King's Fund Emergency Bed Service

The Emergency Bed Service, often called the EBS for short, is available to general practitioners for arranging urgent admissions to hospital,
mainly in the Greater London area. It is administered by King
Edward's Hospital Fund for London as agent of the four metropolitan
regional health authorities, and it supplements the normal practice
whereby the general practitioner makes arrangements direct with the
hospital of his choice. The EBS operates continuously day and night,
throughout the year, and arranges over 40,000 admissions annually.
It can save time for the general practitioner and his patient, and can
ensure that the nearest suitable hospital accepts responsibility for the
patient, by means of a procedure devised in co-operation with the
regional health authorities, involving medical referees appointed with
districts. Though not an information bureau for the general public,
the EBS is also a source of information for anyone responsible for a
matter concerning the admission of patients to hospital.

Other NHS Services

There are a number of other important NHS services that are linked
with the regional, area and district services, such as the Public Health
Laboratory Service, which provides a network of bacteriological and
virological laboratories to help in the diagnosis, prevention and control
of infectious diseases, and the Blood Transfusion Service, which is
organised regionally to collect blood from voluntary donors and supply
it to hospitals (no fee is paid to the donor; no charge is made to the
recipient).

Community Participation

Community Health Councils

A completely new feature of the reorganised NHS is the establishment
of Community Health Councils (CHCs). These CHCs are intended to
represent the views of the consumer. There is one for each of an area's

health districts. Half the members of the council are appointed by the
local authorities of which the area, or part of it, is included in the
CHC's district, at least one-third by voluntary bodies concerned locally
with the NHS and the remainder by the RHA after consultation with
other organisations. The number of members varies according to local
circumstances, but there are usually between 20 and 30. Members are
unpaid, but entitled to travelling and other expenses. Councils appoint
their own chairmen from among their members, and employ a paid
secretary and supporting staff.

The council's basic statutory job is to represent to the AHA the
interests of the public in the health service in its district. Councils have
powers to secure information, to visit hospitals and other institutions,
and have access to the AHA and in particular to its senior officers
administering the district services. Councils may bring to the notice of
the AHA potential causes of local complaints, but their function is
distinct from that of the AHA's complaints machinery and of the
Health Service Commissioner. The AHA is required to consult the
council(s) on its plans for health service developments — e.g. closure
of hospitals or departments of hospitals, or their change of use — and
may put forward alternative plans. The full AHA meets representatives
of all its councils at least once a year. The council publishes an annual
report (and may publish other reports) and the AHA is required to
publish replies recording action taken on the issues raised.

Voluntary Services

Under the new arrangements, voluntary bodies, which have always
played an important part in the development of the health and
welfare services, are being encouraged, in close co-operation with
the area health and local authorities, to increase and extend their
activities. Membership of Community Health Councils helps to
provide another way in which volunteers and other members of the
community can help to influence the way in which the health services
are developed. The recent growth in the number of organisers co-
ordinating voluntary help in hospital will continue and this method of
co-ordination is being extended to the wider field of voluntary work
in the community. The RHAs and AHAs are able to make grants in
support of voluntary bodies which provide and promote services
within the general scope of the authorities' responsibilities. Financial
help for national activities continues to come from the central
DHSS. As all this voluntary activity develops, it is important to
emphasise that the role of volunteers is no longer seen as being to plug

gaps in the welfare state, but rather to complement and enrich the quality of life for people in need, whether they are living in their own homes or in hospital or in any form of residential care, and also to pioneer new ideas and to develop in the hospital and its neighbourhood a real sense of community involvement in the services which as tax-payers or ratepayers they largely finance.

Finance

Costs and Charges

The facilities and services provided under the NHS in London and the rest of the country are financed by the government through the DHSS. The money to pay for the NHS is raised mainly through general taxation on the whole population. Patients using the services of the NHS make no direct payment to the doctor at any time, but there is a small charge paid by most patients for prescriptions for medicines, etc., and for dental treatment and spectacles: only about 5 per cent of the cost of the NHS is recovered from patients in this way.

Budgeting

There is an annual cycle of estimating and budgeting to meet the cost of the NHS. Each district is responsible for preparing annual estimates of the funds required to run its health services. These estimates are collated and vetted first at area level and then at regional level before being submitted to the DHSS. Each year the government decides at national level how much money is to be allocated to the DHSS for the NHS as a whole. Once that decision is taken, the DHSS then allocates funds to each region in relation to its estimates, and each region then makes allocations to areas and thence from areas to districts. It is largely through this well-defined system of annual allocation and budgeting control that the government exercises over-all authority over the pace and direction of the development of the NHS.

Payment of Doctors and Other Staff

Doctors in London and elsewhere in the country are paid either on a capitation basis in the case of GPs, or on a full-time or part-time salaried basis in the case of hospital doctors. There is very little fee-for-service method of payment within the NHS. The rates of pay for doctors are determined by review and negotiation at national level and are applied nationally. Most other Health Service staff are paid salaries or wages on a full-time or part-time basis. As in the case of

doctors, their rates of pay are determined at national level and applied
nationally, although for most staff working in London there is a special
extra allowance made to compensate for the higher cost of living in
London.

Private Medical Services

General practitioners and part-time hospital consultants working for
the NHS may have private practice as well, and there are over 3,000
private beds in London (compared with a total of 75,000 NHS beds).
There are also a number of private insurance schemes providing cover
mostly for short-term acute illness. About 2 per cent of the population
are insured under such schemes giving limited coverage to about 4 per
cent of the population, and the benefits provided amount to about 1
per cent of the total expenditure on the NHS.

Planning

The Planning Cycle

The proposed planning cycle over one financial year is divided
notionally into four quarters. The first involves a flow upwards from
district level of information on patterns of need and opportunities for
change; the second period is used to pass down formal planning guidelines from DHSS and RHA to AHA and to set forward planning
allocations; in the third period, AHAs and DMTs prepare plans in the
light of the guidelines and allocations, and the fourth and final period
is used to pass these plans upwards for review, approval and consolidation by RHAs and the DHSS into the national NHS plan. Through the
mechanisms of financial authority over capital and revenue spending
by the DHSS and the regional and area authorities, there is close control
over the preparation and implementation of policies and plans for the
development of buildings and distribution of staff.

Distribution of Staff

About 70 per cent of the total cost of health services in London goes
on staff of all categories. For doctors, a reasonably fair distribution
has been achieved through the control of the number and allocation of
hospital doctors by RHAs and of GPs by the Family Practitioner
Committees of the AHAs, which have powers to bar doctors from
moving into relatively over-doctored areas and to offer incentives for
additional doctors to move into relatively under-doctored areas. For
other staff, numbers and allocation are agreed annually as part of the

planning and budgeting process.

Epidemiology, Statistics and Social Medicine

Successful planning depends increasingly upon the provision of accurate epidemiological information and statistical and other data on a wide range of topics. A wealth of such material is regularly collected through the official channels of the DHSS, Greater London Council (GLC) and health and social service authorities in London, including medical schools and university departments. Much remains to be done to ensure the effective use of all this material for the purposes of planning, management and research, but a significant trend of recent years has been the growth and development of departments of epidemiology and social medicine in London and elsewhere, and of statistical/intelligence departments in the DHSS, GLC, RHAs, AHAs and the London boroughs. Such departments are likely to become increasingly important in relation to health planning and management in London and else-where.

Health-Related Agencies

Standards of Health

It is recognised that the improvement of health standards depends upon many things besides the development of health services. Political, social and economic change will often have far greater effect in improving health standards than changes in the organisation and management of health services. Housing, sanitation, nutrition, transport, education, wage-levels and pensions are just some of the factors that have a pro-found influence upon the health of any population. In London, some of these health-related factors come within the orbit of the GLC and the London boroughs.

Greater London Council

The GLC is the strategic planning authority for Greater London as a whole, working closely with the 32 London borough councils and the City of London Corporation which are the local planning authorities for their own areas. Boroughs draw up local plans and review applications for development within the context of the Greater London Development Plan, the strategic plan for which the GLC is responsible. There are no formal consultative links between the GLC and DHSS, though in the preparation of the Development Plan there were informal consultations between the two bodies.

The GLC is also an executive authority at the strategic level, for example, providing a regional refuse disposal service, being responsible for the London Fire Brigade, and managing a stock of 200,000 dwellings. The Inner London Education Authority is a special, virtually autonomous committee of the GLC, and the GLC is responsible for the policy and financial control of the bus and underground services operated by the London Transport Executive.

Other London Authorities

There are a number of other authorities that have responsibility for matters having a direct or indirect bearing on standards of health, such as the Thames Water Authority, Port of London Authority and the British Airports Authority. Likewise there are a number of central government departments whose policies have a direct influence on the well-being of Londoners, such as the Department of the Environment, on housing, transport or pollution; the Department of Employment and Productivity, on health and safety at work; the Department of Education and Science and various other departments. These bodies have informal links with each other and with the GLC and DHSS, but there is no formal consultative machinery between them specifically related to the preparation of over-all policies and comprehensive plans aimed at improving the standard of health of the population of London.

London Boroughs

The most obvious efforts to integrate health services with health-related services occur at AHA level. Figure 1.2 shows the advisory link with local authorities (or London boroughs) at this level through the Joint Consultative Committees whose job it is to co-ordinate policies. The London borough services represented at this committee are the Social Services and Environmental Health Services. AHAs have obligations to the Inner London Education Authority and individual boroughs in relation to such fields as education and housing, and therefore also participate mutually in policy-making. There is also an indirect promotion of co-ordinated policy-making in the form of appointments: some AHA members are London borough appointees and there are community physicians attached to the borough Environmental Services, which have a very important part to play in monitoring and improving standards of health.

Particularly important are the formal and informal links between AHAs and health districts on the one hand and the social service departments of the London boroughs on the other. Under the new arrangements of the reorganised NHS, as under the old, health service costs are met mainly through central government funds from tax revenue. Social services, on the other hand, are planned and controlled by local government authorities and their costs are met mainly through local government funds. Although separately financed, it is very important that health and social services should be planned jointly, particularly for the old, the mentally ill and mentally handicapped. There is therefore under the 1973 Act a statutory responsibility for area health authorities to collaborate in planning with their corresponding local government authorities. Co-operation in this field is vital to the success of the reorganised NHS.

B. THE FUTURE DEVELOPMENT OF HEALTH SERVICES IN LONDON: THE IHF PROJECT

1. The Preparation of the Survey

Following the launching of the International Hospital Federation 'Big Cities' project in November 1974, Mr John Lloyd, at that time a health services planner with the firm of Llewelyn-Davies Weeks, Forestier-Walker and Bor, was appointed as a project officer on a part-time basis for the first stage of the project, and a small steering committee (see Appendix B) was appointed to help guide the London study.

At an early meeting, the steering committee agreed that the London study should start with a Delphi-style* survey involving a number of people, inside and outside the National Health Service (NHS), with knowledge and experience relevant to the problems of London. At the time the project started, the NHS in London, as in the rest of Britain, was in the throes of adjusting to major reorganisation. It was therefore recognised that particular tact and understanding would be needed to secure the co-operation of overburdened staff at every level of the NHS, and that every effort should be made to explain and ensure that the results of the survey should eventually be of real practical value to patients and staff in London. For the same reason it was agreed that the questionnaire to be used in the survey should be as simple and

---

* The Delphi technique aims at co-ordinating the opinions of a group of experts on the likely direction of future development. The technique employs the following features: anonymous replies from a group of experts whose members should have no contact with each other while the survey is being conducted; systematic processing of the replies; feedback of analysis of replies to the panel in one or more subsequent rounds; production of final report.

painless to fill in as possible.

In pursuit of this policy, an initial approach was made personally by telephone to a handful of contacts at the Department of Health and Social Security and Greater London Council and at regional, area and district level in the London area. This was followed up by a letter explaining the project in more detail, enclosing first drafts of the questionnaire and supporting papers, and arranging for a meeting with the project officer to discuss the drafts. These meetings proved to be very useful and constructive. After hearing a report on them from the project officer, the members of the steering committee decided to make substantial revisions to the draft questionnaire and then agreed to try to write replies to the revised version themselves. The answering of this pilot questionnaire also proved to be a very valuable exercise: first, the answers given by each member from his or her own particular viewpoint provided a wide variety of constructive comments about London that helped to convince the steering committee of the potential usefulness of the whole project; and second, the experience of trying to answer the questions themselves led the members to agree on a further revision of the questionnaire and supporting papers for use in the next stage of the study. For the final version of the main questionnaire (see Appendix C), three main headings were chosen and the questions themselves were made open-ended:

(a)   What are some of the *main problems* that seem to you to be currently affecting the planning and provision of health services in London?

(b)   What are the *good ideas and practices* in London that you think other big cities might usefully study, adopt or adapt for themselves?

(c)   What *changes in planning and provision*, or what *studies and experiments*, do you think might most usefully be undertaken to promote improvement in health standards and health services in London?

Selection of Participants

With the preparation of the main questionnaire completed, the next step was to decide who was to be invited to participate in the Delphi survey. It was agreed that the aim should be to get replies from a panel of about 80 people: it was felt that this number should provide for a fair spread of opinion without making the task of collation and analysis too daunting. It was also agreed that the participants should comprise a balance of representatives between five main categories:

(1)   official NHS authorities;
(2)   central and local government authorities outside the NHS;
(3)   voluntary organisations and consumer groups;
(4)   academic departments and research organisations;
(5)   other individuals thought likely to offer a useful viewpoint.

The panel was chosen by the 'expanding nucleus' technique used in earlier Delphi surveys, starting with a small number of people from the different categories known to have expert knowledge and to be generally forward-looking. These were invited to participate and to suggest others who might also be invited. These were approached in similar fashion and the process continued until it was clear that the panel was becoming sufficiently large and representative. Eventually about 110 people were listed of whom 83 agreed to take part and 76 completed the questionnaire. A draft report was prepared and circulated to the participants for comment, and in the light of these comments a final report was prepared in February 1976.

2. The Conclusions of the Survey*

Problems

Structure. 'A communications chart for the reorganised NHS structure in London is a systems analyst's nightmare' was the bruising comment made by one respondent, and this feeling was reflected in a high proportion of the questionnaires. After more than 25 years' experience of the NHS, and after several years of discussion and debate on reorganisation, it is saddening to find that the new structure should be causing so many problems to so many people. Allowance obviously needs to be made for the aches and pains that usually accompany any reorganisation, but to judge from this survey, it looks as if it will be an unhappily long time before any benefits of the new structure will begin to outweigh its disadvantages so far as London is concerned. And there are clearly some who feel that it is unreasonable to expect a single management pattern to fit the whole country and that it would have been better to have devised a separate structure altogether for London. As it is, London could hardly stand the strain of yet

* This section was prepared by the author as a commentary on the summary of replies received in the questionnaires.

another reorganisation so soon after the last one. Consequently for planners and managers in London, the prospect is probably one of rather greater frustration for rather longer than elsewhere in the country as the new structure sorts itself out.

Finance. Every administrator or treasurer can usually give many good reasons why his district, area or region should be spared the pruning knife compared with other parts of the country. Cynics will say that Londoners are as skilled as any in this art, but the questionnaires did present many eloquent and telling comments about the special problems of London, and particularly of the declining parts of inner London: the nature of its population and disparities in its social conditions, concentration of services, high costs and other factors that some would say have been given insufficient weight in the debates on the reallocation of resources. There were also comments, many of them applicable to the rest of the country as well, about the problems caused by the demarcation between capital and revenue expenditure; the unbalanced distribution of funds between hospital and primary care and the difficulty of reallocating them; and the division of responsibility between NHS authorities and local boroughs for financing health and social services.

Primary Care. 'While hospital services in London are over-doctored, general practice is neglected' was the comment made in the questionnaire returned by a doctor, and it is significant that the problems of primary care in London were mentioned more often than any other topic except that of the new NHS structure. Comments about the relatively low quality of many inner-city general practices were matched by those that questioned whether the conventional pattern of the family-doctor style of general practice is appropriate throughout a big city. Likewise comments about primary care being left to the hospitals, without them being explicitly geared to the task, were matched by those that argued that the ready availability of these hospital services encouraged the atrophy of GP skills. So far as the patient's well-being is concerned, the problem of primary care emerged as being perhaps the single most important topic of all those mentioned in the survey.

Acute Hospital Services. Criticisms about the quality of acute hospital services in London were few compared with those about primary care. The comments were related more to over-provision and the large number of acute and teaching hospitals serving areas of declining population in inner London; the familiar conflict between teaching commitment and service needs; and the concentration in teaching on the clinical spectacular rather than on primary care. Despite the progress made in recent years in strengthening the role of general practice, social medicine and other hitherto neglected specialties in the teaching of medical students, it is clear that many people feel there is still much more that needs to be done to strike the right balance in medical education.

Geriatric and Psychiatric Services. The comments in the preceding paragraph were confirmed by many respondents who referred to the over-concentration, both in teaching and service, on acute services and the relatively poor standard of care for the chronic sick, elderly, mentally ill and mentally handicapped, with many psychiatric hospitals too distant from the population they are supposed to serve. The inadequacies of preventive and other services in the community were criticised, as were the problems caused by the division of administrative and financial responsibility between health and social services — problems common to the rest of the country, but exacerbated in London by the confusion of borough, district and area boundaries. Along with primary care, these services appear to be amongst those causing deepest worry.

Planning and Information. Planners in London have to wrestle with the problems caused not only by the structural and geographical anomalies of the reorganised health and social services, but also by the untypical nature of London; its role as the capital city, and its population with its variety of transient, elderly, single, immigrant, commuter, tourist, homeless, rootless and destitute, and the general shift of population from the centre to the periphery. Some respondents emphasised the dangers of impersonal and bureaucratic planning in a big city; some felt that the absence of any strong co-ordinating planning responsibility for London's health service makes matters worse, whilst others hope that the London Co-ordinating Committee may adequately fill the gap, particularly if given greater executive powers. But at present it certainly seems to be a matter of concern that neither information nor planning is organised on an all-London basis so far as health services are concerned.

Staffing, Training and Attitudes. A wide variety of difficulties were mentioned by many people under this heading, with particular reference to staff shortages and high turnover caused by problems of the high cost and/or inadequacy of housing and transportation; the unsatisfactory environment in parts of London; and the more attractive employment opportunities outside the NHS. These shortages in turn lead to a greater use of agencies and deputising services, and to a greater dependence on immigrant staff (particularly medical) than perhaps in any other 'developed' country. Reference was also made to deficiencies in training programmes and to the attitudes of some staff, who seem to lack a sense of commitment to the health service.

Socio-Economic Factors. As mentioned earlier, standards of health depend upon much else besides health services. Many replies re-emphasised this point very forcibly. Particular reference was made to poor standards of housing and social conditions, especially in parts of inner London, and to the fact that although Greater London as a whole has about the highest average earnings in the country, it does contain pockets of very low pay. There is also an inadequate supply of sheltered housing, hostels and other categories of accommodation that could help to improve the quality of life and to relieve the isolation and loneliness of many in the community, and the unnecessary institutionalisation of many in hospital. Many respondents also referred to the difficulties caused by London acting as a magnet for people with problems and the consequent overburdening of the services dealing with the urban problems that cross health/social service boundaries — and not least those services caring for children and young people and immigrants. Some argued that when the national cake starts to get larger again, increased expenditure on relieving all these problems will contribute at least as much to improving health standards as increased expenditure on health services.

Participation and Self-Help. A variety of comments were made that can best be classified under the general heading of participation and self-help. The need for health education, and encouragement to look after oneself — and one's neighbour; the need for still greater deployment and development of voluntary services; the need for greater consumer involvement and participation in the planning and operations of health and social services. In times of financial strain, these needs assume an even greater significance, but in good times and bad alike their importance has been too little heeded.

Good Ideas and Practices

In keeping with the well-known British capacity for masochistic self-deprecation, it was not surprising to find that the number and length of comments about the problems and difficulties of the NHS far exceeded those about good ideas and practices, and one suspects that the over-all response to the questionnaire underrated the benefits of the NHS system. This feeling was confirmed by some of the comments made about the draft report: a few people expressed strongly the view that compared with most other big cities in the world, London is relatively well off in most respects, with many advantages deriving from its concentration of high-quality services. One reason for the apparent preoccupation with problems may be that many of the good points relate to the health services on a national scale rather than just to London, so that many respondents did not dwell at any length on the national scene and concentrated on the much smaller number of factors affecting London alone. In the analysis, an attempt has been made to differentiate between the national and the London scene.

Structure, Finance and Management. Under this heading, virtually all the comments referred to the over-all concept of the NHS rather than to any factors relating specifically to London. The fundamental principle of free (at time of use) access to the NHS for everyone, and the ready availability of its services is obviously highly regarded, as is the basic system of financing the health service from taxation rather than insurance. As regards the 1974 reorganisation of the NHS, many emphasised the potential benefits that might arise from the new integrated management structure and the establishment of community health councils, health care planning teams and joint consultative committees. But it was also pointed out that these benefits were as yet far from being fully realised.

Services. Many of these comments related to services inside and outside London, some of which are generally available throughout the country, whilst others have as yet been introduced only on a local or limited scale and could perhaps be much more rapidly and widely adopted. Reference was made also to the value and importance of voluntary services and self-help groups — developments which should be encouraged at all times, but which have particular significance, and hazards, in the present difficult economic situation. As regards London alone, the London Ambulance Service and the King's Fund Emergency Bed Service were the two features most frequently mentioned as being particularly worth while.

Planning and Information. As was the case with the new structure of
the NHS, comments about the new planning system related more to
hopes for tomorrow than to the realities of today. However, there is
clearly strong support for the potential effectiveness of the basic
NHS system for the planning and control of the distribution of staff,
services and facilities throughout the whole country. Within London
itself, reference was made to the value of the Greater London
Council's statistical and other intelligence functions and to the role of
the London Co-ordinating Committee, as well as to a number of useful
surveys in particular boroughs or areas.

Staffing and Attitudes. Despite the well-recognised difficulties of the
Whitney Council system and the dangers of bureaucratic over-
centralisation, many comments referred to the over-all benefits derived
from the nation-wide pattern for the recruitment, training, deployment and payment of NHS staff through NHS authorities. London is
known to have particular difficulties over staffing, and a few respondents mentioned some ideas to deal with these problems, such as
special induction courses for staff from the provinces and overseas,
courses in English for foreign staff, and help over accommodation
and transport.

Socio-Economic Factors. Some respondents referred to the high
standards of the basic environmental and public health services of
London — sanitation, water supply, clean air, parks, etc. These are all
factors which one tends to take for granted here, but which are still
the source of major problems in many other big cities, particularly in
the developing world. A wide variety of other good ideas and practices
were mentioned in fields such as housing, transport, nutrition,
community development schemes, youth services and voluntary help.
Many of these topics had also been mentioned in the 'Problems'
section of the questionnaire as being areas of activity where too little
was being done, which gives a good indication of the potential for
improvement of the situation in London.

Changes, Studies and Experiments
In analysing this section it proved difficult to differentiate clearly
between proposals for changes and proposals for studies or experiments.
For example, a number of people advocated the establishment of one

all-London region, whilst others suggested a study on the feasibility
of setting up such a region. In the event, the replies were classified
under the same topic-heading whether they were put forward as
proposed changes or studies. In commenting on the draft report,
several respondents emphasised the immediate need to encourage
practical improvements in communication and collaboration and
to apply more widely the ideas already shown to be effective, rather
than to embark on numerous new studies.

Structure. 'It was a fundamental mistake to leave London to be
administered by four regional health authorities . . . change in London
must be radical, and what is needed is a complete reassessment of
London government with a view to all services being co-ordinated by
one agency.' Thus replied one senior NHS officer, and just as the
problems of the structure of the reorganised NHS evoke more
comments than almost any other topic, so changes or studies on the
structure were mentioned more frequently than any other topic in
this part of the survey. Whether or not immediate change is practicable
or desirable, there is clearly a strong body of opinion that the present
structure is by no means ideal for London and that there is a great
need for studying how it can be improved in both the short-term and
the long-term future.

Finance. On finance, the main proposals were for more studies and
experiments on the problems and possibilities of joint or cross-
financing between health and social service authorities, particularly in
the fields of the elderly and mentally disordered. This is a nation-wide
problem, but exacerbated in London by the confusion of the NHS
and local authority boundaries. Frequent mention was also made of the
need for more studies on the cost effectiveness of different types of
care, particularly in relation to health centres and general practice.

Services. Proposals for changes and studies in primary care were very
numerous, and reflected the concern shown in the first part of the
survey. The functional interdependence of primary health care and
hospital-based services was emphasised. There was also clearly a strong
feeling that the patterns of general practice, especially in the inner
city, need to be critically reviewed and that there is a great scope for
fresh initiatives to try out new methods of providing integrated primary
care at neighbourhood level in both health and social services —
including new ways of using nurses, auxiliaries and non-professionals

in the team. After primary care, services for the elderly and mentally ill were those most frequently mentioned, with particular emphasis on the need for innovation and development in community services, co-operation between statutory and voluntary agencies and support for those caring for elderly or disabled relatives at home. Many other topics were mentioned, ranging from acute hospital services to health education, family planning and occupational health, and it seems that many changes, experiments or studies could be undertaken at relatively little cost.

Planning and Information. With the revised NHS planning procedures still in embryonic stage at the time of the survey, it is not surprising that many of the comments under this heading reflected the widespread concern felt about current deficiencies in planning and information, both nationally and in London. With so much uncertainty and ignorance about what information is needed at what levels, and about the most effective planning procedures, it is clear that many feel there is a great need for further studies and experiments before a uniform pattern of planning is imposed on the whole country. There is also concern about the need to make greater use of the epidemiological and other technical skills available through appropriate university departments, research and consultancy organisations, and the Greater London Council; about the methods of achieving effective involvement and participation by consumers and the public in the planning process; about the importance of planning and organisation of comprehensive services at street or neighbourhood level as well as on a broader scale; and last but not least, the need for monitoring and evaluation of structures and services.

Staffing, Training and Attitudes. Proposals under this heading covered a broad spectrum, from studies on the role of the nurse in primary care to the need for more language training for foreign staff. Emphasis was also given to the importance of encouraging attitudes of self-help and autonomy of individuals in health care. Most suggestions were of national relevance, rather than London-only, but several respondents emphasised the need for studies and experiments on ways of attracting staff to work and/or live in deprived areas — a problem that is of major and increasing importance in London and other big cities.

Socio-Economic Factors. Easily the most frequently mentioned topic under this heading was that of housing — ordinary housing, sheltered

housing, hostels and other forms of residential accommodation. One of
the strongest impressions from the whole survey is that of very deep
concern over the need to improve standards of accommodation at
every level — for patients and public whose low standards of housing
may force them to become unnecessarily heavy consumers of health
and social services; for NHS staff and other community workers, who
so often find it difficult to get reasonable accommodation at reasonable cost close to their place of work. Of all the socio-economic factors
mentioned, this is the one that most people feel to be most in need of
action.

3. Summary

The survey showed that London has some advantages compared with
other cities and that it shares many problems with the rest of the
country. But, equally, it has other problems that are peculiar to the
big city itself. Particularly in inner London, poor housing and social
and environmental conditions cause special strains on health and
social services alike, as does the untypical nature and scale of London's
population; the structure of the reorganised NHS causes more anomalies
and difficulties in London than elsewhere; the problems of planning
and information are more complex, as are those of consumer
involvement and participation; the deficiencies in primary care in inner
London are serious, as are those of the services for the elderly and
mentally ill; staffing difficulties are more acute and less easy to resolve:
these are but some of the main points that were repeatedly mentioned
in the questionnaires. It is hoped that the results of this survey may
help policy-makers, planners and managers to clarify some of the issues
and identify some of the priorities for further study and action on an
all-London basis.

When invited to comment on the draft commentary, respondents
were also asked to suggest which three topics they thought might
most usefully be the subject of particular attention at the IHF congress
in Tokyo. Priorities for discussion at the congress may not necessarily
be the same as priorities for action in London, but it may be of interest
to note that although many different topics were mentioned, easily
the most frequent were:

(1)   Patterns of primary care, including 24-hour services, self-
care, health education and the prevention of illness.
(2)   Structure and organisation for management, planning and
information, including the role of the consumer.

(3)   Co-ordination of health and social services and their relationship with housing, environmental and other services.
(4)   Services for the mentally ill and the elderly, both in hospital and community.
(5)   Allocation of finance and resources, and measures of cost-effectiveness and evaluation of services.

In many respects the picture of London that emerges from the original replies to the questionnaires was not a very cheerful one. The response to the draft report helped to lighten the gloom by focusing more attention on some of the advantages that London enjoys in comparison with other parts of the country and with big cities elsewhere in the world. It was also clear from the questionnaires that much could be done to improve the situation by extending more widely the good ideas and practices that are already in use in some parts of London or outside. Many such developments would involve little new thinking, and in many cases little new money either, but they would perhaps require some changes in attitudes and call for a greater willingness to accept other people's ideas as well as one's own. A readiness in fact to conquer the familiar NIH syndrome (Not Invented Here) which is probably as widespread in Britain as it is in other countries. Another impression is that there are probably many more good ideas and practices in use than were actually mentioned in the responses to the questionnaire. Quite apart from this survey, it might be no bad thing if someone in each area and district, and borough, could once each year or so list the facilities or services of which it is particularly proud, and the good ideas that have been introduced or developed in the previous year in the planning and operation of the local health and social services — the things that one would be pleased to show to visitors, and that other areas, districts or boroughs might be encouraged to adopt or adapt for themselves. The collection (perhaps by Community Health Council members and/or young administrators or trainees?) and exchange of such information and ideas might well help to improve London's health and social services at relatively little cost. It might also help to improve morale by concentrating more attention on what is going well in London — and despite our infinite capacity for talking ourselves into gloom and despondency, there are many good ideas and practices in health care of which London can be proud.

Appendix A: Health Statistics of London 1974

Table 1.1: Population of Greater London by Age and Sex, 1974

Age	Males Number	Per cent	Females Number	Per cent	Totals Number	Per cent
0–4	241,000	3.4	230,800	3.2	471,800	6.6
5–14	519,800	7.3	497,600	6.9	1,017,400	14.2
15–44	1,443,400	20.1	1,441,400	20.1	2,884,800	40.2
45–64	863,700	12.1	922,800	12.9	1,786,500	25.0
65 and over	375,000	5.2	632,100	8.8	1,007,100	14.0
Total	3,442,900	48.1	3,724,700	51.9	7,167,600	100.0

Table 1.2: Population Density, 1974

Population	7,167,600
Area	1,580 sq km
Persons per sq km	4,537

Table 1.3: Vital Statistics, 1974

	Number	Rate
Live births	90,512	12.6 per 1,000 population
Still births	944	10.3 per 1,000 live and still births
Infant deaths	1,439	15.9 per 1,000 live births
All deaths	83,741	11.7 per 1,000 population

Table 1.4: Mortality — First 10 Causes of Death by Rank, 1974
(by WHO 'B' List, Numbers and Per Cent)

	Males	%		Females	%
Rank	Cause	%	Rank	Cause	%
1	Ischaemic heart disease	28.3	1	Ischaemic heart disease	20.8
2	Malignant neoplasm — lung and bronchus	10.8	2	Cerebrovascular disease	14.0
3	Pneumonia	8.0	3	Pneumonia	11.4
4	Cerebrovascular disease	7.9	4	Other malignant neoplasms	6.4
5	Bronchitis and emphysema	6.9	5	Other forms heart disease	5.8
6	Other maligant neoplasms	5.8	6	Other circulatory diseases	5.1
7	Other circulatory disease	3.7	7	Malignant neoplasm — breast	4.2
8	Other forms heart disease	3.2	8	Malignant neoplasms — lung and bronchus	3.1
9	Malignant neoplasm — stomach	2.4	9	Malignant neoplasm — intestines	3.1
10	Malignant neoplasm — intestine	2.4	10	Bronchitis and emphysema	2.7
Per cent of all deaths		79.4	Per cent of all deaths		76.6

Table 1.5: Resources — Number of NHS Staff and Number of
Population per Health Worker

Staff type	Number	No. of population per health worker
General practitioners	3,692	1,941
Hospital doctors	8,756	819
Total doctors	12,448	576
Hospital nurses	57,100	125
Community nurses	4,800	1,493

Table 1.6: Resources — Hospital Beds, 1974

	Number	Rate/1,000 population
General medical	8,207	1.1
Paediatric	1,271	0.2
Other medical	3,694	0.5
Geriatrics	7,677	1.1
All surgical	14,079	1.9
Gynaecology and obstetrics	5,962	0.8
Mental handicap	3,954	0.6
Mental illness	21,984	3.1
Other	3,056	0.4
Total	69,884	9.7

Table 1.7: Utilisation of Hospital Beds, 1974

Discharges (including deaths) from hospital —
Number and rate/1,000 of population

Hospital in-patients 1974	Non-psychiatric			Mental illness	
	Number	Rate	Mean length of stay	Number	Rate
Greater London	928,328	130	14.2 days	33,178	4.6
England and Wales	5,296,720	108	13.3 days	184,201	3.7

Table 1.8: Finance — Expenditure on the National Health Service, 1974/5

	Greater London		England and Wales	
	£ million	£ per head	£ million	£ per head
Hospitals	447.0	62	1,951.2	43
Community health	38.9	5	198.2	4
FPC	125.2	18	717.1	15
Other	40.4	6	205.4	4
Totals	651.5	91	3,071.9	66

Appendix B: Steering Committee

The following people served on the steering committee for the initial stages of the project: most had previously taken part in the comprehensive health planning seminars organised by the King's Fund Centre in 1971-3 and were chosen for that reason.

Mr S. Argyrou, Area Administrator, City and East London AHA.
Dr P. Draper, Senior Lecturer, Department of Community Medicine, Guy's Hospital.
Dr D.G. Gooding, Area Medical Officer, Brent and Harrow AHA.
Mr A. Griffith, Lecturer, Department of Community Health, London School of Hygiene and Tropical Medicine.
Mr M.C. Hardie, Director, King's Fund Centre (until July 1975, subsequently with International Hospital Federation).
Mr B. Langslow, Associate Partner, Llewelyn-Davies Weeks, Forestier-Walker and Bor.
Mr D. Plank, Intelligence Unit, Director-General's Department, Greater London Council.
Mrs S. Thorne, Secretary, Lambeth CHC; Research Officer, Department of Community Medicine, St Thomas' Hospital.
Mr J. Lloyd, Project Officer.

Appendix C: Questionnaire

(A) Problems

(i) *What are some of the* main problems *that seem to you to be currently affecting the planning and provision of health services in London?*

(Please concentrate on those problems in which you have particular interest or expertise, or feel most strongly, either as national issues or special 'Big City' London issues. For some you may want to answer in a few words; for others you may prefer to write a paragraph or more. The following are some of the headings under which your answers may eventually be collated: structure, organisation and management; finance; staffing and attitudes; planning and information; socio-economic factors, including any comments about factors affecting standards of health generally, such as housing, employment, pensions, social services, transport, etc.; any other problems.)

(B) Good Ideas and Practices

(i) *What are the* good ideas and practices *in London that you think other big cities might usefully study, adopt or adapt for themselves?*

(Please mention any good ideas and practices in any field relating to London. As in question (A), please feel free to include reference not only to special 'Big City' factors peculiar to planning and provision in London, but also factors that affect health standards and health services in the rest of the country as well as London. Or putting the point another way, if talking to a 'Big City' audience overseas, what would be the good points about the NHS and London's health services that you would want to emphasise? The following are some of the headings under which your answers may eventually be collated: structure, organisation and management; finance; staffing and attitudes; planning and information; socio-economic factors, including any comments about factors affecting standards of health generally, such as housing, employment, pensions, social services, transport, etc.; any other good ideas and practices.)

(ii) *Have you seen or heard of any good ideas and practices in other big cities that you think could be usefully studied, adopted or adapted for use in London? If so, please give brief details.*

(C) Changes, Studies, Experiments

(i) *What* changes in planning and provision, *or what* studies and experiments, *do you think might most usefully be undertaken to promote improvement in health standards and health services in London?*

(Please suggest any changes, studies or experiments, at national or local level, that you consider would be relevant to the problems of London. As with the first two questions, the following are some of the headings under which your answers may eventually be collated: structure, organisation and management; finance; staffing and attitudes; planning and information; socio-economic factors, including any comments about factors affecting standards of health generally, such as housing, employment, pensions, social services, transport, etc.; any other changes, studies or experiments.)

(ii) *Do you know of any current studies in your own or any other organisation that you think are particularly relevant to the 'Big City' aspects of London's health services? If so, please give brief details.*

(iii) *Do you know of any studies or experiments in other big cities that you think are relevant to London? If so, please give brief details.*

2 NEW YORK CITY

John C. Rossman and S. David Pomrinse*

A. THE PATTERN OF EXISTING SERVICES

This chapter attempts to give a factual description of the very complicated and diverse health services which are provided to the 7.6 million
residents of New York City and to the more than six hundred thousand
non-residents who work in the city. The attempt is complicated by
the diversity of the population and its health needs. It is further
complicated by the multipartite structure and financing of health care.

Demographic and Other Basic Data

New York City consists of five boroughs: Manhattan, Brooklyn, the
Bronx, Queens and Richmond, covering a land area of approximately
300 square miles with a waterfront of over 550 miles. Two of the
boroughs, Manhattan and Richmond, are islands, and Brooklyn and
Queens are part of Long Island. NYC is the largest municipality in
New York State and has 42 per cent of the total population of the
state.

The population density exceeds 25,000 residents per square mile.
This ranges from a concentration of over 64,000 per square mile in
Manhattan to approximately 6,000 per square mile in Richmond.
The population is diverse ethnically, racially and in language.
Immigrants constitute 18.2 per cent of NYC's population; Spanish is
the mother tongue of approximately 10 per cent. About 77 per cent
of the population is white, and 23 per cent non-white, with blacks
constituting over 90 per cent of the non-white category. Thirty per
cent of the population is under 20 years of age and 12.4 per cent is
over 65.

* The paper was prepared, under the aegis of the Hospital Association of
New York State and the Greater New York Hospital Association, in
co-operation with the International Hospital Federation's 'Big Cities' project.
Any limited success this paper has in providing a useful overview of New
York City's health services is due to the materials, both published and
unpublished, made available by the many individuals in governmental agencies,
university and research organisations, and voluntary organisations who co-
operated with the project.

Health Status

Significant differences between locations and groups exist which are
masked in the over-all vital statistics. The infant mortality rate for
the non-white population is 23.7 per thousand as compared to that
for the white population of 15.8 per thousand. The rate varies
substantially between boroughs, from a low of 14.6 in Queens to a
high of 20.9 in Brooklyn. The crude mortality rate of NYC exceeds
the national average, but the age-adjusted rate, based on the age
distribution of the US population in 1970, is slightly below the
national level. The age-adjusted mortality rate also varies significantly
between the boroughs, with Queens having the lowest and Brooklyn
having the highest. The variations between the 33 health planning
districts are even greater, both in respect to infant mortality and the
age-adjusted mortality rate. The variations in infant mortality between
districts are from a low of 10.8 in a district in Queens to a high of 41.1
in a district in Manhattan. The age-adjusted mortality rate ranges from
6.7 in one Queens district to over 17.0 in a Manhattan one.

A number of key factors relating to health are only partially or
tangentially affected by the health care system. Data endorsing this
are plentiful. Accident and homicides both rank among the first ten
causes of death. The communicable diseases with by far the largest
number of reported cases are gonorrhoea and syphilis. An estimated
175,000 persons are addicted to 'hard narcotics', such as morphine
and heroin. There are more than 400,000 alcoholics in the city.
Respiratory conditions, induced by air pollution, are the most prevalent
of acute conditions. (Statistical data and references as to source are
provided in the appendix and reference list at the end of this chapter.)

Structure

Much of the governmental authority and responsibility with respect
to health care is at the state and local levels. Over-all control of
expenditure has, however, been vested in an Emergency Control Board,
dominated by state officials, as a result of the near-bankruptcy of the
municipality. The structure of health care and its financing are multipartite and diverse. Three levels of government, numerous voluntary
and proprietary organisations, and tens of thousands of individual
providers are part of the health care 'system'. Community boards, in
some cases policy-making, in some cases advisory, play a role in the
governmental and voluntary sectors.

The financing also involves three levels of government as well as
private insurers and direct payment, thus increasing the complexity,

since services, in many cases, are furnished by one type of provider
(e.g. proprietary) but financed, in total or in part, by other sectors
(e.g. one or more levels of government). The federal government,
directly or indirectly, funds and controls a number of key health
programmes, with the state being delegated to administer many of
the key ones, such as the responsibility for the licensing and inspection
of health facilities. In addition the municipality has substantive public
and environmental health responsibilities, and is the direct provider
of a variety of services.

Planning

Federal legislation passed in 1974 mandated the replacement of pre-
decessor planning agencies by a single local agency to be responsible
for all health planning: the Health Systems Agency (HSA) for the
City of New York. The responsibilities of the HSA are: to improve
health status, increase accessibility, acceptability, continuity, and
quality of health services, restrain increases in cost, and prevent
unnecessary duplication of health resources.

A majority of its Governing Board are 'consumers'. The HSA of
the City of New York has designated 33 local districts, each with their
own council and with representation in the main governing body of
the HSA which itself has a membership of over 90. The prime
administrative and executive responsibilities are exercised in an
Executive Committee with a membership of 25. Local government
providers, labour and consumer groups are represented both on the
Governing Board and on the Executive Committee. A majority of
both the Governing Board and the Executive Committee are consumers, as required by the legislation. Governmental officials, depending on their specific official function, may be designated either as
consumers or providers.

The HSA has a responsibility for developing a health plan for
New York City based on criteria developed by the state. This Health
Systems Plan is reviewed by the State Health Planning and
Development Agency prior to integration into the State Health Plan
by the State Health Co-ordinating Council. The HSA has direct
decision-making powers to approve specified public health services,
certain community mental health and mental retardation programmes,
and alcohol abuse programmes and projects. Approval of health
facility construction and most new services involves a parallel process
where separate recommendations are made by the HSA and the
responsible state programme agency, i.e. the NYS Department of

Health or Mental Hygiene, for review by the State Hospital Review and
Planning Council. Final approval is a prerogative of the New York
State Commissioner of Health or Mental Hygiene, with the exception
of the establishment of a newly sponsored facility. The final
establishment decisions are made by the State Public Health Council
(see Figures 2.1 and 2.2).

Financing

Total NYC fiscal 1975 expenditures for personal health care, including
the cost of public health programmes and the costs of prepayment,
are estimated at $6.7 billion. The NYC 1975 *per capita* expenditure
was $885, constituting over 13 per cent of *per capita* income, com-
pared with a US expenditure of $514, constituting approximately
9 per cent of US *per capita* income.

Sixty per cent of NYC's personal health care expenditure is directly
or indirectly financed by the public sector, and 40 per cent by the
private sector, almost an exact reverse of the general US ratio, 61 per
cent private, 39 per cent public. Federal government funds constitute
44 per cent of governmental expenditures, state funds 26 per cent, and
city funds 30 per cent. Personal health care services constituted 23.6
per cent of the municipality's total expense budget in 1975, as
compared to 13 per cent in 1961. This does not include over $370
million spent by the Environmental Protection Administration in
1975.

Hospital care, in-patient and ambulatory, accounted for 53 per cent
of the 1975 expenditure, physicians' services 13 per cent, dental
services 7 per cent, nursing home care 6 per cent, and drugs 5 per cent.
Other professional and health services accounted for the remainder.
Personal health care expenditure in NYC has almost tripled since 1966.
The cost of hospital care, in-patient and ambulatory, has more than
tripled within the last nine years (cost in 1975 was $3.5 billion). The
cost of physicians' services during the same period increased by 50 per
cent (1975: $900 million). The cost of drugs almost doubled (1975:
$324 million). The cost of nursing home care, the most rapidly rising
component of health care, almost quadrupled (1975: $387 million).
These increases have occurred despite a 5 per cent decrease in the
population of NYC within the last nine years.

Insurance Programmes: Medicare, Medicaid, Private Insurance

The federal Medicare programme was introduced in 1966. Coverage
includes almost all persons over 65 years of age and certain categories

Figure 2.1: Planning Process

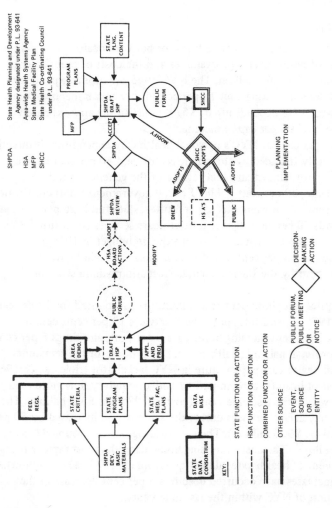

Source: Modification of a chart prepared by New York State Health Planning Commission, 1976

Figure 2.2: Certificate of Need

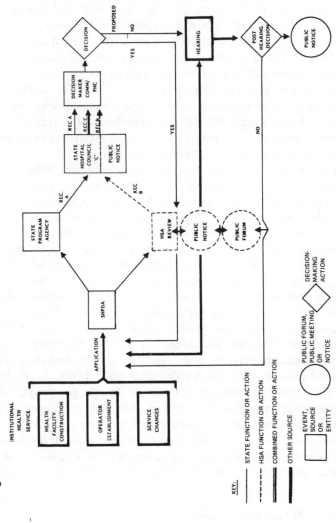

Source: Modification of a chart prepared by New York State Health Planning Commission, 1976

of the disabled; 12.5 per cent of the NYC population. It provides for payment of in-patient hospital services, and of physician and certain other medical services. A small deduction applies to both in-patient and out-patient services and a 20 per cent co-insurance applies to physician services. Limited coverage with respect to skilled nursing-home care and home nursing care is also provided. This programme meets close to 95 per cent of the cost of in-patient hospital care of those covered. The proportion of the cost of physician services, including both hospital and non-hospital care covered by the programme, is estimated as being close to 75 per cent. The Medicare programme is financed primarily through a payroll tax on employed workers, although there is also a general tax subsidy. This federal programme liaises with non-governmental health insurers to perform claims processing and specific administrative activities.

The federal Medicaid programme, also implemented in 1966, covers recipients of public assistance and certain other persons deemed medically indigent: 15.1 per cent of the NYC population. The programme covers virtually all in-patient and out-patient services, including physician services and care in nursing homes. It is state-administered with certain functions pertaining to eligibility, control and payment delegated to the municipality. Approximately half of the expenditure is paid from general federal tax funds, with the remaining costs being divided between the state and the municipality.

Close to 75 per cent of the population not covered by federal programmes have some coverage for hospital care through private insurance. Blue Cross/Blue Shield (BC/BS), a non-profit organisation, is the predominant insurer for in-patient hospital care. Most emergency care is also covered by BC/BS. A majority of subscribers to BC/BS are covered through their employment when usually, but not always, the employer pays part or all of the premium. Relatively few individuals, not covered by governmental programmes, have coverage for non-emergent ambulatory care. The major exception consists of the close to seven hundred thousand individuals covered under a large prepaid insurance programme, the Health Insurance Plan of Greater New York (HIP).

Financing of Physicians' Services

Payment for physician services is predominantly on a fee-for-service basis except for those rendered at clinics and to enrollees by physicians of the major prepaid group health insurance plan (HIP). Physicians under the Medicaid programme, although operating on a fee-for-service basis, are paid according to a schedule that is considerably below the usual charges. Medicare pays the usual and customary fee of the physician, if reasonable, subject to co-insurance.

Financing of Hospital Services

The total of $3.5 billion spent for hospital in-patient and ambulatory care includes $600 million spent on veterans' hospitals and other federal facilities, and state mental health facilities. The voluntary municipal and proprietary hospitals account for $2.9 billion. The voluntary non-profit hospitals receive approximately 26 per cent of their revenues from Medicaid, 27 per cent from Medicare, 25 per cent from Blue Cross, with the remainder from other sources. Blue Cross is the most significant source of income for proprietary hospitals, with direct payments from patients and Medicare providing most of the remainder. The majority of the income of the heavily subsidised municipal hospital system is derived from Medicaid.

The high rate of increase in the cost of hospital care is partly due to increased usage. The predominant reasons for the increase are, however, higher prices of the goods and services purchased by hospitals and changes in the quantity and quality of the goods and services required to produce hospital care.

The shift in financing towards the public sector and the sharp increases in expenditure for hospital care have created a strong impetus towards governmental control. Reimbursement to hospitals under Medicaid, as well as the rates paid to hospitals by the key private sector insurer, Blue Cross, are stringently controlled by the state government under a prospective reimbursement formula. The Medicare programme has less stringent controls, reimbursing under a retroactive system, on the basis of reasonable costs of hospital services. There is also a special programme whereby city and state funds are made available to voluntary hospitals for the expansion of ambulatory services to the economically disadvantaged. State legislation has also been passed requiring Blue Cross/Blue Shield partially to compensate hospitals for certain deficits incurred in providing ambulatory care.

Financing of Long-Term Care

The explosive increase in the cost of nursing-home care, the largest percentage increase in any sector, is primarily due to increases in utilisation, with a secondary impact from inflation and quality change factors. Most long-term in-patient care is financed through the Medicaid programme, and is subject to stringent constraints similar to those affecting hospital reimbursement. The Medicare programme has very limited benefits, private insurance does not usually provide such coverage, and the costs over time are such that few individuals can pay for this care through their own resources. Thus approximately 90 per cent of nursing-home expenses were paid from public-sector sources.

Home care benefits under the Medicare programme are severely limited. Private payments and the Medicaid programme are the sources of most funding for home care with some free or reduced-rate services offered by voluntary organisations.

Financing of Other Health Services

Dental services are paid for mainly on a fee-for-service basis with, however, the fees paid under the Medicaid programme being more restrictive than the usual and customary charge. There is very limited private insurance coverage in respect to dental insurance. The public sector of dental expenditure, including governmentally funded clinic services, was 9 per cent. The predominance of payments for drugs and other special health services is made directly by the patient, except for those covered by Medicaid, which has a fee schedule which is below the usual charges of the suppliers and, of the total New York City drug expenditure, approximately 25 per cent is covered by Medicaid.

Resources, Delivery and Utilisation

Primary Care and Preventive Health Services

The physician/population ratio for physicians directly involved in the delivery of patient care services is 2.5 per thousand. Approximately 8.7 per cent of physicians are engaged in general practice, although substantial 'general practice' is also conducted by physician specialists. Over half of the active physician population is in the borough of Manhattan where the physician/population ratio is more than four times that of the boroughs of Brooklyn and the Bronx, and more than three times that of Queens and Richmond. The 8.7 per cent of the physicians engaged in general practice account for 26.5 per cent of all private physicians' office visits; 67 per cent of primary care visits are to private physicians' offices. The out-patient departments of hospitals account for 21 per cent; the emergency rooms of hospitals for 9 per cent; and ambulatory care centres, including neighbourhood health centres, account for the remainder.

The mode of delivery of primary care differs by socio-economic status. The predominant method for the upper- and middle-income groups is the private physician, whereas for Medicaid recipients principal modes are the hospital out-patient departments and emergency departments, ambulatory care centres and neighbourhood clinics, and physicians specialising in rendering care to Medicaid patients. There were more than eight million visits to out-patient departments of hospitals and more than three million visits to emergency departments of hospitals in 1974. The *per capita* usage of out-patient departments and emergency departments has increased at a rate of approximately 9 per cent per year.

The municipality has the prime responsibility for all public health matters, including the compilation of vital statistics. City agencies also operate a variety of primary care service programmes. The 30 district health centres throughout the city provide immunisation services, dental clinics, venereal disease clinics, maternal and child health services, nutrition clinics, family planning clinics, public health nursing, social work consultation and health outreach activities. Glaucoma, lead poisoning and sickle cell anaemia detection clinics are additional special services.

School health services include examinations by school physicians, special immunisation programmes, health education, accident prevention and safety, and first aid. Special programmes are provided including those for the mentally retarded, the visually handicapped, the deaf and the socially maladjusted.

Secondary Care

NYC has 117 general care hospitals with 38,012 hospital beds (5 beds per 1,000 population). The heaviest concentration of general care beds is in Manhattan, 12.3 per thousand, with the fewest beds per thousand, 3.3, in Queens. Two-thirds of all general care patients are hospitalised in voluntary non-profit institutions. Municipal hospitals provide care for 19 per cent of the patients admitted, with proprietary hospitals admitting 14 per cent. The average length of stay of NYC short-term stay general acute care hospitals (1973) was 10.9 days. This average stay was above the national average and also the highest of the six US cities with a population of more than a million. The occupancy rate of NYC hospitals, 83.1 per cent, was the second highest of these six cities. NYC hospitals had the second-highest daily cost ($154), ranking below only Los Angeles ($177). The case cost of NYC, due to the longer length of stay, was the highest at $1,682, with

Detroit a distant second with a case cost of $1,262. This is due mainly
to high pay rates and staffing ratios, although the high concentration of
teaching hospitals is also significant.

Almost 46 per cent of physicians engaged in patient care have
hospital-based practices. Most specialists have admitting privileges at
one or more hospitals. A substantial portion of hospital physician
care in teaching hospitals is rendered by over 8,000 residents and
interns. The large teaching hospitals have a number of full-time and
part-time highly qualified salaried specialists employed in both teaching
and patient care activities. Many non-teaching institutions employ
'house physicians', often graduates of foreign medical schools, to
supplement coverage provided by the visiting staff. The municipal
hospitals system (Health and Hospital Corporation) contracts with
various voluntary hospitals to provide medical services and supervision.

Rehabilitation and Physical Medicine

There are 774 beds devoted to physical medicine and rehabilitation
with the heaviest concentration in Manhattan. Most of the larger
general hospitals offer out-patient rehabilitation services. Skilled
nursing facilities are required to offer in-patient rehabilitation services.
Home care programmes usually provide for the availability of
rehabilitative and physical therapy.

Long-Term Care

NYC has 30,550 skilled nursing care beds, of which nearly two-thirds
are in proprietary institutions and most of the remainder in voluntary
non-profit institutions. There are, in addition, 8,593 beds in health-
related facilities providing services for patients requiring less intensive
care. There are close to 8,700 domiciliary care beds. The heaviest
concentration of nursing-home and health-related facility beds in
relation to the population over 65 is in the boroughs of the Bronx and
Richmond. Manhattan has the lowest ratio. This contrasts sharply with
the distribution of general care beds and rehabilitative beds.

Home care services are provided by a variety of agencies, both
governmental and non-governmental. The Visiting Nurse Association,
a voluntary agency substantively supported by government funds,
is the largest organisation providing home nursing service. Other
programmes, many conducted by voluntary bodies, provide hot meals,
homemaker services, and a telephone reassurance programme as well
as necessary medical care, psychiatric and rehabilitative services. Many
home care programmes are hospital-based.

Mental Health

There are 8,918 mental health care beds in NYC (1.2 per 1,000) with the heaviest concentration in Manhattan. Eighty-five per cent of these beds are in state and local governmental facilities with almost all of the remainder in voluntary non-profit institutions. Most hospital out-patient departments and a variety of non-profit and government-financed clinics provide mental health services to the population. There are over 1.8 million visits each year to the offices of private psychiatrists.

The NYC Department of Mental Health and Mental Retardation has the responsibility of planning and co-ordinating local, municipal and voluntary non-profit mental health, mental retardation and alcoholism services. This agency contracts with voluntary agencies for the provision of a variety of services.

Ambulance Services

The municipal hospitals provide an emergency ambulance service. Approximately 30 per cent of the ambulances active in NYC are part of this system, with proprietary companies operating 40 per cent of the remainder. Others are operated by voluntary hospitals and, primarily in the boroughs of Queens and Richmond, by voluntary organisations.

Addiction and Alcoholics Services

The municipal Addiction Services Agency (ASA) funds, monitors and evaluates treatment programmes, school-based prevention programmes, hospital referral projects and emergency treatment. Methadone maintenance, drug-free therapy and ambulatory detoxification are among the services provided. There are over one hundred agencies offering services to addicts, including specialised services for such groups as youths and pregnant women.

There are 48 treatment and rehabilitation agencies serving alcoholics in New York City, including 20 clinics in hospitals and many half-way houses. They provide meals, beds, employment, religious services, medical and psychiatric treatment and counselling, detoxification programmes, outreach services and vocational and recreational facilities. One of these voluntary agencies, Alcoholics Anonymous, acts as a contact for over 500 local groups.

Quality and Utilisation Control

There are parallel systems for utilisation review for in-patient hospital care by the state of New York and by the federal government. The federal government programme, Professional Standards Review Organization (PSRO) provides for the review of all direct patient services funded by federal programmes by what is essentially peer review. The New York State programme, while also based on initial peer review primarily by hospital utilisation review committees, is subject to a final determination by state officials as to the necessity of care.

Quality and utilisation control in out-patient services has been implemented only in a very limited way with respect to certain governmental programmes. It is the expressed intention, however, to make such controls a part of all governmentally funded programmes in the future.

Education and Research

There are seven medical colleges in NYC (five of these in Manhattan) graduating 1,003 students per year. More than 8,000 residents and interns are being trained in NYC hospitals each year. NYC schools have education and training programmes for over 600 health and health-related occupations. Almost all major teaching hospitals in NYC have major medical research programmes. This research is most often supported by federal government funds, and by private and foundation sources.

Administrative and systems research is conducted under the auspices not only of specialised research organisations and universities, but also under the auspices of governmental and non-governmental operating agencies.

Environmental Health

The Environmental Protection Administration (EPA) co-ordinates and plans environmental control programmes in sanitation, water supply, water and air pollution control and noise abatement. It enforces the NYC Air Pollution and Noise Control Codes, monitors air and noise pollution levels and carries out research, planning and public education programmes. NYC, in co-operation with New Jersey, Connecticut and the federal government, operates an air pollution warning system. The agency is also responsible for testing emission control devices on motor vehicles for compliance with applicable laws.

Voluntary Organisations

In addition to voluntary hospitals and other health care facilities discussed previously, there are over 1,700 social and health agencies providing various types of assistance and services. The Community Council of Greater New York is a voluntary city-wide central resource providing information about the health and social service programmes offered by all agencies, governmental and non-governmental. The council promotes research and develops policy alternatives in the field of human services.

The variety of services offered by voluntary agencies spans the entire health spectrum. These include services for specialised groups, e.g. the aged, unmarried mothers, and services for patients suffering from specific diseases such as cancer and arthritis, as well as broad-spectrum service programmes. The role of these voluntary organisations in the health care spectrum of NYC is crucial, and their variety and scope of activities are such that no short description can do them justice.

B. PROBLEMS, SOLUTIONS AND SUGGESTIONS FOR CHANGE

The authors, acting under the aegis of the Hospital Association of New York State and of the Greater New York Hospital Association, adopted a two-pronged approach. One approach involved an analysis of a considerable body of recent reports, statements and other publications issued by various governmental, planning, academic and research and consumer organisations. This information source was particularly useful since a fiscal crisis affecting both the city of New York and the state of New York has focused very sharp attention on the health care system of the city. The second approach involved interviews with 31 persons knowledgeable about health care in New York City. Efforts were made to select individuals with varying backgrounds and interests. Those selected included government officials with key positions in city and state agencies, planning agency officials, physicians, administrators of health care institutions, representatives of provider groups, academics and individuals active in consumer organisations. The questions asked, with minor modification, duplicated the main questions utilised in the IHF's London survey. The format, however, was an open-ended interview, with confidentiality assured.

The reader may be puzzled by the appearance, in some cases, of a particular item both in the section on 'problems' and in the section on 'good ideas and practices'. This contradiction is the result of a divergence of opinion among respondents with 'one man's good idea sometimes being another man's problem'. It is furthermore indicative of the financial crisis in which New York City now finds itself that

responses were plentiful in respect to problems and relatively sparse
in respect to solutions and in respect to 'good ideas'. It may be possible,
however, also to learn from others' problems.

Problems

General Comments

Individual Social Responsibility. 'People have to take more responsibility for their own health status' was a comment by one of the
respondents. Another respondent commented, 'People's expectations
are unrealistic when it comes to what health care can do for them.'
These respondents emphasised that many health problems had their
origin in personal behaviour. Poor nutritional habits and the abuse of
drugs, alcohol and tobacco were given as examples.

The same general theme was cited in relation to certain social,
economic and environmental conditions. Examples included the social
and economic isolation of the elderly in our society, the effects of poor
nutrition, inadequate housing and air and noise pollution. The prevalence of venereal disease was seen in large part as a result of present
social attitudes. The presence of violence and accidents among the
leading causes of death was cited as a particularly clear example where
the effect upon morbidity and mortality of health services was
secondary to the effect of social, economic and environmental factors.

Balancing Perceived Needs against Community Resources. Expansion
in health care programmes and consequent increases in health care
expenditure were seen as having been made without adequately balancing the benefits to be obtained against the effect upon the community
of having to muster the resources to pay for the resulting expenditure.
This was particularly the case with costly technological innovations,
currently being adopted by the large teaching hospitals. Short-term
political considerations and the pressures exerted by specific groups,
both consumer and provider, were seen as often being the basis for
decisions.

Imbalance between Curative and Preventive Care. Excess emphasis on
curative care as contrasted to preventive care was seen by several
respondents. The public's perceived need for curative health services
was seen as being very strong, whereas its interest in preventive health
services was seen as relatively weak. The view expressed by one
consumer respondent was that most providers and public officials had

passively accepted the resulting imbalance in the health care system, and that some of them had helped to foster this imbalance.

Structure

Several published articles and several of the respondents termed the health care system in NYC a 'non-system'. A lack of co-ordination was seen as resulting in a maldistribution of resources and a duplication of services which is not only wasteful but leads to inadequate service to some segments of the population. There appeared to be no effective relation between the governmental voluntary and proprietary sectors of the health economy. Individual institutions and groups within each sector were seen as pursuing individual goals without much regard to consideration of the impact upon other parts of the health system or upon the population as a whole.

Planning

Consumer, government official and provider respondents all saw problems with the planning process, but emphasised different aspects.

The provider viewpoint, as excerpted from a report made by a committee of the Hospital Association of New York State, is as follows:

> The Health Systems Agencies (HSA) have a broad mandate for planning, resource development, and review. However, many of these agencies have only a fraction of the budget of the predecessor CHP/RMP agencies. As a result they can only carry out minimal activities.
>
> There has been little net change in the system to date, except for an increase in the role and influence of the New York State Department of Health.

Another problem noted by providers was duplication in the planning process, especially the parallel roles of the HSA and the State Department of Health or of Mental Hygiene, in approving hospital construction and new services.

Critical comments by government officials related primarily to the prior planning process, which they saw as ineffective in controlling the bed supply.

Consumer respondents expressed the strong view that, in the past, the planning process had been dominated by providers, in particular the large teaching hospitals. One consumer respondent expressed the very strong view that the process had been used to benefit unduly the voluntary teaching hospitals at the expense of the municipal hospital system.

Government Programmes

Medicare. The comments with respect to the Medicare programme were, in general, few and relatively mild. Gaps, particularly with respect to long-term care coverage, were pointed out. The failure of the programme to provide adequately for homemaker services as well as the severe limitations on the provisions of skilled nursing care at home, were noted. The very limited coverage provided by Medicare for institutional care was seen to be throwing an undue burden on the state and city since most long-term care consequently became a responsibility of the Medicaid programme which is in substantial part financed by state and local funds.

Medicaid. There is no health care issue which generated more comments and controversy than Medicaid, the programme that covers public assistance recipients and the medically indigent. Much published material and more than one half of the respondents mentioned one or more problems relating to this programme. The problems pointed out should be viewed in the context of general agreement, supported by statistical and financial data, that the programme has substantially increased access to health care for those covered by removal of financial barriers.

Medicaid Administration. Several respondents suggested that the programme is mismanaged both at the state and local levels. A quote from a former state medicaid official, made recently when the state made cutbacks in services and in payments to providers, may be used to summarise the widely shared point of view:

> I must agree with statements by the State Hospital Association, Medical Society and others that the Medicaid program has been mismanaged. Most of the cutbacks proposed would not have been necessary if the management systems were in place to control the program, and if the state could point to one agency and one person as being responsible and accountable for the $3.5 billion Medicaid program.

Medicaid Delivery of Care. Comments from consumer, governmental and institutional provider respondents also found problems in respect to health care as delivered under Medicaid.

Primary care. A physician respondent gave the opinion that, as presently designed, the programme should never have been instituted; that it provided enrollees with a 'blank check' and provided every incentive towards over-utilisation. He also expressed the view that the programme, by limiting payment to providers to a level below that charged for the same services to other segments of the community, resulted not only in inequity to the providers, but adversely affected the quality of care given to enrollees. He noted that, other than care provided at clinics, hospitals and free standing, a significant number of enrollees were accepted for treatment by a small minority of physicians. Several respondents in this connection mentioned the problem of 'Medicaid mills', proprietary clinics specialising in the delivery of primary care to Medicaid patients. This type of medicine, according to the critics, emphasises high volume, particularly in ancillary pro- cedures with the providers more than compensating for relatively low fees by unduly increasing the volume of services.

Secondary care. Hospital in-patient care is also seen as presenting a problem for the Medicaid enrollee. The key point given is that, because Medicaid recipients most often do not have a private physician or have a private physician who does not have admitting privileges at the local hospital, there is no continuity of care.

Long-term care. The administration of the programme and quality of care given were subject to particularly harsh criticism in respect to long-term in-patient care. Several recent reports do document quality deficiencies in these institutions. There have been several court cases lately which resulted in the jailing of proprietary nursing-home operators for multimillion-dollar frauds against the Medicaid programme.

Over-all comments. A consumer representative stated the opinion that Medicaid recipients often receive 'assembly line' care and stated that 'more consideration of patients as human beings is needed'. A quote, again from the former Medicaid official, may serve to summarise the points of view expressed by a number of respondents:

The mismanagement of the Medicaid program in New York State is perhaps only a reflection of basic flaws in the program itself. Medicaid is a health care program foundering in a welfare environment. It is a poor program for poor people, and this basic

flaw in concept will not be changed until some form of national
health program is established which treats all people equally.

Financing

The comments in respect to financing must be considered in the light
of a situation where the municipality of NYC has been and still is on
the thin edge of bankruptcy and has been forced drastically to reduce
its expenditure. The state government, in part because of the financial
problems of NYC, has also been and still is under strong pressure to
curtail expenditure.

> We are expending more than we can afford on health care. We, in
> the last decade, have made tremendous progress in removing
> financial barriers to health care. We now find that we cannot afford
> the price of the problem of the programs we instituted.

This view, expressed by a government official, typifies the views
expressed by several respondents. One respondent (not a state official)
indicated that the state should bear a larger share of the governmental
burden. Several respondents (including state officials) suggested that
the problem was that the federal government was not bearing a larger
share of the cost. The costs of the Medicaid programme and the costs of
operating the municipal hospital system were seen as central to the
financial problems.

In the context of payment to providers, respondents produced
a number of diverse, strong, and at times contradictory views. These
comments should be considered in the light of the fact that a number
of major lawsuits have been brought and are in the process of being
brought by institutional providers against New York State with respect
to methods of determining payment and rates of payment. Provider
respondents, pointing out that a majority of NYC hospitals have
incurred both operating and bottom line deficits over the last several
years, termed the present methods of payment inequitable and
destructive. Specific aspects of the payment system were commented
on, including: a 'freeze' imposed by state government on out-patient
rates paid by Medicaid and Blue Cross; ceilings on reimbursable cost
which inevitably penalised at least half of the hospitals; delays in the
promulgation of prospective rates which prevented effective
budgeting; and counter-productive facets of the system which resulted
in the penalisation of a hospital which shortened its length of stay
or reduced occupancy by more thoroughly screening admissions.

The comments of state government officials focused on their perception that hospitals were not being responsive to the need for economy and were continuing to adopt expensive new procedures and services. One consumer respondent gave the view that even the stringent controls imposed were inadequate to control inefficiency on the part of some hospitals and that an inordinate share of the penalty burden was being borne by the municipal hospital system.

Resources

Ambulatory Care. Several of the respondents saw problems with respect to ambulatory care, especially through the maldistribution of physicians. Problems in respect specifically to access to care included transportation difficulties and differences in language. Excessive waiting time, particularly for those who went to clinics for care, was also mentioned. A lack of continuity of care was seen as a particular problem for patients receiving care under the Medicaid programme. A problem was seen resulting from fewer persons having family physicians, a problem which resulted in both a decrease in the 'humanness' of care and the continuity of care.

Secondary Care. Most respondents mentioned the maldistribution of hospital facilities as a problem. Many, especially governmental and planning officials, expressed the view that there was an excess bed capacity. Reports issued by various planning bodies, state agencies and municipal agencies indicate that from 4,000 to 5,000 hospital beds should be considered 'surplus'. Some respondents consider these findings in themselves a problem. They express the opinion that the findings are politically motivated and based, at least in part, on questionable assumptions such as a 90 per cent average rate of occupancy and a substantial decrease in the average length of stay.

A problem that several respondents mentioned is what they consider an undue emphasis on curative care and especially on some of the more expensive facets of in-patient care. A primary cause of the problem is seen as a mixed product of the large teaching institutions which '. . . dominate the hospital scene in NYC'. These critics contend that physicians of these institutions have a substantial impact on the institutions' priorities and 'too often place undue emphasis on teaching and research'.

Long-Term Care. The lack of care beds was here seen as problematic. Several respondents pointed out that the length of stay in acute general hospitals could be decreased if long-term beds were readily available to accept transfers. The predominance of proprietary institutions in the long-term care area was noted as one cause of problems of fraud and low quality. One respondent, however, pointed out the relatively higher cost of voluntary nursing homes as a point in the proprietary institutions' favour.

Furthermore, a consumer respondent suggested that the high cost of long-term care forced many requiring such care, in particular the elderly, to deplete their life savings and then have to accept benefits as medically indigent. This is seen as psychologically traumatic and destructive to dignity.

Other Health Resources. Specific problems mentioned in respect to other sectors of health care resources were:

(1)   A shortage of rehabilitation beds.
(2)   The discharge of mentally retarded persons from state institutions without adequate facilities and resources being available to help integrate these persons into the community.
(3)   A forthcoming decrease in the availability of ambulance services furnished by the municipality resulting from a lack of funds without additional services becoming available from the proprietary or voluntary sectors.
(4)   A reduction in the funding for methadone treatment clinic for narcotic addicts is resulting in a larger number of known addicts not receiving any treatment.

Health Service Education and Human Resources

The dependence on foreign medical graduates (FMGs) to render physician services was seen as a key problem. A task force of the Regents of the State University of New York in a recent report expressed concern about the US's and New York State's dependence on FMGs. The task force expressed concern not only with respect to the impact on medical care and organisation within New York State and New York City, but also on the impact of this 'brain drain' on foreign nations and, in particular, developing countries.

A recent change in federal law provides that foreign medical graduates will be required to pass a special examination, equivalent to that given to US medical students, in order to obtain immigrant status. This change is seen as resulting in a major reduction in the number of FMGs admitted to the US. This will alleviate considerably the 'brain drain' impact on other countries. Many hospital administrators believe, however, that this will also result in serious disruptions in the operation of some hospitals in NYC and other parts of the US.

Concern was expressed by respondents that medical education programmes did not relate adequately to the type of physician (family and general practice) needed by society. Financial barriers to medical education were seen as excluding some who, if given the opportunity, would be most likely to become the type of physician needed. In addition, many comments were made about the necessity of removing legal barriers to encourage a larger role for para-professionals.

Other Comments

Malpractice Insurance. The high cost of malpractice insurance, both to physicians and to institutional providers, was pointed out as a major problem by several respondents. The necessity of practitioners consequently practising 'defensive medicine' was pointed out with one respondent commenting, 'Defensive medicine is expensive medicine.'

Consumer Participation. A consumer respondent expressed the view that consumer participation in policy-making is most often just a facade. The problem of effectively involving consumers in a meaningful way was seen as most significant.

Environmental Problems. The air and noise pollution programmes of New York City were deemed ineffective by several respondents. 'Exhaust fumes from internal combustion engines pose a major public health problem in our urban environment. Present pollution control programs are mostly public relations,' was one of the views expressed. Indeed, several respondents noted that New York City is still polluting its waterways by dumping raw sewage.

Solutions and Suggestions for Change

General Comments

(1)   Improved public education is seen as a main avenue to improve health care with respect to problems that centre upon individual behaviour. Emphasis was placed on such education starting with children in school.

(2)   The responsibility of the health professional to get actively involved in advocating and working for positive changes in social, economic and environmental factors which detrimentally affect health

was emphasised by several respondents.

(3)   'We have to relate inputs to outputs in the health field,' one respondent said. A most important area of research and experiment is the attempt to ascertain the effect of changes in specific health resources upon morbidity and mortality.

Structure and Planning

The suggestions for solutions and for change in respect to structure were somewhat contradictory. Several respondents suggested that there should be one type of hospital system in New York City rather than the multipartite spectrum which currently includes municipal, voluntary and proprietary institutions. There was no consensus, however, on how this should be done or which sectors should be eliminated.

The new planning process, based on the local Health Systems Agency, was seen as providing an acceptable solution by a large number of respondents. There were several suggestions, however, that the HSA should be given more funds and more independent authority if it is to function effectively.

Governmental Programmes

A substantial majority of respondents saw a national health insurance programme as the best solution to the problems currently encountered by the Medicaid programme. One respondent suggested that the Medicaid programme be abolished and that a new programme, in which a health insurance policy from an insurer such as Blue Cross/Blue Shield was purchased for the benefit of the medically indigent, be substituted. Others suggested specific reforms such as a review mechanism whereby utilisation and quality would be more closely monitored as, at least, a partial solution.

The effective implementation of an information system which would supply adequate and timely data with respect to Medicaid recipients and the services they utilise was also pointed to as a partial solution. (Such a system is in the process of development.)

Financing

National health insurance, federally financed, was mentioned by many as a solution to the present problems of state and local financing. A federal programme, with a broader tax base, would relieve the municipality and the state of a major financial burden. The federal take-over of the financial responsibility for Medicare was also suggested as an alternative.

As for payment of providers, a variety of suggestions for solutions was given. These included the establishment of a quasi-independent state health services commission which would, among other tasks, set rates to providers. Several specific methods for hospital reimbursement, including a budget review approach, were suggested.

Health Service Education and Human Resources

Solutions ranging from an increase in medical school enrolment to a re-evaluation (downward) of the appropriate physician/population ratio were suggested. There was a consensus that para-professional personnel acting as 'physician expanders' could help provide a solution to the physician resource problem.

Good Ideas and Practices

(1)   The new planning process based on the local Health Systems Agency.

(2)   The Professional Standards Review Organization's system of utilisation and quality review.

(3)   The 'Physician's Associates' programme whereby para-professional personnel are being trained to supplement the supply of physicians.

(4)   The training of para-professional health workers drawn from a specific ethnic or racial neighbourhood to work in health programmes, including outreach programmes, within their own neighbourhood.

(5)   Crisis therapy clinics for persons with psychiatric problems, the emphasis being on helping the individual to meet effectively his *immediate* problems.

(6)   The active vital roles of numerous voluntary health agencies.

(7)   An active Hospital Association-sponsored programme for improving hospital efficiency by measuring and improving productivity of individual institutions.

(8)   Affiliation agreements between medical schools and major teaching hospitals and community hospitals.

(9)   An inter-hospital kidney transplant network.

(10) Joint purchasing and shared services, such as joint laundries and shared computer systems.

One respondent suggests that health workers in other cities '*can also learn from our mistakes*'.

Appendix: The Health Statistics of New York City

Table 2.1: Population of New York City by Age and Sex, 1975

Age group	Male Number	Male Per cent	Female Number	Female Per cent	Totals Number	Totals Per cent
0–4	295,000	3.9	283,000	3.7	578,000	7.6
5–19	892,000	11.7	865,000	11.4	1,757,000	23.1
20–39	1,085,000	14.3	1,170,000	15.4	2,255,000	29.7
40–64	930,000	12.2	1,138,000	15.0	2,068,000	27.2
65 and over	372,000	4.9	573,000	7.5	945,000	12.4
Total	3,574,000	47.0	4,029,000	53.0	7,603,000	100.0

Table 2.2: Population Density by Borough

Borough	Total population (thousands)	Land area (square miles)*	Residents per square mile
Bronx	1,403	41.2	34,000
Brooklyn	2,467	70.3	35,000
Manhattan	1,451	22.7	64,000
Queens	1,958	108.0	18,000
Richmond	325	57.5	6,000
Total NYC	7,604	299.7	25,000
Total USA	213,137	3,536,855.0	60

* 1970 land area

Table 2.3: Vital Statistics, New York City, 1973

Birth rate per 1,000 resident population	13.1
Infant mortality rate per 1,000 resident live births	19.0
Mortality rate per 1,000 population	10.4
Total deaths	82,319

Table 2.4: Mortality — First Ten Causes of Death by Rank, New York City, 1973

Rank (all persons)	Cause	Rank White		Rank Non-white	
		Male	Female	Male	Female
1	Diseases of the heart	1	1	1	1
2	Malignant neoplasms	2	2	2	2
3	Cerebrovascular disease	3	3	5	3
4	Influenza and pneumonia	4	4	6	6
5	Cirrhosis of the liver	5	8	4	4
6	Total accidents	6	6	8	9
7	Diabetes mellitus	7	5	10	5
8	Homicide	8	18	3	8
9	Other diseases of circulatory system	9	7	11	10
10	Other diseases of digestive system	12	9	12	11

Table 2.5: Patients Discharged from Short-Stay Hospitals by Highest Ten Categories, 1972, North-East US

		Number	Per cent
1	Complications of pregnancy, childbirth and the puerperium	977,000	13.72
2	Diseases of the digestive system	935,000	13.13
3	Diseases of the circulatory system	925,000	12.99
4	Diseases of the genito-urinary system	776,000	10.90
5	Accidents, poisonings and violence	659,000	9.26
6	Diseases of the respiratory system	630,000	8.85
7	Neoplasms	571,000	8.02
8	Diseases of the musculoskeletal system and connective tissue	279,000	3.92
9	Mental disorders	265,000	3.72
10	Diseases of the nervous system and sense organs	255,000	3.58

Table 2.6: Number of Acute Conditions per 100 Persons per year,
July 1973 to June 1974, North-Eastern US

Infective and parasitic diseases		23.3
Respiratory conditions		75.3
Upper respiratory conditions	47.9	
Influenza	24.0	
Other respiratory conditions	3.4	
Digestive system conditions		7.6
Injuries		25.5
Fractures, dislocations, sprains and strains	7.2	
Open wounds and lacerations	6.9	
Contusions and superficial injuries	6.2	
Other current injuries	5.2	
All other acute conditions		21.1
All acute conditions		152.8

Table 2.7: Facilities Summary, New York City, January 1975

Type of facility	Number of facilities	Total bed capacity	Beds/1,000 population
General care	117	38,012	5.0
Physical medicine and rehabilitation	16	774	0.1
Mental health care beds	44	8,918	1.2
Nursing home beds	168	30,550	4.0
Health-related facilities	56	8,593	1.1
Tuberculosis beds	7	492	0.1
Domiciliary care bed*	71	8,702	1.1**

*   Based on 1972 bed capacity and population (last available figures)
** 9.2 for over age 65

Table 2.8: General Care In-Patient Hospital Statistics, by Ownership,
New York City, 1974

	Discharges	Patient days	Average stay (days)
Voluntary hospitals	743,228	8,086,172	10.9
Municipal (local government) hospitals	211,701	2,217,253	10.5
Proprietary hospitals	157,598	1,325,996	8.4
State hospitals	8,871	93,254	10.5
Total (all hospitals)	1,121,398	11,722,675	10.5

Table 2.9: Total Out-Patient Visits, New York City, 1974

Type of visit	Number	Per cent
Private physicians' offices	26,999,660	67
Hospital emergency room	3,429,562	9
Out-patient department	8,244,354	21
Ambulatory care centre	1,304,714	3
Total visits	39,978,290	100

Table 2.10: Number of Physicians and Number of Population per Physician, New York City, 1974

Type of physician	Number	Number of population per physician
General practice	1,684	
Medical specialties	3,298	
Surgical specialties	2,862	
Other specialties	2,609	
Hospital-based practice	8,838	
Total patient care	19,291	394
Total others	5,166	
Grand total	24,457	311

Table 2.11: Patient Visits to Private Physicians' Offices by Characteristic and Specialty, New York Metropolitan Area, 1974 (per cent)

By sex		By race	
Male	38	White	90.3
Female	62	Black	8.3
		Other	1.4

By age		By specialty	
Under 15	18.0	General practice family	26.5
15–24	14.4	Internist	14.1
25–44	28.9	Paediatrician	9.6
45–64	23.0	Gynaecology and Obstetrics	12.4
65 and over	15.7	Surgeons	7.4
		Psychiatrists	6.7
		Other	23.3

Bibliography

American Hospital Association (1974). *Hospital Statistics, 1974 Edition.*

Community Council of Greater New York, Inc. *Directory of Social and Health Agencies of New York City 1975-1976.* Columbia University Press.

Health and Hospital Planning Council of Southern New York, Inc. (1975). *Hospitals and Related Facilities in Southern New York, 1975.*

――― (1974). *Hospital Statistics of Southern New York, 1974.*

――― (1975). *Ambulatory Visits by Hospital, Southern New York Region 1973 and 1974* (1 November).

Health Services Administration, Bureau of Health Statistics and Analysis (1973). *Service and Vital Statistics by Health Center Districts, New York City, 1973.*

Health Systems Agency of New York City (1976). *Grant Application for Conditional Designation* (January, rev. 2 December 1976).

Jamison, Conrad C. (1976). *The Decline of Employment in New York City: A Lesson To Be Heeded.* (Revised for the NY State Department of Labor, 2 March.)

National Center of Health Statistics, Washington, DC (unpublished information).

New York State Department of Labor (1973). *Commutation in New York State, 1960 and 1970.* Report No. 6 (February).

New York State Department of Social Services. *Statistical Supplement to Annual Report for 1974.* Publication No. 1053.

New York State Economic Development Board (1975). *Projection Summary: Population Projections for New York State Counties, 1970-2000.*

Piore, Nora and Lieberman, Purlaine (1973). *Changes in the Scope, Characteristics and Role of Public Expenditures for Personal Health Care, New York City, 1961, 1966, and 1971.* Center for Community Health Systems, Columbia University Faculty of Medicine.

――― and Linnane, James (1976). *Health Expenditures in New York City: A Decade of Change.* Columbia University Faculty of Medicine.

Roback, Gene and Mason, Henry R. (1975). *Physician Distribution and Medical Licensure in the US, 1974.* American Medical Association,

Center for Health Services Research and Development, Chicago.
United States Bureau of the Census, Washington, DC (1975).
  Statistical Abstract of the United States, 1975. Library of Congress
  Card No. 4-18089.
———— (1973). *County and City Data Book, 1972.* Library of
  Congress Card No. 52-4576.
United States Department of Health, Education and Welfare, Health
  Resources Administration. *Acute Conditions: Incidence and
  Associated Liability United States July 1973 – June 1974.*
  Series 10, No. 102, DHEW Publication No. (HRA) 76-1529, Vital
  and Health Statistics.
———— *Inpatient Utilization of Short Stay Hospitals by Diagnosis
  United States 1972.* Series 13, No. 20, DHEW Publication No.
  (HRA) 76-1771, Vital and Health Statistics.

3 PARIS

The Hospitals in the Paris Conurbation
Eve Errahmani

The problems concerned with the planning and organisation of the
health services of Paris are so numerous and so complex that it
seemed sensible for the purposes of this study to consider only general
hospital care. This part of the chapter will therefore deal with the
subject as a whole and will also describe the way in which it is linked to
the development of the conurbation of Paris and the Ile-de-France
region; while Monsieur Jean-Marc Simon's section, which follows, will
examine the specialist care, teaching and research services provided by
the Assistance Publique in Paris.

Before going on to the main features of the present hospital
provision, I should like to describe the framework in which it has
developed, highlighting the features that are specific to the Paris
conurbation. For the hospital policy of Paris has to be defined in terms
of the organisation of health services in the whole Ile-de-France region.

1. Paris and the Ile-de-France Region

The Geographical Context of Paris

The city of Paris is the centre of one of the largest conurbations in the
world, having today some 10 million inhabitants. With about 5,000
inhabitants per square kilometre, it is the most densely populated
metropolis after Tokyo. In less than 1 per cent of the land area of
France, Paris contains 19 per cent of the total population of France
and 26 per cent of its urban population. If we consider that France's
second-largest city, Lyons, is about a seventh of the size of Paris, we get
a better idea of the exceptional demographic and economic importance
of Paris.

The conurbation has spread rather like an oil-slick, pouring out
from Paris's historical boundaries at the end of the last century and
extending along the valleys of the Seine and the Marne and the main
axes of communication.

To overcome this anarchic growth and the attendant problems
of increasing distance between jobs and services in the centre and the
residential suburbs, the French government set up in 1961 the District

of the Paris region, today called the Ile-de-France Region.

The region is made up of 1,300 communes grouped into eight departments. Paris is both a commune and a department, and, together with the three departments that surround it, forms the central core of the conurbation. In an attempt to come to grips with the growth of the conurbation and to achieve more organised development the Regional Prefect had a 'Master Scheme for Organisation and Town Planning' drawn up in 1965, updated in 1975 and approved in July 1976 by the relevant Ministers after consultation with the regional assemblies. This scheme, which now constitutes the 'charter for regional organisation', lays down two axes for urbanisation, running parallel to the Seine and the Marne, on which the main points for private- and public-sector development are indicated. With a view to restructuring the inner suburbs situated mainly to the east, eight key poles have been selected. The most important of these are the five new towns situated further from Paris: Cergy-Pontoise and Marne-la-Vallée on the north-east axis and Saint-Quentin-en-Yvelines, Evry and Melun-Sénart on the south-west axis.

These new towns will each have about 300,000 inhabitants before the end of the century; they have already about 120,000. They are intended to take most of the overspill of the region and aim to be real towns, providing jobs of all kinds and services of a high standard, so that the regional tendency to monocentrism can be ended.

Demographic Aspects of Regional Development

Since the beginning of the century, the population of the region has increased by 5 million, of which more than 3 million has occurred since the Second World War. But in the last ten years, this increase has slowed down, mainly because of a reversal of population movements between Paris and the rest of France, with more Parisians leaving the area than provincials coming to settle in Paris. Between now and the end of the century, the region should probably not grow by more than 2 million inhabitants, and the aim of the government is for the population of the Ile-de-France to be 12 million in the year 2000. But this over-all increase masks a development that in fact varies considerably from area to area. The population of Paris, which has remained almost static for sixty years, is now undergoing a marked decrease: the population of the three departments of the inner ring increased by 50 per cent between 1946 and 1968, but has since then settled down; and the four departments of the outer ring have been growing rapidly over the past ten years and will from now on absorb almost the entire population increase of the region.

Thus at the beginning of the century, out of every five inhabitants of the region, three lived in Paris, one in the inner ring and one in the outer. At the end of the Second World War, of every five inhabitants, there were just over two in Paris, almost two in the inner ring and still only one in the outer ring. Now, the distribution is one in Paris, two in the inner ring, and two in the outer ring, which by 1985 will contain 43 per cent of the population of the region.

Of course, the distribution of jobs and services — especially health services — reflects the past population distribution — and this is one of the major problems of regional organisation. A striking example of these distortions may be found in medical demography. In 1975, Paris had proportionately twice as many general practitioners as the rest of the region. The imbalance is much worse with regard to specialists: per 1,000 inhabitants, Paris has 3.3 doctors, of whom 30 per cent are specialists, whereas the outer ring has 1.0 doctor, of whom only 20 per cent are specialists.

2. Hospital Provision in the Ile-de-France Region

The Number of Hospitals and the Number of Beds

The Number of Institutions. In January 1977, the Ile-de-France region had 569 institutions for general hospital care with 81,192 beds. This represents about a fifth of the national hospital supply.

One of the unusual features of the French hospital system, and particularly in the main metropolitan region, is that only 19 per cent of these institutions (106 of the 569) are *public* hospitals. These comprise the 44 teaching hospitals of the Regional University Hospital group, all under the control of the Assistance Publique,* 42 communal, intercommunal or departmental hospitals, 9 national or special category hospitals, and 11 small rural or local hospitals. The role of the public hospitals is to respond to the health needs of their local area without regard to the social, economic or health status of individual inhabitants. They are obliged to admit any patient and provide continuity of care without regard to cost. They also provide some teaching and research.

On the other hand, the 370 private commercial clinics, providing two-thirds of the hospitals in the region, are free to limit their services to a particular clientele.** Of these, 361 are basically short-term

---

* For details of this, see M. Simon's section of this chapter.
** Most of these clinics are 'contracted', i.e. they charge patients fixed fees

institutions and only 9 are convalescent homes or rehabilitation centres, but in fact about 30 establishments have an average length of stay of more than 30 days.

The third category of the hospital service in the region consists of the 93 private non-profit hospitals, more akin to the public hospitals than the clinics, in that two-thirds of them fulfil the public service function but with more flexible management than the public hospital. They represent one-sixth of the hospitals and they are more numerous in Paris than in the rest of France, although less common than in Holland and Germany. The provision of hospitals in France and in the Ile-de-France region is thus very different from other European countries where nearly all the hospitals belong either to the public sector or to foundations, religious orders, and non-profit lay organisations.

The Number of Beds. However, the distribution of beds is rather different from the distribution of the hospitals. The average size of the Assistance Publique hospitals is around 650 beds and of the other public hospitals about 300, whereas the private non-profit hospital hardly ever exceeds 110 and the private independent clinic 60. Thus the public hospitals contain 59 per cent of all the beds, the private non-profit 13 per cent and the private clinics 28 per cent.

The distribution of 1,000 beds in the Ile-de-France region in January 1977 would have been as follows:

180 beds in hospitals of less than 80 beds, nearly all independent;
166 beds in hospitals of 80-150 beds, again mainly independent;
103 beds in hospitals of 150-300 beds distributed in a more
    balanced way over the three types;
142 beds in hospitals of 300-500 beds, nearly all public but some
    private non-profit; above this threshold of 300 beds there are
    no private independent clinics;
153 beds in hospitals of 500-750 beds, all public and nearly half of
    them Assistance Publique;
115 beds in hospitals of 750-1,000 beds, two-thirds of which belong
    to the Assistance Publique, the remainder shared between other
    public hospitals and the private ones;
141 beds in hospitals of over 1,000 beds, all belonging to the
    Assistance Publique.

under contract with Social Security and the patients can claim the same reimbursement as in the public hospitals. A few clinics (37 throughout the region) are only 'approved' and their patients cannot claim the difference between their charges and those in the 'contract' clinics.

Number of Beds by Category. In January 1977, the Ile-de-France region had 81,192 general hospital beds, of which 11,570 were for medium- and long-stay cases. Just less than half of these were occupied by convalescent patients or patients undergoing rehabilitation, the remaining half being devoted to chronic patients. Seventy-five per cent of these beds are public and scarcely 3 per cent in private independent clinics. This leaves almost 70,000 beds for active treatment divided into 31,215 for surgery, 31,297 for medicine and 7,110 for obstetrics/gynaecology.

However, the distribution by specialty varies considerably according to the type of hospital: in the public hospitals, the medical beds account for 62 per cent of the active treatment beds and the obstetrics/gynaecology beds for about 7 per cent. In the private commercial sector, medical beds represent only 16 per cent of the total, about the same as for obstetrics/gynaecology, whereas surgery accounts for 68 per cent of the beds. In the private non-profit sector, the distribution is close to the average for all types taken together. Thus, whereas in medicine more than three-quarters of the beds are public, in surgery half of the beds belong to the private commercial sector and in obstetrics/gynaecology the preponderance in this sector is even more marked.

The fact that the private hospitals tend to prefer the more profitable specialties results in an imbalance between supply and need.

The official ratios for the provision of hospital beds are:

3.0 beds per 1,000 inhabitants in medicine;
2.6 beds per 1,000 inhabitants in surgery;
0.65 beds per 1,000 inhabitants in obstetrics.

These ratios will, moreover, soon be revised downwards by the Minister of Health. However, when we relate the number of beds in January 1977 to the estimated population of the region we find:

3.13 beds per 1,000 inhabitants in medicine — a very slight excess of only 4 per cent;
3.12 beds per 1,000 inhabitants in surgery — here a surplus of 20 per cent over the norm;
0.71 beds per 1,000 inhabitants in obstetrics/gynaecology — a surplus of about 10 per cent.

From this it would appear that the needs of the region are largely covered. However, this estimate does not take into account the fact that about 6,200 beds — nearly 10 per cent of the total — are used for patients coming from outside the region, the rest of France, or abroad. This strong attraction for people outside the region stems from the specialised nature and the high reputation of many of the departments in Paris.

Geographical Distribution

Paris contains 35 per cent of the active treatment beds for 23 per cent of the population, the inner ring departments 37 per cent of the beds for 40 per cent of the population and those of the outer ring 28 per cent of the beds for 37 per cent of the population. On the other hand, only 3 per cent of the medium- and long-stay beds are situated in Paris, whereas 45 per cent are to be found in the inner ring and 52 per cent in the outer ring. The present geographical distribution of the beds for acute cases reflects more or less the distribution of the population twenty years ago.

In relation to the average bed-population ratios, the over-all surplus in the region, therefore, varies from between a 30 per cent surplus at the centre in Paris and the inner ring of suburbs, and a 13 per cent deficit on the periphery — i.e. to the detriment of the 3.5 million, rising to 4.5 million, inhabitants of the outer-ring departments.

This imbalance is, however, much worse in specialist care: for 60 per cent of the population, the centre of the region contains 66 per cent of the general beds, 76 per cent of the normal specialist beds and 87 per cent of the specialised and highly specialised beds. In surgery, the figure is as high as 96 per cent.

But this imbalance of the concentric distribution of services is accompanied by differences between north and south. For all the active treatment beds, the provision in the south-west of the region — relative to the population — is 20 per cent higher than in the north-east. The specialised beds are concentrated in the south of Paris and its immediate suburbs; this area, a very small proportion of the region, contains one-third of all the specialist beds and two-thirds of the beds for major surgery (neurosurgery, thoracic surgery and cardiovascular surgery). Of course, patients travel to be hospitalised and many of the patients for major surgery come from other parts of the region and also from the rest of France and abroad. However, the flow of patients does not compensate entirely for the basic geographical imbalance.

Admissions and Activity

The most recent statistics available for the *whole* of the general public and private hospitals are for 1973 and are given here only for the active treatment departments.

Between 1962 and 1973 the admission rate increased by almost 50 per cent, passing from 112 admissions per 1,000 inhabitants in 1962 to 156 ten years later. In 1973, 35 per cent of admissions were to the Assistance Publique hospitals, 20 per cent to the other public hospitals, 8 per cent to the private non-profit hospitals and 37 per cent to the private clinics. Between 1973 and 1976, the number of admissions to Assistance Publique hospitals increased again by 23 per cent.

The average bed occupancy rate increased from under 80 per cent in 1962 to 83 per cent in 1973, but it was higher than this in the private and in the Assistance Publique hospitals; although, since then, it has remained at about 84 per cent in the Assistance Publique hospitals. The average length of stay has decreased very rapidly: for all hospitals it fell from 17.1 days in 1962 to 12.5 in 1973 and in the Assistance Publique hospitals it had dropped to 10.2 days in 1976. Thus patient turnover is 40 per cent higher than it was ten years ago; in 1973 one active treatment bed was used on average by more than 24 patients instead of 17 in 1962.

The pressure for hospitalisation seems to be greater in the Paris conurbation than in the rest of France where the admission rate is lower, the length of stay longer and the average occupancy near the 80 per cent optimum. Many of the hospitals of the region are over-crowded at certain times of the year in conditions prejudicial both to the patients and to the staff looking after them.

The geographical variations in hospital admissions have been examined in depth, commune by commune, by the Regional Health Observatory. It has been ascertained that 4 out of every 5 patients are admitted to a hospital near their home. For three-quarters of the outer-ring communes, one single hospital attracts more than half the patients, whereas at the centre of the region where hospitals are more numerous and situated closer to each other, admissions are dispersed among several hospitals.

Distance is therefore really a fairly important deterrent to hospitalisation. Despite the fact that the Assistance Publique hospitals have much better specialised departments than the hospitals on the periphery, they draw most of their patients from the heart of the region. In the outer ring — except in some areas served by particularly unattractive or far distant hospitals — only 6-7 per cent of all admissions go to specialised departments in the centre. In the outer ring transportation is the critical factor: the areas which use one particular hospital more than any other are those that are most conveniently linked to it.

Qualitative Aspects

Great efforts have been made to modernise and humanise the region's public hospitals, thanks mainly to funds provided from within the region. Fifteen years ago, the average age of hospital buildings was 66 years, with 17 per cent of the beds in buildings more than a hundred years old and 30 per cent in buildings over eighty years old. No completely new hospital had been opened between 1935 and 1962. Between 1962 and 1977, ten new hospitals were set up, nine by the Assistance Publique, of which four were exclusively for convalescents and chronics. The six new acute hospitals were all built within the inner ring of suburbs to meet the needs of the million additional inhabitants who settled there between 1946 and 1962, i.e. during the period of greatest population growth in this part of the region. Also between 1962 and 1977, eight old hospitals were completely rebuilt and many other hospitals were partly modernised.

At present around forty hospitals have still to be renovated, most of them completely or nearly completely. In addition, four new hospitals should soon be built in the new towns of Evry, Saint-Quentin-en-Yvelines, Marne-la-Vallée and Cergy-Pontoise. Finally, the Assistance Publique proposes to build three new hospitals in Paris, two of which are intended to replace old hospitals.

Within the public hospitals, the number of beds in open wards has been reduced over the last fifteen years from 25,000 to 10,800. But despite these improvements relating to patient comfort, the technical level of care provided varies considerably from hospital to hospital.

In the private clinics, in 1971, almost 7,000 beds were in units considered too small for patient safety.* Thanks to extensions, and hospital amalgamations encouraged by the authorities, and finally to the closure of many unprofitable clinics, by 1977 this figure had been reduced to only 3,500 private beds and it is likely that these remaining 3,500 beds will disappear even more quickly in the present economic climate.

In the public hospitals, in 1971, there was an average of 14 doctors

* The minimum levels for a unit are: medicine 50 beds, surgery 30 beds, maternity 15 beds if the clinic also has a surgical department, and 25 beds if not.

per 100 beds, varying from a minimum of 3 to a maximum of 44. So, too, the ratio of medical procedures per 100 beds varied from 1 to 44 depending to a large degree on the level of medical staffing. Non-medical staffing averaged 95 employees per 100 beds, but varied from 21 to 207. Finally, out-patient visits were sometimes very few; the average was only one out-patient visit for every four patient days. Between 1971 and 1975, in the Assistance Publique hospitals, the number of medical procedures undertaken increased by almost three-fifths and the number of out-patient visits by nearly a quarter.

Admissions for less than a day (day hospitals, dialysis sessions, chemotherapy sessions, etc.) have increased by about 30 per cent per year. Despite this rapid development, these out-patient treatments without actual admission still represent only about 1 per cent of the hospital's output. In the other public hospitals, out-patient services are even less developed and the various indicators of medical productivity are all much lower, particularly for the hospitals in the outer ring.

Thus, the quantitative inequalities in the geographical distribution of hospital provision are further reinforced by qualitative anomalies. It was this general imbalance in hospitals which led to the definition of the objectives of a regional hospital policy.

3. Objectives and Tools of a Regional Hospital Policy

The Objectives

The imbalance in hospital provision led to a series of problems — probably shared to some extent by most of the old cities in free market economies — which may be summarised under three main headings:

(1)   to reconcile the geographic redistribution of the hospital provision with its over-all quantitative stabilisation and qualitative improvement;
(2)   to ensure that the public hospitals and the private ones properly complement each other;
(3)   to improve the medical productivity of the hospitals by reducing admissions in favour of ambulatory care.

In an attempt to achieve these objects, certain measures have been taken over recent years — the main ones stemming from the law on hospital reform dated 31 December 1970.

The Tools

In order to control the quantitative growth of the hospital services and to bring some order to their geographical distribution, a 'health map' was drawn up.

The health map divides the region into health sectors — 20 at present in the region — and lays down for each sector the type, size and position of the services, with or without beds, that are required to fill the needs of the population. These needs are at present estimated in terms of bed population. Changes in the capacity of hospitals are submitted for approval and must comply not only with a set of technical standards but also with these quantitative needs; that is to say, if current needs are considered to be covered using the official bed-population ratios, additional beds will not be authorised. Thus the health map provides a compulsory framework not only for the planning and programming of public hospitals, but also for the extension or creation of private hospitals, which cannot be done without permission.

The health map is reviewed on consultation with many bodies representing, at sector, regional and national levels, public hospitals, private hospitals, the medical unions and the health insurance funds, as well as with various individuals who are invited to give their opinion. At the technical level, in the Ile-de-France region, it is the Regional Health Observatory that is responsible, under the Regional Prefect, for deciding the sectors by monitoring patient flow and determining the multi-sectorals' need for certain medical and surgical specialties. It also undertakes special studies of the need for expensive medical hardware (radiotherapy equipment, renal dialysis sets, scanners, etc.).

In fact, the simplified bed-population ratio is inadequate on two counts: (1) the use of the bed as a unit expresses only the hotel capacity of the hospital and not its capacity for producing care; (2) it does not take account of the structural components of the population which have as much influence on the size and the type of hospital needs as its over-all quantity. Epidemiological studies, still too few and inadequate, are essential in estimating the number of patients and their probable distribution by types of disease, the optimal average length of stay for each type of illness and the average number of medical procedures during this length of stay.

The implementation of the health map is a function of the Regional Hospitalisation Commission which gives an opinion on private as well as on public projects. This is almost always accepted by the competent authority (the Regional Prefect for private projects, and the Minister

of Health or the Departmental Prefects for public projects). In the
Ile-de-France region, since March 1973 when this Commission was set
up, the growth in hospital provision has been slowed down and quite
considerable spatial redistribution has taken place.

Whereas between 1968 and 1972 about 8,000 new private beds were
authorised in the Paris region, less than 2,000 have been authorised
between March 1973 and March 1977 — an average of only 500 per
year. So too there have been many closures, cancellations of permits
and abandoned projects in the private sector, and in the public sector
many public hospital programmes have been revised downwards. Since
the end of 1975 existing hospital capacity has dropped by 1,500 beds
and the future capacity by 2,000.

The geographical distribution of future hospital provision will differ
considerably from the present one. With the projects under way,
including the Assistance Publique Master Plan which is described in
the second part of this chapter, Paris will contain only 31 per cent of
the active treatment beds (as against 35 per cent at present), the inner
ring 36 per cent (37 per cent at present) and the outer ring 33 per cent
(28 per cent at present). This distribution is nevertheless still very far
from reaching the population distribution, which in 1985 is expected
to be 19 per cent in Paris, 38 per cent in the inner ring and 43 per cent
in the outer ring.

In fact, to correct the geographical imbalance properly, we would
have to relocate some of the hospitals due for demolition and
modernisation in the outer ring and the new towns instead of rebuilding
them on their old sites. But this solution, for various reasons, seems
rather difficult to apply at present. For this reason the critical issue
of humanising the hospitals is in contradiction to the problems of
providing services in the places they are most needed.

The complementing of public and private hospitals is ensured both
by control of new projects under the health map and by the 'public
hospital service' also instituted by the law of 31 December 1970.
Alongside the public hospitals, this public service can be provided not
only by the private non-profit hospitals which are *entitled* to participate
simply on request, but also the private commercial clinics which may
be admitted to the public service under contract. Lastly, the private
clinics, other than those providing this public service, may, by
agreement concerning all or part of their activity, become *associated*
with the functioning of the public hospital service. These hospitals
must then receive any patient and provide continuity of care, and are
expected to make some contribution to teaching, research and

preventive medicine services. Since the decree of 3 November 1976, 51 private non-profit hospitals have been taking part in the public hospital service in the Ile-de-France region. On the other hand, very few private commercial clinics have so far shown any interest in contracts or agreements of association with the public service.

Finally, to maintain the medical activity of the hospitals at the centre of the conurbation at a steady level by reducing their number of beds in favour of out-patient treatment, the Assistance Publique has drawn up a draft 'Master Plan'. In the outer ring, and more particularly in the new towns, studies have been undertaken to design hospitals that will be better integrated into the community they are to serve and into the health system as a whole; out-patient services especially will have a very important part to play in these hospitals whose work will be reinforced, in direct contact with the population, by setting up neighbourhood centres for mental health and social services.

New ideas for the role of the hospital in the health care system are still being elaborated. The last quarter of the twentieth century will probably be a time of far-reaching change in the French hospital services, particularly at regional level.

The Role of the Teaching Hospitals in Greater Paris and the Ile-de-France Region

J.-M. Simon

In Paris, specialist hospital care, teaching and research in the hospital environment come under one public institution, the Assistance Publique of Paris, which administers 44 teaching hospitals, 24,000 short-stay beds and 14,000 medium- and long-stay beds. The organisation requires an administrative system on several levels, which may appear rather cumbersome compared with that of the small autonomous institutions. On the other hand, its power to take action is considerable and its techniques of investment and management are often more highly developed than elsewhere.

But the distribution of health care in the Paris conurbation is being subjected to far-reaching changes, certain elements of which are contradictory. The population, which used to be concentrated in the centre of the conurbation, is now growing on the periphery, whereas the city of Paris is tending to depopulate. The conurbation itself is now part of a larger entity, the Ile-de-France region, the policy for which is based on the creation of new towns. Finally, the demographic evolution leads us to expect a relative ageing of the population, which will have obvious consequences for the morbidity pattern of hospital care. Nevertheless, the existing hospitals seem to be sufficient although in some cases poorly distributed. Consumption of hospital care by the population is already at a high level and costs of hospitalisation are rising steeply. Lastly, certain factors suggest that the techniques of hospitalisation are going to change radically in the coming years and will perhaps require a different provision.

How can the Assistance Publique of Paris anticipate and measure these changes and foresee their consequences? How can it adapt to them? These are the questions which my paper will try to answer, by developing three themes:

(1)   the situation concerning the distribution of hospital services in Paris and the Paris region in the seventies and the traditional role of the Assistance Publique;
(2)   current and possible future changes;
(3)   the possible adaptations due to a redefinition of the role and the organisation of teaching hospitals in Paris.

1. The Position and Role of the Assistance Publique in the Paris Conurbation

The origins of the Assistance Publique go back to before the tenth century, to the first Hôtel-Dieu of Paris. Other hospitals were set up later, mainly from the sixteenth to the eighteenth century, and these were run, from 1801, by a single council. The general administration of the Assistance Publique was finally formed in 1848.

This historical background is necessary for an understanding of the present position and role of the Assistance Publique. In fact the original purpose of setting up a single administrative body for all the Paris hospitals was to simplify their management, to put an end to certain private interests and to co-ordinate a hospital organisation which was taking on social welfare responsibilities as well. But it also resulted in the creation, within the French hospital system, of an entity of exceptional size, with its own means of development and diversification and the ability to make its influence felt very strongly on the organisation of medical care in Paris and the surrounding region. The position of the hospital services in Paris and the Paris region is thus quite unique. One can, in fact, distinguish three types of hospital services:

(1)   The Assistance Publique, which has 44 hospitals, about 30 of which are short-stay teaching hospitals and 15 medium- and long-stay hospitals.

(2)   The public communal or intercommunal hospitals set up on the outskirts of Paris and, within Paris, some large private non-profit hospitals. Although they have a different legal status, these hospitals have much in common: they generally have several hundred beds, departments of medicine and surgery, together with their own technical services (mainly X-ray and laboratories). Furthermore, several of them play some part, by special agreement, in the teaching hospital programme of the Assistance Publique.

(3)   The private establishments, commonly known as 'private clinics', with hardly ever more than 100 beds, oriented particularly towards surgery, obstetrics and convalescence.

About ten years ago, with its 23,850 short-stay beds out of a total of 57,500 beds for the whole of the Paris region, the Assistance Publique owned about 41 per cent of the total capacity of the hospital departments for acute patients.

But, since then, all other types of hospital services have increased their number of beds while the Assistance Publique has concentrated on reconstruction and modernisation, while maintaining a constant number of beds. As a result, each of the broad categories of service today represents about one-third of the hospital provision for the region (see Table 3.1).

Table 3.1: Number of Beds in the Three Types of Hospital Services

Assistance Publique		23,450 beds
Public communal hospitals	16,310 beds	
and private non-profit hospitals	7,740 beds	24,050 beds
Private clinics		23,250 beds

Nevertheless, the Assistance Publique is still highly effective because although the bed capacity has not varied, the funds assigned to these beds have been increased considerably and at the same time the hotel side has been improved, the technical equipment of all short-stay institutions has been increased and new hospitals have been built to compensate for the reduction of beds in the old hospitals. Total staff, excluding doctors, has increased from 46,000 in 1968 to 61,500 in 1977, and the number of senior medical staff from 1,400 to 2,300 in the same period. The latter increase has been made exclusively in full-time staff, who today number just over 2,000, while the number of part-time medical staff has been constantly decreasing. These senior doctors are supplemented by 1,200 interns, 1,100 specialists in anaesthesiology and haemobiology and just over 4,000 doctors with visiting privileges who spend three or four half-days a week at the hospitals. Thus with this considerably increased operational funding, the medical activity of the Assistance Publique hospitals has been able to develop and reach a high level of technical efficiency.

This improvement has shown itself in various ways. There has been a diversification of diagnostic and treatment services, particularly in biology and radiology. New clinical specialties have come into being, like haematology and nephrology, or have been developed, like neuro-surgery and cardiovascular surgery. Finally, for the most seriously ill patients, medical, human and material resources are densely concentrated in the new intensive care or constant supervision units. Table 3.2 illustrates the extent of the Assistance Publique's efforts to raise the level of care.

Table 3.2: Constant Supervision and Intensive Care Units

	1965	1975
Percentage of total short-stay beds	0.8	8
Percentage of total acute patients	0.8	10
Percentage of total short-stay costs	1.7	15.2

Furthermore, the Assistance Publique has made every effort to improve its hospital distribution on the periphery of the conurbation, within the limitations set by the land and buildings it owns and its legal status of providing services for Paris. From 1965 onwards, it undertook a medium-term programme designed to build several modern teaching hospitals outside Paris in order to relieve the burden on the Paris hospitals, which was at that time a prerequisite to modernising them.

This policy made it possible to build five hospitals of 500-1,200 beds on the periphery of the Paris conurbation (i.e. in the first of the two 'rings' of the Ile-de-France region). The result was to move 3,000 beds towards the periphery (see Table 3.3).

Table 3.3: Number of Short-Stay Beds in Assistance Publique Hospitals

	1968	1976	
Short-stay beds in Paris	18,500	15,400	−3,100
Short-stay beds in the inner ring	5,000	8,000	+ 3,000

In addition, in the same period, it built four new medium-stay hospitals in the inner and outer rings, totalling almost 3,000 beds. With these changes, the Assistance Publique has been able to continue to play a major part in the distribution of hospital care in the Paris region, while the other types of hospital service have been increasing their bed capacity considerably, but have not made the same improvements in staffing or medical technology. In fact the number of in-patients in Assistance Publique hospitals increased by 20 per cent between 1970 (406,000) and 1976 (486,000), whereas the average length of stay (if more than 24 hours) decreased from 16.3 to 13.6 days.

2. Changes Occurring in Hospital Care

French hospital organisation is at present undergoing certain changes which will in future call for a different policy of hospital siting and development. Some of these changes are deliberate, others have been imposed. They are particularly noticeable in regions that are already heavily urbanised and well endowed, such as Paris.

As pointed out in the first part of the chapter, the population of the region will increase in the coming years, but rather slowly; and the population of Paris, which has already lost half a million people in ten years, is likely to diminish still further while that of the inner ring (of the periphery) will stabilise and only the population of the outer ring will increase considerably, by about one million inhabitants (see Table 3.4).

On the other hand, it has been mentioned that the number of beds has increased considerably in less than ten years, to such an extent that, after the relative shortage of beds in the sixties, we are now passing through a period of financial retrenchment which is already affecting the small clinics in the centre of the region.

Now, a number of public or private institutions are still in possession of permits to build extra beds: about 6,000 for the public hospitals, 800 for the private non-profit hospitals and 1,800 for the private clinics. Of course, these permits will not all be used, particularly for

Table 3.4: Population Estimates

	(million inhabitants) Census 1975	Estimate 1986
Paris	2.3	2
Inner ring	3.9	4
Outer ring	3.6	4.6
Total for the region	9.8	10.6

the public hospitals, in as much as the Ministry of Health and Social Security may introduce cuts in the public hospital programmes. But some of the new towns of the region which are being developed are naturally enough eager to have their own public hospital and are tempted to blame the Assistance Publique for the present concentration of hospitals in the centre of the conurbation. It must, however, be realised that this concentration is only partly due to the Assistance Publique and that, merely by completing the projects already authorised, the outer ring of the region will have approximately 24,600 beds, which is probably excessive if it is accepted that the dispersion of certain forms of specialised care impairs quality.

Two other developments will influence the future of hospital care in France generally and in the Paris region particularly. These are the growth of hospital costs and the probable development of different types of care.

The increase in hospital costs is a major preoccupation in France, as it is in many other countries. It is particularly felt in the Paris region where it is obvious, from the refunds made by social security, that if the costs are increasing at a fast but bearable rate in those types of hospital services where the total capacity is stabilised, they are increasing at a disturbing rate for hospitals which are continuing to grow. Thus in 1974/5, a period during which the rate of hospital cost inflation reached 20 per cent, hospital expenditure borne by social security increased by a national average of 33 per cent, and by 34 per cent in the Paris region. The Assistance Publique costs reimbursed by social security increased by only 26 per cent, whereas those of the other public hospitals of the region increased by 44.8 per cent and those of the private hospitals by 33 per cent. One can see, therefore, how much more it would cost if the hospital services on the periphery of the conurbation were to continue to develop without taking account of the existing services.

New types of care are appearing in the teaching hospitals of the Assistance Publique and it is likely that in the next few years these types of care will cease to be experimental and will become routine in most hospital departments. These new types of care either permit very short stays (4 to 5 days) or they dispense completely with the need for hospitalisation (day hospital).

Thus, at the Assistance Publique: in 1976, the number of patients staying less than ten days increased by 9 per cent over 1975, and that of those staying for more than ten days decreased slightly; between 1970 and 1976 the number of out-patient visits increased from 2 million to 2.75 million; in the same period, the number of treatments limited to a day or a half-day went up from 2,200 to 62,000. The provision of additional beds is therefore now no longer the primary objective. Current attention must instead be focused on the adaptation of existing facilities to novel modes of treatment.

3. The Assistance Publique and the Future

Faced with an unpredictable future, the Assistance Publique is anxious to define its role by developing its forecasting tools and fixing the direction it will follow so as to fit in with its internal constraints and the general interests of the Paris region.

It has adopted three forecasting strategies:

(1) Over a ten-year period it is evaluating the hospital care needs of the population of the region. These needs are assessed for each specialty, a specialty corresponding either to a specific group of diseases (neurology, cardiology) or to a certain type of medical activity (paediatrics, general surgery). These forecasts are adjusted to the limitations of the Assistance Publique within the framework of a general masterplan which is also established for a sliding period of ten years and brought up to date every year.

(2) Over an indeterminate period the hospital master plans, which prescribe capital investment, lay down the changes in buildings on the basis of the facts already known. These plans may have several stages: those which can be completed in a short time are quite specific, whereas those that are longer-term than the general master plan are naturally more schematic. In the latter case, it is essential to set out clearly the hypotheses which make them at present desirable so that they may be subsequently revised. In the master plans, the choice of medical assignment for the hospital and the

organisation of the medical services required for its successful execution are essential factors. The architectural side and the technical services are designed as a result of this choice and not as predetermining instruments.

(3)   Over a shorter period, the creation of highly technical ward units (constant supervision, intensive care, etc.) and the installation of the most highly developed medical equipment are being subjected to analyses of medical and economic expediency, carried out both by the planning departments and the medical team who put forward the request. The development of these forecasting and classifying tools has led to the opening up of the Assistance Publique administration to doctors, epidemiologists, economists and organisation experts.

As a result of these plans, certain orientations are already clear and tend to confirm that the future role for the Assistance Publique is in the existing specialised teaching hospital. It is not to be primarily concerned with geographical or quantitative expansion. In this way the Assistance Publique is making a distinction between its general and specialist hospital services. As far as general hospitalisation services (which include medicine, surgery, orthopaedics and maternity hospitals, with about 8,600 beds admitting 175,000 patients per year) are concerned, the Assistance Publique intends to use these beds to serve only the local population. The breakdown of patients at present is shown in Table 3.5.

Table 3.5: Breakdown of Patients in Assistance Publique Hospitals

	Per cent
Paris	47.2
Inner ring	37
Outer ring	7.6
Outside the region	8.2

The figures for the outer ring and outside the region could be reduced by half. In addition, we foresee the stabilisation of the population of Paris and the inner ring, another reduction in the length of stay and the development of very short-term admissions (less than 24 hours). The number of beds could thus be reduced progressively by 1,200 to 1,500 between now and 1985. On the other hand, for its specialist services, which are being used more and more every year, with an average increase of 5 per cent per annum (310,000 patients admitted in 1976 to the 15,000 beds), the Assistance Publique is of the opinion that grouping and co-ordinating is appropriate because these specialist services have the backing of a strong teaching and research structure, which constitute a unique guarantee of quality of care while avoiding unnecessary costs. The areas from which the in-patients come are very different, and the number of patients coming from the periphery of the region, the rest of France and other countries is increasing, thus confirming that the medical environment has more influence on the patient's choice of hospital than the distance from his home. However, in the case of these services, it does not seem at present as if the reduction in the length of stay and the new types of care can reduce the number of beds required by more than a few hundred.

The Assistance Publique intends to undertake two additional specific tasks:

(1)   to set up, in each acute hospital, polyclinics and day hospitals accessible to the community and to the doctors working in individual or group practice who would be able to make use of the medical and technical facilities necessary for detailed investigations and complicated types of treatment;

(2)   to organise rehabilitation centres (with or without beds) near to the teaching hospital complexes.

The policy of the Assistance Publique of Paris therefore appears to be both conservative and innovative. It seems conservative to advocate the grouping and limitation of the specialist services when local authorities and many doctors argue in favour of the extension, even the general introduction, of the highly technical services. But is it not unreasonable to keep on increasing specialist provision without having either to justify the costs borne by the community or to prove that it is being put to good medical use? On the other hand, if it is true that the exposure of the hospitals to external factors and the extension of hospital involvement to the patient's rehabilitation is now favourably regarded, then it is a pity that this need to justify their existence and costs has not always been the case.

There is no question that the crisis through which hospitals in all countries are now passing is not merely an economic one; it is also to some extent a crisis of confidence between the hospital and the community. It is by opening their doors and possibly by reducing their provision that both kinds of crisis may be survived. The Assistance Publique hopes that in this way it will be able, with all its peculiarities, its weaknesses and its advantages, to continue making a useful contribution to the organisation of health care in the Paris region.

4 SYDNEY

Anthony I. Adams*

A. PATTERN OF EXISTING SERVICES

Demography

The 2.9 million people in metropolitan Sydney are spread over an area of 4,077 square kilometres, ranging from the densely populated inner city suburbs (almost 6,000 people per square kilometre) to the newly developing areas in the north, south and west (less than 150 people per square kilometre in some areas). Although Sydney occupies only a small fraction of the area of New South Wales, more than 60 per cent of the population of the state resides in Sydney.

As the spread of population to the outer areas has occurred in comparatively recent years, the health services of Sydney have been concentrated mainly in the inner-city areas and have not expanded rapidly enough to keep pace with the distribution of population. While only 18 per cent of the city's population now resides in the inner area, the specialist teaching hospitals, together with a large proportion of general hospital and medical practitioner services, are situated in the inner city. The northern and southern areas of Sydney, each with approximately 25 per cent of the city's population, have suffered to a lesser extent from the inner-city concentration of health services than the western area, which now has one million people over a large area with scarce health services, and where distance adds to the accessibility problems.

Over-all, more than 50 per cent of Sydney's population is aged less than 30 years, 40 per cent from 30 to 64 years and 9 per cent aged 65 years or more (see Table 4.1). However, an uneven age distribution throughout the city has resulted from the drift of young marrieds and their families to newer areas in the north, south and especially the west, where 32 per cent of the population is aged less than 15 years, while the inner-city areas are largely young singles and elderly people. Housing varies from old established homes and high-rise buildings, creating their own health problems, in the areas close to the

* This report on the complex mixture of government, private and voluntary organisations which comprise Sydney's health services was produced by Dr Adams and his colleagues in the Health Service Research Division of the Health Commission of New South Wales.

101

city centre, to conventional bungalow-style housing in the outer areas. In general, the standard of housing is commensurate with the relatively high standard of living but, as in most big cities, pockets of low-standard housing exist in the inner-city areas.

The public hospitals in Sydney treat approximately 425,000 in-patients annually (146.6 per 1,000 population) and almost 1,500,000 out-patients. However, because of the location of the major specialist teaching hospitals, people from all over the state receive hospital treatment in Sydney. Approximately 22,000 people are treated each year in psychiatric and mental retardation hospitals in Sydney; a rate of 7.6 per 1,000 population. Private health organisations, hospitals, nursing homes and medical practitioners add considerable resources to the city's health services and without them the public health system would be strained to meet demand (see Table 4.7).

Planning and Organisation

The health services for the Sydney Metropolitan Area are in the main provided by the three levels of government: federal, state and local, giving rise to both a complicated and confusing picture of the health care scene. A private sector, providing health services, adds even more to this complexity.

State Government

The main burden for the organisation and planning of the city's health services falls on the state government through the Health Commission of New South Wales. The Health Commission was formed in April 1973 from the amalgamation of two state government departments: the NSW Department of Health and the Hospitals Commission of New South Wales. The Health Commission is headed by a chairman who is responsible to the state Minister for Health and four Commissioners. The organisational structure of the Commission comprises four bureaux, each responsible to a Commissioner. These bureaux are: (1) Personal Health Services: general administration of public hospitals, development of hospitals and allied services, maternal and child health services, mental health services, paramedical and other specialised health facilities; (2) Environmental and Special Health Services: health education, public health activities, private hospitals, pathology, radiology and scientific services and other special health services; (3) Manpower and Management Services: staff development, industrial relations, manpower planning and other staff services; (4) Finance and Physical Resources: collection of revenue, budgeting, building and equipment and other financial matters. A Division of Health Services Research services the whole Commission and is responsible to the chairman (see Figures 4.1 and 4.2).

In addition to the above structure, the state is divided geographically into 14 health regions. Each region has a Regional Director of Health, together with a deputy and assistant Regional Directors and supporting staff, and is directly responsible to the Commission (see Figure 4.3). The administrative authority for all health services within each of the regions' geographical boundaries has been delegated to the regions. Within each region it is planned to have a Regional Advisory Committee drawn from both professional health workers and representatives of the community.

The Sydney Metropolitan Area is divided into four health regions: Inner, North, South and West, each with administrative authority for health services within its boundaries (see Figure 4.4). The central office of the Health Commission thus has the ultimate responsibility for over-all co-ordination, policy-making and arbitration of standards while the day-to-day administration of the city's health services is the responsibility of the regions. The decentralisation of administration to regional levels enables closer contact with the community and their requirements and input from the regional level provides informed opinions on which the decisions regarding policy and standards can be based.

Federal Government

The federal government through, particularly, the departments of Health, Social Security and Repatriation, administers various health and health-related services in the city. Important among these services are age and invalid pensions, sickness benefits and child endowment and maternity allowances, while the Repatriation Department provides health and related services to ex-servicemen and their dependants. One of the most significant aspects of the federal government's role in the operation of the city's health services is its administration of the National Health Insurance Scheme (Medibank) which provides financial protection against the costs of medical, optometrical and hospital care. The federal government also plays an important role in providing much of the financial resources necessary to improve and maintain the city's health services.

Local Government

Local government authorities are concerned mainly with environmental

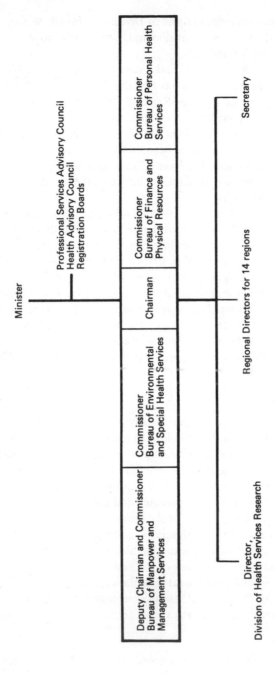

Figure 4.1: Health Commission of New South Wales: Organisation Chart — Central Administration (Present)

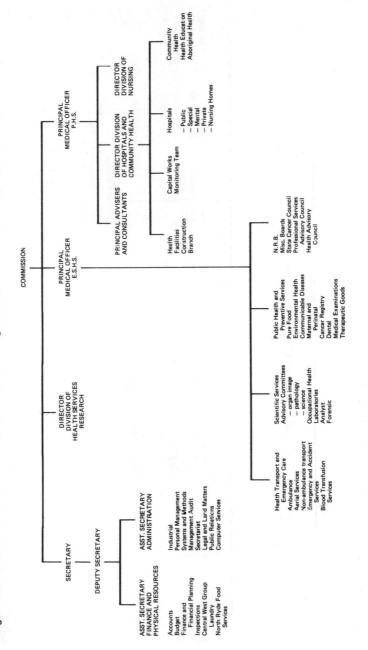

Figure 4.2: Health Commission of New South Wales: Organisation Chart — Central Administration (Proposed)

Figure 4.3: Health Commission of New South Wales: Regional Administration

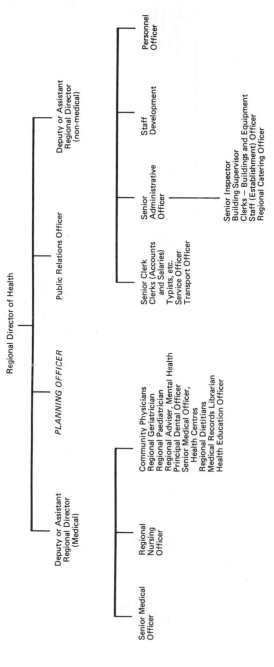

Figure 4.4: Sydney Metropolitan Area: Health Regions

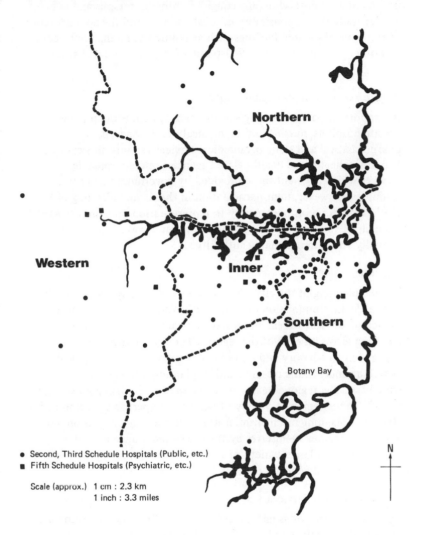

Northern

Western

Inner

Southern

Botany Bay

- Second, Third Schedule Hospitals (Public, etc.)
- Fifth Schedule Hospitals (Psychiatric, etc.)

Scale (approx.) 1 cm : 2.3 km
                 1 inch : 3.3 miles

N

control and a limited range of personal health services. Immunisation programmes against whooping cough, diphtheria, tetanus and polio are generally the responsibility of local councils and the administration of some health-related facilities such as public swimming pools, parks and other recreation services is also one of the roles of local government.

Private and Voluntary Organisations

An important part of the city's health care system is the private sector. Private hospitals, nursing homes, medical practitioner, dental, pharmaceutical and some paramedical services fall into this category. Voluntary health and health-related agencies operate valuable services which augment those provided by government and private resources. However, their participation in the formal planning of the city's services is confined mainly to representation on committees and councils of various kinds along with representatives of the more formally structured planning authorities.

Planning

Formal planning of the city's health services is largely the responsibility of the Health Commission of New South Wales through the Division of Health Services Research, located centrally, and research and planning teams, in each of the regions. The central division is engaged in an advisory and participatory capacity to the regional teams as well as undertaking research and/or planning projects on an area-wide basis. The regional teams are concerned with planning exercises specific to the region. A variety of skills and expertise are combined to effect the planning mechanism, not only in the central division, but within the regions themselves by the use of planning committees, offering an even larger variety of skills, and which may operate in both an executive and advisory capacity.

Access to Health Services

Primary medical care is mainly the province of general practitioners. The general practitioner is usually the first point of contact for patients seeking medical attention and if necessary he may then refer patients to other services for appropriate attention. However, in some areas of the city, general practitioners are in short supply and there may be difficulty in attracting them to these areas. Where this is the case they are supplemented with a community nurse who acts as the first contact with the sick patient. The nurse treats those that she can and refers the remainder to a general practitioner. The community nurses are based at health centres which may also be used as a source of primary care. In the larger centres a team of health professionals, such as community nurses, psychologists, physiotherapists, social workers and other paramedical staff support general practitioners who may have rooms at the centres as well as their private surgeries. Some areas of the city have an adequate number of general practitioners, although health centres are maintained in these areas to provide the range of supportive services.

Although the provision of health centres has helped, to some extent, to provide primary care in areas where shortages of general practitioners are evident, the casualty departments of hospitals are used by some as a source of primary care. Even in the inner-city areas, where general practitioners are numerous, casualty departments are used for primary medical care, particularly for services required 'out of hours'.

The casualty departments form one of the ways in which patients gain access to hospital in-patient care. The majority of people treated as in-patients are referred to the hospitals by private practitioners, either general or specialist. Patients may be referred to hospitals for in-patient treatment by a variety of sources; in addition to private medical practitioners, welfare agencies, community centres and nurses, nursing services and other health and related agencies, both voluntary and government, all participate in the referral of patients to hospitals.

Distribution of Doctors and Staff

The distribution of doctors in the private sector of the city's health services has been influenced largely by the location of hospitals, particularly the specialist teaching hospitals. Formal controls over the distribution of private medical practitioners do not exist and the lack of controls has had some effect upon the maldistribution of doctors. This is particularly evident in the new developing areas of generally low socio-economic status, where severe shortages of doctors exist. A similar situation exists for nursing and other paramedical staff with severe shortages in the outer areas of Sydney. The Health Commission of New South Wales offers subsidies to attract medical practitioners to areas where there are shortages, although this applies mainly to the rural areas of the state.

The only formal controls over health manpower are statutory registration boards which have the power to register personnel, depending upon their qualifications. These boards have no controls

over the distribution of manpower. Manpower within the public health
sector is controlled by the Health Commission of New South Wales.
The Health Commission is responsible for the determination of the
numbers of staff in all categories — medical, paramedical, administrative
— employed in all public hospitals, nursing homes, health centres and
other public health services. (For distribution data on general
practitioners and other health personnel in the Sydney area see Table
4.9.)

Community Participation and Voluntary Organisations

Community Participation

Community participation in the planning and operation of the city's
health services is part of the over-all philosophy and aim of the Health
Commission of New South Wales. However, at present, real community
participation is an ideal still to be attained. Hospital boards of
management and advisory committees of various kinds provide some
contact with the people.

In each of the city's health regions it is planned that there should
be a Regional Advisory Committee to be made up of representatives
of the community as well as health professionals. These committees
are intended to advise the regional health authorities of the requirements of all health services of the community. They will provide to the
Commission the formal input and feedback from workers in the health
field and consumers of health care in order to communicate the needs
of the people and the practicality of policies. Similar functions to those
of the Regional Advisory Committee are provided by a Health Advisory
Council of community representatives and a Professional Services
Advisory Council of health professionals, which were established to
advise the Commission itself.

Participation by members of the community through informal
channels is also encouraged and suggestions for the improvement of
health services may be received by letter, telephone or informal
contact with staff members. Letters of complaint also help to highlight
deficiencies or breakdowns in the provision of services.

Voluntary Organisations

Voluntary organisations provide invaluable input in the communication channels to the health authorities. Although there are no formal
lines of participation by voluntary organisations in the planning of the
city's health services, their involvement in a wide variety of areas

connected with health and health-related services often enables early awareness of existence of problems and possible solutions.

Voluntary organisations form a very important element in the city's health care system by providing a multitude of services which in some cases augment those provided by government authorities, but which in further cases are not otherwise available. In some cases these services are better provided by these organisations than by government. Some important areas of activity of the voluntary organisations include supportive medical care — rehabilitation, training, after-care, health education, recreational facilities, fund-raising, research, 'pressure group' activities and supportive activities for 'underprivileged' and minority groups.

Finance

Sydney's health services are financed by a multiplicity of sources. The largest proportion of finance is provided by federal and state governments by means of taxation. This is supplemented by funds from local government authorities, via council rates, compensation insurance, voluntary insurance, patients' fees as well as minor contributions from grants, donations and investments. Public hospitals and health services receive the major portion of their income for maintenance and capital expenditure from state and federal governments either directly or in the form of benefits for occupied hospital bed days. Private organisations, both profitable and non-profitable, chiefly hospitals and nursing homes, contribute valuable resources to the health services of the city and these services again receive a large proportion of their finance from the federal government (see Table 4.10).

Expenditure on institutional care consumes the largest proportion of finance allocated to health services while pharmaceutical goods, medical appliances and private medical and dental services use a sizeable amount of the remainder. Public health services, teaching and research consume only a small fraction of the total. Since the introduction of national health insurance (Medibank) in July 1975 the federal government contributes a considerable amount towards meeting the cost of primary medical and optometrical as well as hospital care.

Due to the limited taxing powers of the state government, much of the funds committed by the state to the city's health service have first been collected by the federal government before being allocated to the state. Capital works programmes for public hospitals and institutions are also heavily dependent on federal government financing, either directly or via state government. While conventional health services consume the largest proportion of health finance, the voluntary health agencies also have an important role to play and, although they rely heavily on public donations, financial assistance from government funds is essential to some for the maintenance of their operations.

Estimating Expenditure

In the public health sector, annual estimates of expenditure are prepared by all public health organisations receiving monies from state government for maintenance costs. These estimates are submitted by the 'institutions' first to the regional offices of the Health Commission which then forward these together with estimates of expenditure for the community health service and the regional administration itself to the central office of the Health Commission. Allocation of funds to the public health services from state government resources is based upon these estimates.

Expenditure in the private health sector is difficult to estimate. Little information is available from private hospitals and nursing homes regarding their sources of income and sites of expenditure. However, the regulations under the Private Hospitals Act which specify the terms of licensing and monitoring these institutions could be adapted to allow a freer flow of information to those involved in the financing of health services. The Health Commission of New South Wales has the responsibility for expenditure in the public sector and thus estimates for the government sector are more reliable than those for the private sector. In addition to the estimates of expenditure required by the state government, the introduction of the National Health Service, which involves payment by the federal government to hospitals on the basis of occupied bed days, requires that the Health Commission submit estimates of expenditure on hospitals for three periods of the year to the Federal Government

Payment of Doctors

Private medical practitioners are paid on the basis of fee for service; they may receive full payment for service direct from the patient; they may bill the patient the full amount, but receive 85 per cent of the 'scheduled' fee direct from the Health Insurance Commission (Medibank) and the remainder from the patient; or they may 'bulk bill' the Health Insurance Commission and accept 85 per cent of the scheduled fee as full payment. The same arrangements apply for the payment of medical practitioners in private hospitals. Within the public hospital system medical staff may be salaried staff paid by the hospital or they may be visiting medical officers paid on the basis of fee for service by the patient as above or on a sessional or contract basis and paid by the hospital. In determining the scheduled fees for medical services, the Australian government accepted the independent findings of the Medical Fees Tribunal and of private fee enquiries conducted in December 1974 and May 1975.

Patient Payments

Under the Health Insurance Act, medical benefits are payable in respect of fees charged by medical practitioners, certain dentists and participating optometrists for specified services. In general, benefits payable are 85 per cent of the scheduled fee, with the proviso that the difference between the scheduled fee and the benefit payable for any service does not exceed $5. The Health Insurance Programme automatically covers all residents of Australia, without payment of any premium or contribution, in respect of services received.

Thus, under the National Health Insurance Programme patients are required to pay, at the most, 15 per cent of the scheduled fee for medical and optometrical and some dental services. They may pay these fees either by: (1) direct payment of the full fee to the provider of the service and then recoup the benefit from Medibank; or (2) payment of the difference between the fee charged and the Medibank benefit, to the provider of the service; or (3) no payment at all if the provider of the service agrees to accept the Medibank benefit as full payment for the service. Should the patient contribute to a voluntary health insurance fund he may also be refunded his out-of-pocket expenses caused by differences between fees charged and the Medibank benefit.

The National Health Insurance Programme also pays benefits to patients for treatment in hospitals. Patients may receive free accommodation (excluding medical treatment) in standard wards of public hospitals or, if the patient prefers treatment as a private patient, he receives a subsidy from Medibank towards the hospital fees charged. Private patients treated in public hospitals have their charges substantially reduced because of the Medibank payments direct to the hospitals while patients treated in private hospitals receive cash benefits from Medibank and these benefits are deducted from the daily fees charged to them. The fees charged for medical attention received from their own doctors by private patients in both public and private hospitals are also subject to the benefit from Medibank as above.

Should patients contribute to a voluntary health insurance fund they may also receive benefits from the fund in respect of out-of-pocket expenses for hospital care. Patients receiving other health services provided by organisations on other than a fee-for-service basis may also have their payments subsidised under Medibank subject to the approval of that service by the National Health Insurance Commission.

Health Standards and Health-Related Agencies

The Health Commission of New South Wales has the main responsibility for the formation of policy and plans and the setting of standards to improve the quality of life for the people of Sydney. Many other agencies, mainly government or semi-government, are involved in activities related to maintaining and improving the quality of life of the people. Some of the state government departments involved in this sphere are those concerned with planning and environment, pollution control, youth, ethnic and community affairs, education, housing, roads, transport and water, sewerage and drainage. All make contributions to policies, plans and standards of services related to the health of the people. In addition to the state governments, several federal government departments are also concerned with issues related to health matters. Some of these departments are: Social Security: concerned with pensions, family allowances, unemployment benefits, health benefits and many welfare services; Repatriation: health and related services to ex-servicemen and their families; Health: pharmaceutical benefits, quarantine services, and other health services and the National Hospital and Health Services Commission. Both state and federal government treasuries have considerable influence on the implementation of policies and plans. The financial constraints imposed by these two bodies encourage the formation of policies and plans that can reasonably be expected to be achieved. Similarly the respective Public Services Boards do much to influence the staffing structures of any public health service.

The fragmentation of responsibility between federal, state and private organisations as well as separate departments and organisations within each of these spheres makes the process of rational policy-making extremely difficult. The planning process also becomes extremely complicated when such a multitude of organisations are involved, and consultation and co-operation is essential to co-ordinate and rationalise all the different policies and plans that evolve.

Collection of Data

The variety of organisations involved in the management of health and
health-related services entails that there is a diversity of information
collected. The collection of data is fundamental to the planning of
health services by providing the foundation for objective planning
decisions. The Health Commission of New South Wales, through its
central and regional offices, has the prime responsibility for the
collection of information relating to public health services. An ongoing
collection of patient data from psychiatric hospitals in the Sydney area
(undertaken as a joint venture by the Health Commission and the
Australian Bureau of Statistics) provides basic morbidity data to the
Health Commission on the use of public and psychiatric hospitals.
Attempts to evaluate and monitor the use of community services have
necessitated the collection of data from these services by the Health
Commission, but despite their early conception these ongoing data
collections are still in their infancy and require continual upgrading and
adjustment to meet the ever-changing needs of planners, researchers
and managers.

Apart from the Health Commission, the numerous government
agencies listed above collect and collate data relevant to their own
fields and consequently related to the health field. University departments, private health/welfare organisations as well as hospitals and
health facilities themselves collect information pertinent to research,
planning and management of the health services. The information
collected by all these sources covers a wide spectrum of health and
social aspects of the community. However, the diversity of organisations involved limits the effective use of the wealth of information
collected. To a large degree reliance is placed upon the individuals
involved to communicate with others in the field and to pass on the
relevant information.

Co-ordination between Organisations

The many organisations concerned with health and health-related
services makes co-ordination between them extremely difficult.
Consultation and co-ordination between the different bodies is usually
achieved by the formation of committees, councils or conferences.
At the highest level a conference of premiers of all states of
Australia takes place annually and similarly there is an annual conference of all state Ministers for Health and their senior officers.

At state government level committees of senior officers
representing various government departments are formed to consult,

advise or resolve issues of common interest to them all. These
committees may be long-standing, interdepartmental committees or
they may be *ad hoc*, convened to advise on specific areas or problems.
Similar committees may comprise representatives of government
bodies, community groups and voluntary organisations.

Interdepartmental committees also exist to co-ordinate the activities
of federal government departments and there are committees or
councils with representatives from both federal and state government
organisations. The Hospitals and Allied Services Advisory Council, for
example, is made up of state and federal Health Administrators with
the aim of providing information on which the annual Health Ministers'
Conference can make decisions of national importance. These
committees or councils are not confined to health matters alone but
may be formed by representatives of health-related departments and
their members may then report back to the various interdepartmental
committees at state level. Some of the federal-state councils may also
include representatives from non-governmental bodies. The National
Health and Medical Research Council comprises government representatives as well as representatives of various medical bodies and
schools and lay people appointed to the Council by the federal
government. The Council advises both federal and state governments
on general health matters and on medical research grants. A number of
committees have been appointed by the Council, and these committees
also have representation from experts outside government to advise on
specialised aspects of health matters.

The secondment or exchange of officers between departments and
organisations encourages the exchange of information and aids in the
co-ordination process, as do the informal contacts between officers
engaged in the same or similar field of activity.

B. PARTICULAR ASPECTS OF PLANNING AND PROVISION

1. Problems Affecting Planning and Provision of Health Services

Maldistribution and shortage of services, rising cost, unco-ordinated
effort and limited finance are just a few of the many problems facing
the city's health administrators. Such problems are not confined
to Sydney alone but are common to New South Wales and Australia
generally.

These problems give rise to the urgent need for more objective
health planning with the ultimate aim of making available to all
sectors of the community the highest possible level of health care,

and the most economic use of the resources available.

To be successful, the planning process should be flexible so as to meet continually changing needs brought about by medical, demographic and social changes in the community. A combination of diverse disciplines can offer expertise essential to health planning and a multidisciplinary team representing hospital, medical, government and other groups would be able to make the most effective use of the skills available.

The rising demand on the city's health facilities accentuated by the advent of national health insurance (Medibank) and the increased benefits offered by the voluntary health insurance agencies is expected to have a profound impact on the utilisation of present and future health services. However, effective health planning has been handicapped to some extent by several important problems, common to most large cities.

Maldistribution of Population, Services and Manpower

Population. The rapid growth of population in the outer areas of Sydney, particularly the west, has resulted in an uneven and continually changing age distribution of the city's population. Within the inner-city areas there is now a strong concentration of young single and aged people while young marrieds and their families have drifted to the expanding outer areas of Sydney. The city's health services have not changed or expanded rapidly enough to be able to meet this demand in the outer areas and thus access to appropriate services is not always easy.

Certain segments of the community such as low-income earners, migrants, aborigines, homeless and destitute give rise to special areas of concern.

Services. Hospitals and health-related facilities within common geographical boundaries often develop plans independently of each other. This lack of co-ordination and co-operation makes the task of rationalising services all the more difficult.

The main teaching hospitals are located near the universities and the policies of medical faculties have influenced the hospital services provided. In addition, some of these large teaching hospitals have their own Acts of Parliament and are thus largely independent of outside influence.

A major problem, particularly for the older hospitals in the inner city, is obsolescence, but the movement of population to new localities places doubt upon the replacement or upgrading of out-of-date facilities. Another compounding factor is the high cost involved in developing and redeveloping facilities on difficult sites.

Manpower. At present there exists a shortage of all types of health professionals in the outer districts of the metropolitan area. This problem is made worse by the predilection of doctors, particularly specialists, to live or practise near the hospitals.

The more affluent suburbs of Sydney naturally attract a greater proportion of health professionals to the disadvantage of the lower-status suburbs. Socio-economic aspects tend to have a detrimental influence on the distribution of health manpower, particularly in the fast-growing outer suburbs and areas inhabited by minority groups.

One effect of the introduction of Medibank and the consequent lowering of the financial barrier to medical care for many people is the increased work-load of the private practitioner and other health manpower. In this regard the increased effort may affect the standard and quality of health care.

Structure and Administration

Although the concept of regionalisation is commendable and forms the basis of the administrative structure of the Health Commission of New South Wales, there are certain administrative problems and other difficulties that regionalisation entails.

(1)   Overlapping services, facilities in close proximity to regional boundaries and heterogeneity of population within defined geographic boundaries are some important problems facing regional administrators.

(2)   Channels of communication between the community, the health services, the regional administration, the Health Commission and federal government authorities are complex, confusing and not clearly defined.

(3)   The federal/state dichotomy whereby both governments provide finance and services often creates confusion and uncertainty not only amongst users of the services but also those providing, co-ordinating and planning services.

(4)   The current division between Health and Social Welfare Services is sometimes frustrating, particularly when several services required cannot be supplied by the one authority.

Finance

The fragmented and complex process of financing the city's health
services suggests that a properly defined funding mechanism is required
before effective planning can be implemented. The financial constraints imposed by the present funding system, annual budgeting,
funding for specific projects, have hampered the implementation
of some plans while this delay has made other forward plans
inappropriate to changing needs of the community.

The funding mechanism lacks flexibility for new innovative projects
when the funds are allocated in a 'piecemeal' fashion or for single
purposes. Similarly, the financial constraints imposed by annual
budgeting can lead to a lack of continuity in making long-term planning
decisions. The present system of annual budgeting makes no allowance
for the most economic use or supply of services. In this regard over-
spending usually results in the government paying for the excess while
underspending can lead to the loss of finance or, worse, the incentive to
spend the money wastefully.

Plans have been implemented in haste to avoid problems caused by
rising costs and shortages of materials. Combined with the limited
method of budgeting this has resulted in some instances in a lack of
proper evaluation and management of certain projects and to irrational
decisions in spending funds as well as a lack of adequate documentation
of new programmes.

There are many agencies which contribute greatly to the health and
welfare of the community but because of the diverse nature of their
work are given low priority in terms of finance by the federal and state
governments. Without proper finance many of these agencies will
disappear, further increasing the heavy burden now carried by government authorities.

Hospital Boards of Management

The governing bodies of the city's major hospitals are composed of
respected and influential members of the community who naturally
retain a keen interest in maintaining the prestige and tradition of their
respective hospitals. However, this attitude of independence by these
hospitals, some within common geographical boundaries, can adversely affect over-all planning strategy and hence place constraints on
the implementation of services. This problem is particularly evident
with the inner-city specialist teaching hospitals, partly because of their
separate Acts of Parliament and University affiliations. Such hospitals
can make planning largely ineffectual when they bypass or ignore

regional authorities. By comparison, although district hospitals have autonomous boards of management they have a lesser effect on the over-all planning mechanism.

Attitudes of Private Practitioners

The medical profession can strongly influence the course and behaviour of medical care, particularly when organised into strong professional associations. These groups can exert powerful pressure-group and political activity, especially when their interests diverge from those of the government.

Private medical practitioners can affect the extent of utilisation of hospital services as well as the nature of cases treated. They can also determine the time spent by patients in hospital and consequently influence the financial resources required to meet hospital costs. The system of referral of patients by doctors also determines the sources of in-patient care.

The acceptance of new types of services, particularly community centres and community nurses, by doctors also influences the degree to which they are used as well as the acceptance by the community of the services provided.

Information

The basis of any sound planning is adequate factual data. However, the complex mixture of organisations involved in the provision of services results in a variety of non-standardised data with many large gaps. Even within the field of public health services, the collection of data relating to hospital use and financial sources often needs to be supplemented by special studies to obtain the necessary information.

The private sector leaves even more gaps in the information system on which to base sound planning strategies. The very nature of it being private implies no routine requirement to collect and submit information.

Although the necessity for adequate information is well recognised, attempts to institute collections of relevant data have been slow to progress. The rapidly changing health services now require different and modified data on which to base evaluation and monitoring of these services.

In the past the planning of health services was given a low priority and often seen as an expensive luxury when direct patient services were lacking and finance for health limited. As a result of this, planning techniques and related expertise were given little chance to develop.

Planning of health services was generally carried out on an *ad hoc* basis, particular problems were solved as they arose, in isolation from the total health care system of the city. The resulting 'hotch-potch' and maldistribution of services has made rationalisation throughout the city extremely difficult.

The recognition of the need for forward planning by the Health Commission of New South Wales has led to the establishment of the Division of Health Services Research and regional planning/research teams.

2. Good Ideas and Practices

Regionalisation

Although regionalisation of health services within the city has certainly had its share of 'teething' problems, over-all it has had a significant effect upon the supply and management of all types of services. The complexity of services and organisations involved and the geographical size of the area make central administration unwieldy and often apt to neglect areas of low political concern. The regional authorities have been able to concentrate on problems and needs specific to their regions and are aware of the local requirements of the community and can thus provide and improve services at a faster rate. Health services or areas which have been given low priority in the past because of more pressing problems centrally have been able to receive the attention they deserve.

The delegation of authority to administer health services at the regional level has in many ways shortened the traditional bureaucratic process, by allowing decision-making at the local level to be thus more responsive to the community needs. The many frustrations of dealing with a large organisation have been lessened and the community now has relatively easy access to the decision-makers.

Staffing of health services and the regional administration itself has become easier by selection from the local population as well as enabling staff to reside closer to their place of work. Staff satisfaction is more evident because of the possibility of more rapid promotion both within the regional administration as well as the patient treatment centres and the ability to see their own contributions to the planning and management of health services materialise.

Planning

The regional setting has promoted more successful planning. The establishment of regional planning/research teams has facilitated the acquisition of information pertinent to local needs and thus the policies and plans produced, relevant to the community's needs. The central research/planning team acts as co-ordinator between the regional teams as well as participating in and advising on specific projects.

Many of the planning exercises undertaken by the regions have used a 'committee' technique, bringing together expertise from various professions within government organisations as well as from hospitals, universities, management consultants and the community itself. The involvement of a multidisciplinary group as well as those likely to be directly affected by the plans has facilitated the implementation of projects by changing attitudes during the planning process rather than imposing uninformed material change.

The use of private consultants and university groups as part of the planning committee has linked government and private enterprise personnel with a consequent exchange of ideas and expertise and has also provided a link with modern business techniques.

The involvement of outside bodies in the planning process has placed the Health Commission in the role of the 'client' and as such it has the power of approval of the final plans. Duplication of services, particularly those overlapping or close to regional boundaries, has been avoided by the inclusion of representatives of the central research team as well as the regional planners. The role of the Health Commission as client has to some extent aided in controlling costs of the planning itself as well as the implementation of plans.

The multidisciplinary and multi-organisational approach to planning has resulted in well-developed plans which have had some effect on decreasing the influence of powerful hospital boards and other political pressures.

Building Programmes

The implementation of building projects has been facilitated by the appointment of Project Managers who represent the Health Commission as client. The Project Manager, in consultation with architects, hospital boards and others involved in the construction and design process, has authority over events and the timing of such, and by reporting at regular intervals to his client, the Health Commission, allows it control over construction progress as well as costs.

The limited finance available has often delayed the construction and implementation of deserving projects. Network analysis has therefore been introduced and this has allowed for the staging of building projects, enabling several projects to be commenced within a relatively short period and, although not completed, to be partially used. Where health services have been scarce, this method has provided communities with some services previously not accessible to them.

A concept of 'plan as you build' has been introduced for the construction of one new hospital. This method allows for the commencement of building before plans are finalised and approved. Staging of interior plans permits work to continue on some sections while other sections are still being planned and approved. Thus the time from inception to commissioning of the building is shortened and thereby rising costs are, to some extent, avoided.

Finance

The expansion of community health services was accelerated by provision of funds specifically allocated to the community health programme by the federal government. Although causing many administrative problems, the allocation of finance for specific projects, within a particular area of health or health-related services, has given the opportunity of establishing some services without competition against the more politically powerful bodies or other more popular services.

Other Practices

(1)   Household interview surveys have provided valuable base-line data on which to plan services responsive to the needs and expectations of the community. They have also highlighted areas or populations of special concern and those which require special or intensified health services.

(2)   Community centres and nurses have eased the load on general practitioners and in those areas with severe shortages of general practitioners have made primary medical care accessible.

(3)   Emergency and crisis centres have been established with easy access by telephone.

(4)   In addition to interpreting services provided by some health facilities, a service is also provided by the federal government to assist migrants with all types of enquiries or problems.

3. Research and Planning

A major source for studies concerning the health and well-being of the people of Sydney is the Division of Health Services Research. This Division, along with regional planning officers, has an important role to play in research and developing health services not only for the city but also for the state. The staff of the Division are engaged in a wide range of research projects covering a broad spectrum of the health field.

Emergency Health Care Study

The study was conducted recently in the Inner and Western Metropolitan Health Regions of Sydney and looked at the components of emergency care on a regional basis. The over-all objectives were to improve the provision of emergency care by individual providers, to rationalise resources for emergency care on a regional basis and to develop a plan for co-ordinating all providers of emergency services into a system of emergency care both within the region and within the state. The Bureau of Personal Health Services has been designated the responsibility of implementing the policy of categorisation of hospitals for emergency care as recommended by the researchers.

Inner Metropolitan Health Region – Hospital Services Planning Study

Broadly, the objective of the study is an attempt to rationalise hospital services in the Inner Metropolitan Region. This is a current project and represents one of the most crucial planning exercises to be undertaken in New South Wales. The satisfactory adoption of a plan would influence the provision of hospital services elsewhere in Sydney and the state. The study is a combined effort of members of the Division of Health Services Research, the Inner Metropolitan Regional Planning Team and outside private consultants, and the aim has been to identify those high-cost and high-treatment intensity areas that can best be centralised and rationalised, while leaving lower-level care to district hospitals. A major objective is to change the nature and function (if not to bring about the closure) of ancient buildings that are reaching the end of their functional life.

Western Metropolitan Hospitals Plan

A major study of demand for hospital services by the population of this region has been completed and a comprehensive plan developed for the construction of hospitals throughout the region over the next 15 years. This will do much to reduce the accessibility problems faced by that population.

Childhood Accidents Study

Accidents to all age groups account for approximately one-seventh
of the expenditure on hospital beds in Sydney and the potential exists
for considerable savings through effective prevention programmes.
At present childhood accident statistics are incomplete and difficult to
utilise and thus it is the objective of this study to identify what appear
to be critical variables in accident control and to select those that are
subject to control and manipulation for definition and guidance of
prevention programmes. A comprehensive data collection system has
been introduced into all major casualty departments in Sydney.

Other Studies

Apart from the above projects the Division of Health Services Research
has undertaken a large number of other studies concerning health and
health-related issues. These projects cover a wide field and include
studies concerned with psychiatric patients, public hospitals, nursing
homes, demographic and morbidity data, drug use, Medibank, health
manpower, household surveys concerned with the utilisation of health
services, illness patterns and opinions of health service consumers and
studies on the admission of children to hospital and the utilisation of
baby health centres within a defined geographical area.

In addition, there are many requests for studies by the Division
which arise from problems requiring instant analysis, evaluation and
recommendation. Mention should also be made of the valuable studies
carried out by the regional planning teams which in many ways supplement the studies by the Division of Health Services Research.

Effective decision-making in running a health service for a metropolis demands active and relevant research and planning. Health
administrators must be involved at all stages of a research project from
inception to completion if findings and recommendations are to be
implemented as policy.

Appendix

Table 4.1: Population of Sydney by Age and Sex, 1971

Age	Males		Females		Totals	
	Number	Per cent	Number	Per cent	Number	Per cent
0—4	132,097	4.5	125,569	4.3	257,666	8.8
5—14	258,875	8.8	246,250	8.4	505,125	17.2
15—44	661,068	22.5	635,268	21.6	1,296,336	44.1
45—64	304,806	10.4	315,552	10.8	620,358	21.2
65 and over	99,689	3.4	156,762	5.3	256,451	8.7
Total	1,456,535	49.6	1,479,401	50.4	2,935,936	100.0

Table 4.2: Vital Statistics, 1974

Birth rate	18 per 1,000 population
Infant mortality rate	17 per 1,000 live births
Deaths	28,443
Death rate	9 per 1,000 population

Table 4.3: Mortality — First Ten Causes of Death by Rank, 1973

Rank	Cause	Per cent of all deaths
1	Ischaemic heart disease	30.3
2	Malignant neoplasms	17.7
3	Cerebrovascular disease	16.4
4	Accidents	4.8
5	Other forms of heart disease	4.6
6	Bronchitis, emphysema and asthma	3.6
7	Pneumonia	2.3
8	Perinatal problems	2.1
9	Suicide and self-inflicted injuries	1.7
10	Diabetes mellitus	1.4

Table 4.4: Morbidity — Most Common Causes of Hospitalisation in
   Public Hospitals, 1974/5

Deliveries
Injuries
Symptoms and ill-defined conditions
Heart disease
Investigations
Malignant neoplasms
Bronchitis, emphysema and asthma
Abortion
Disorders of menstruation
Hypertrophy of tonsils and adenoids

Table 4.5: Resources, Number of Staff and Number of Population per
   Health Worker, 1971

Staff type	Number	Number of population per health worker
Medical practitioners	4,759	612
Dentists	998	2,941
Nurses (incl. training)	22,360	131
Professional medical workers	3,953	742
Total	32,070	

Table 4.6: Resources — Number of Hospital Beds, 1974

Type of hospital	Number	Number of beds per 1,000 population
General	14,226	4.8
Psychiatric	4,910	1.7
State	1,575	0.5
Private	4,162	1.4
Nursing home	17,841	6.1

Table 4.7: Utilisation — Use of Hospitals, 1974

Number of hospitals (general)	84
Number of beds	14,226
In-patients — number	422,200
— average stay (days)	9.5
Out-patients	1,428,142

Table 4.8: Finance — Expenditure on Health, 1972/3 (Australia)

	$ millions	Per cent of GDP
Financed from public sector	1,465	3.6
Financed from private sector	1,070	2.6
Total	2,535	6.2

Table 4.9: Number of Medical Personnel Employed at the time of 1971 Census

Statistical division	Sydney	Outer Sydney	New South Wales
Medical practitioners	4,661	98	6,125
Dentists	977	21	1,356
Nurses (incl. trainees)	21,558	802	32,505
Professional medical workers	3,845	108	5,156
Total	31,041	1,029	45,142
Population in thousands	2,807.8	128.1	4,601.2
Number of persons per			
medical practitioner	602	1,307	751
dentist	2,874	6,100	3,393
nurse (incl. trainees)	130	160	142
professional medical worker	730	1,186	892

Source: 1971 Census

Table 4.10: Finance

Health service	Sources of finance
Public hospitals	State government Federal government Patient fees — private insurance funds Compensation insurance Inter-hospital charges Donations
Psychiatric hospitals	State government Federal government
Private hospitals	Patient fees — private insurance funds Compensation insurance Federal government Investments
Nursing homes — charitable and non-profitable	Federal government Patient fees Donations
Nursing homes — profitable	Patient fees Federal government Investments
Ambulance service	State government Patient fees Charges to hospitals
Community centres	State government Federal government
Public health services	State government Federal government Local government Patient fees
Pharmaceuticals	Federal government Patient fees
Private medical services	Patient fees Federal government Private health insurance funds
Private dental services	Patient fees Private health insurance funds

/cont.

Table 4.10—cont.

Health service	Sources of finance
Rehabilitation and paramedical service	Patient fees State government Federal government
Research	State government Federal government Donations

Bibliography

A Community Health Programme for Australia (1973). A report from
the National Hospitals and Health Services Commission: Interim
Committee, June.

Australian Department of Health (1975). *Handbook on Health
Manpower, Part 1.*

Dewdney, J. (1972). *Australian Health Services.*

Forward, R. (1974). *Public Policy in Australia.*

Health Commission of New South Wales (1974). *Corporate Plan 1974-
1984.*

Health Insurance Commission. *First Annual Report 1974-75.*

McEwin, R. and Cahill, N. (1975). *Resources and Hospitals – The
Eternal Carousel.* Health Commission of New South Wales.

McEwin, R. and Gross, P. (1974). *The Reorganisation of State Health
Services in Australia.* Health Commission of New South Wales.

Martins, J.M. (1974). *Expenditure on Health in Australia.* Health
Commission of New South Wales.

Martins, J.M. (1976). *The Financing of Health Services in Australia.*
Health Commission of New South Wales.

Sax, S. (1972). *Medical Care in the Melting Pot.*

Spann, R. (1973). *Public Administration in Australia.*

5 TORONTO

R. Alan Hay*

A. THE PATTERN OF EXISTING SERVICES

Introduction

The purpose of this factual statement is to provide background information about the type of health services being delivered to 2.1 million people in Metropolitan (Metro) Toronto. This region is the most densely populated centre in the Province of Ontario, and shares with Greater Montreal the distinction of being one of Canada's business and commercial capitals.

Canada is a confederation of ten provinces, each province having its own government, and two sparsely populated territories which are administered by the federal government. Health care services throughout Canada are influenced by the existence of a universal insurance plan administered by each provincial government on a centralised cost-sharing agreement with the federal government. This programme ensures virtually all residents in Canada of hospital and medical care services on a prepaid basis.

Municipal affairs in Metro Toronto are administered through a two-tier system of government. The upper tier, the Metropolitan Council, administers such services as transportation, police and social services in the metropolitan area generally. Six area municipalities — the boroughs of Etobicoke, North York, Scarborough, East York, York, and the City of Toronto — which forms the lower tier, administer such services as fire protection and public health in their respective areas. A Royal Commission was established in September 1974 by the government of Ontario at the request of the Metropolitan Council to review, evaluate and make recommendations regarding the organising and financing of local government in Metropolitan Toronto. This Commission is expected to present its report in late 1976.

The Medical School at the University of Toronto is the largest in Canada with an annual intake of 250 students. This yields a medical

* Mr Hay was chairman of the Master Committee that conducted the study of Metropolitan Toronto and which produced the report which forms the basis of this chapter. Six months' study was undertaken by a working committee assisted by a full-time project co-ordinator. The appendix at the end of this chapter lists all those concerned.

teaching load of about 1,000 undergraduate students plus more than
1,200 graduate medical students and house staff. The 11 teaching
hospitals directly affiliated with the University of Toronto, together
with other community hospitals and health care institutions, constitute
one of the most comprehensive groupings of speciality medical treatment and referral centres on the continent.

Demography

Metropolitan Toronto covers a surface area of 241 square miles (624
square kilometres). The 1974 population for Metro is reported to be
2,124,095, distributed by municipalities as shown below in Table 5.1.

Table 5.1: Population of Each Municipality in Metropolitan Toronto

	Population	Per cent of population
City of Toronto	682,252	32.1
East York	106,110	5.0
York	140,401	6.6
Total 3 inner boroughs	928,763	43.7
Etobicoke	288,118	13.6
North York	543,662	25.6
Scarborough	363,552	17.1
Total 3 outer boroughs	1,195,332	56.3
Total for Metro Toronto	2,124,095	100.0

Source: Municipal Directory 1975, Ministry of Treasury, Economics and
Inter-Governmental Affairs, p. 1.

Demographic data based on the 1971 census is presented in Tables
5.2, 5.3 and 5.4. It is seen that the population of Toronto is almost
one-tenth of that of Canada and almost a third of the province of
Ontario. The ratio of male to female is even for the population as a
whole, however, there being twice as many females over 65 years of
age as males. The majority of these elderly people live in the inner
municipalities of the Metropolis.

One-third of all immigrants to Canada, and more than half of the
immigrants to Ontario, come to Metro Toronto (see Table 5.5). This
has given the population of Metro a cosmopolitan mosaic composition.

The distribution of available hospital beds in Metropolitan Toronto

Table 5.2: Population of Metro Toronto by Age and Sex, 1971

Age	Males Number	Males Per cent	Females Number	Females Per cent	Totals Number	Totals Per cent
0—4	82,700	4.0	79,300	3.8	162,000	7.8
5—19	270,900	13.0	264,100	12.7	535,000	25.6
20—64	605,400	29.0	613,200	29.4	1,218,600	58.4
65 and over	67,500	3.2	102,900	4.9	170,400	8.2
Total	1,026,500	49.2	1,059,500	50.8	2,086,000	100.0

Table 5.3: Comparison of the Population of Metropolitan Toronto with the Provincial and National Populations in 1971

Area	Total population (thousands)	Per cent of Canada	Per cent of Ontario
Canada	21,568.1		
Ontario	7,703.1	35.7	
Metro Toronto	2,086.1	9.7	27.1

Table 5.4: Percentage of Population in Metropolitan Toronto by Age Groups 0-19 years and 65 plus in 1971

Area	Percentage of population in ages 0—19	Percentage of population in ages 65 +	Percentage of population in ages Total
Metro	33.4	8.1	41.5
Inner three municipalities (East York, York, Toronto)	28.6	10.8	39.4
Outer three municipalities (Etobicoke, North York, Scarborough)	37.6	5.9	43.5

Source: Demographic Trends in Metropolitan Toronto; The Royal Commission of Metropolitan Toronto, 1975. Data originally taken from the 1971 Census.

Table 5.5: Per Cent of International Immigrations to Ontario by Continent of Last Permanent Residence, 1962-72

Source Area	1962	1963	1964	1965	1966	1967	1968	1969	1970	1971	1972
Europe	76.7	79.2	80.1	80.3	81.9	77.0	71.1	59.7	55.7	47.2	47.6
Africa	1.2	1.4	1.7	1.1	1.3	1.4	1.7	1.5	1.7	2.3	5.5
Asia	2.6	2.5	3.9	5.6	5.5	7.9	10.0	12.2	12.4	16.9	17.3
Australia	1.6	1.4	1.5	1.3	1.4	1.9	1.9	2.2	2.4	2.1	1.6
USA	13.7	10.8	8.7	7.7	6.4	5.9	8.5	10.8	12.6	14.4	14.2
West Indies, Central and South America	4.1	4.6	4.1	4.0	3.5	5.9	6.8	13.5	15.1	17.0	13.7
Others	0.1	0.1	0	0	0	0	0	0.1	0.1	0.1	0.1
Total	100.0	100.0	100.0	100.0	100.0	100.0	100.0	100.0	100.0	100.0	100.0

Source: Ontario's Changing Population, vol. 1, Table 12. Patterns and Factors of Change, 1964-71, March 1976.

Table 5.6: Supply of Active Treatment Beds in Metropolitan Toronto by Type of Care Provided

	City of Toronto	York	North York	East York	Scarborough	Etobicoke	Total	Percentage
Medical surgical	4,504	335	1,361	448	731	449	7,828	73.2
Acute care paediatric	880	78	179	46	209	79	1,471	13.8
Obstetric maternity	506	65	138	67	96	73	945	8.8
Intensive and coronary care	233	25	78	17	62	24	439	4.1
Total	6,123	503	1,756	578	1,098	625	10,683	100.0

Source: Ibid., Table 8.

is influenced by the fact that the majority of hospitals affiliated with the University of Toronto for the purpose of medical education are located close by. This explains the reason for 49.5 per cent of all the beds available in Metro being located in the city of Toronto. Of the active treatment beds in Metro, 73.2 per cent are used for medical/surgical procedures (see Table 5.6).

Finance

Introduction

Over $845 million (the Canadian dollar is approximately at par with the US dollar), approximately 30 per cent of the provincial government's total health budget, was spent by the Ontario Ministry of Health in Metropolitan Toronto during the fiscal year 1975-6, a 14 per cent increase over the year 1974-5 (for which see Table 5.7) which in turn was 22 per cent above 1973-4. That unusually high increase, which occurred across the province as a whole, was largely due to a combination of inflation and large wage and salary adjustments for hospital employees. Just over 60 per cent of the total sum spent by the Ministry on health care services in Toronto in 1974-5 and 1975-6 was for hospital services. The services provided by health practitioners, mostly physicians, under the universal Ontario Health Insurance Plan (OHIP) have accounted for an average of 23 per cent of the cost over the past three years.

Virtually all citizens of the province of Ontario are protected for a full range of hospital, medical, nursing-home care, home care, ambulance, and certain other health-related services through the Ontario Health Insurance Plan (OHIP). In addition, those over 65 and those in receipt of social assistance receive prescription drugs. Dental services, drugs, eyeglasses and other health appliances are not currently included in the universal programme.

This programme is financed on a joint basis between the federal and provincial governments with part of the provincial share being raised through a compulsory premium (tax), which presently is $192 per annum for a single person and $384 for families. This premium is waived for all individuals and families 65 years of age or over, those in receipt of social assistance and those who have declared *taxable* income (after deductions) of $1,534 or less for single persons and $2,000 or less for families. Single individuals with taxable incomes between $1,534 and $2,000, and families between $2,000 and $3,000 pay only one-half the regular premium rates.

Table 5.7: Finance — Expenditure of Ontario Ministry of Health in
Metro Toronto in 1974/5

Type	$	$ per head
Public general hospitals	480,535,000	226
Provincial psychiatric hospitals	21,871,000	10
Ontario Health Insurance Plan (payment to physicians)	175,404,000	83
Others	60,931,000	29
Total	738,741,000	348

In 1976 the sources of financing this programme will be: federal
government (general taxation) 48 per cent; provincial government
52 per cent (general taxation 24 per cent, premiums 28 per cent).

Hospital Services

From the advent of the Ontario Hospital Insurance Plan in 1959,
each public general hospital was required to submit to the Ministry of
Health a budget detailing the hospital's estimate of operating funds
required for the following year. Once the budget had been approved
on a detailed line-by-line basis, the hospital had to contain
expenditures within each cost sector. Starting in 1969, in an attempt
to control the rapidly escalating cost of health care and to permit
hospitals to exercise better internal control of their operations, budgets
were generally switched to a 'global' basis. The formula for the global
budget starts with the previous year's approved expenditures and adds
a variable percentage increase for the budget year concerned. This
system enables hospitals to allocate expenditures within a total allowance providing the expenditures are classified as allowable operating
costs.

The provincial government's health spending was 28.7 per cent
of the Ontario budget in 1975. In 1976 the Ministry declared its
intention to slow the rate of cost increase by reducing the level of
hospital facilities and services.

Physicians' Services

The customary method of remuneration for physicians practising
medicine in Ontario is fee for service. Physicians have the option of
working in the Ontario Health Insurance Plan (OHIP) and 89 per cent
of physicians in Ontario do so. The OHIP fee structure is determined

through negotiation between the Ontario Medical Association (OMA) and the Ministry of Health. Physicians operating under the plan can bill OHIP directly, when they receive 90 per cent of the agreed fee. Physicians operating outside the plan send the bill to the patients. The patient then pays the full cost of the fee charged by the physician and is reimbursed 90 per cent of the regulated OHIP/OMA fee. The services provided by physicians operating within OHIP are monitored by the College of Physicians and Surgeons of Ontario, using information from the plan's computerised billing system.

In the majority of cases there is no direct financial arrangement between the physician and the hospital in which he or she works; however, some physicians, e.g. radiologists, pathologists, or casualty officers, may be employed on a salary basis at some hospitals. In addition, physicians with major teaching commitments receive stipends. As a general rule, remuneration received by a physician for clinical services rendered in hospital is provided by OHIP, and not by the hospital. A hospital medical staff is composed of physicians who have been granted admitting and treatment privileges by the hospital board on the recommendations of the Medical Advisory Committee. These privileges are reviewed annually by the board.

The government of Ontario is currently evaluating a method of primary care delivery which involves the establishment of Health Service Organisations (HSO). These organisations are based on the Community Health Centre concept and attempt to provide a comprehensive health service to the patients registered with them. There are 31 HSOs in Ontario, of which 11 are located in Metropolitan Toronto. Over-all funding is through the Ministry of Health. Methods of remunerating physicians, including some innovative salary schemes, vary according to the arrangements agreed between the medical practitioner and board of the HSO.

Public Health Services

Table 5.8 shows the expenditure by the municipalities on public health in 1973. The provincial government provides 25 per cent of the cost of legally required services provided by the six boards of public health in Metropolitan Toronto. Each board provides a number of additional services which they are responsible for funding, leading to variations in the type of public health programmes being provided. When the board of health provides services on behalf of the province, as is the case with family planning, the province pays the full cost of the programme. The provincial government has been trying to persuade the six boards

Table 5.8: Gross Expenditure per capita for Public Health Programmes by Area Municipalities, 1973

	Population*	Per cent population	Total expenditure (thousands)	Expenditure per capita
East York	105,340	5.0	$ 520	$ 4.94
Etobicoke	286,106	13.6	1,433	5.01
North York	527,564	25.1	2,813	5.33
Scarborough	362,005	17.3	1,593	4.40
Toronto	676,363	32.2	6,399	9.46
York	142,297	6.8	1,021	7.18
Total	2,099,675	100.0	13,779	

* 1971 Census

Source: Social Policy in Metropolitan Toronto, The Royal Commission on Metropolitan Toronto, 1975.

of Health in Metro to amalgamate their services. However, to date, this change has been resisted by the separate boards.

Organisation and Planning

Introduction

The introduction of provincial hospital insurance in 1959 and the cost-sharing programmes developed between the federal and provincial governments stimulated a period of hospital expansion. This encouraged utilisation of costly hospital care rather than alternative types of ambulatory and institutional care. The Ministry of Health then saw an urgent need for rationalising the development and utilisation of health services and has introduced the concept of District Health Councils (DHCs) as advisory bodies. Their primary responsibility is to identify local needs, evaluate alternatives, establish priorities and plan a comprehensive health care programme within the policies, guidelines and standards established by the Ministry. It is claimed that through the formation of District Health Councils, the 'consumer' will have the opportunity, for the first time, actively to shape the delivery of health care on a broad front. Although there are many District Health Councils in the Province of Ontario, no plan has yet been implemented for the development of a DHC in Metropolitan Toronto.

The Planning Process

In the absence of a central body in Metropolitan Toronto to co-ordinate services, health agencies have tended to plan in isolation for increasing effectiveness in their local communities. The Ministry of Health has to approve the development plans from each hospital, and local boards of health are accountable to their respective municipal councils for the proposed cost of their plans. The establishment of special Federal-Provincial funds for health-manpower training has resulted in closer co-ordination of the objectives being proposed by the teaching hospitals. This has resulted in considerable co-operation towards achieving common goals amongst this group.

Health Standards

The government of Ontario, through its Ministry of Health, has over-all responsibility for the standard of health care services within Ontario. In practice this responsibility is delegated to a number of subsidiary bodies. In the public hospitals of the province, the boards of directors are legally responsible for monitoring the health care services being rendered. This ongoing assessment is achieved through regular reports from a number of committees of the medical staff, including those responsible for reviewing audit and tissue, credentials, admission and discharge, and records. On a broader perspective, the Canadian Council on Hospital Accreditation provides a periodic evaluation of the hospital's general organisation, care and physical resources. The Hospital Medical Records Institute, a non-profit organisation, provides computerised monthly analyses of hospital records to assist medical and administrative staff in assessing the quality and effectiveness of patient care being provided.

Under the Health Disciplines Act of the Province of Ontario, 1974, five health professions — medicine, dentistry, nursing, pharmacy and optometry — are governed by their own Colleges, with power to impose fines or withdraw the right of a member to practise. This Act makes provision for the participation of lay persons in this process. The Ontario government has stated its intention of extending the Act to other health professions in due course.

Health Care Services

First Contact (Primary Care)

Primary care in Toronto is administered mainly through the offices, or clinics, of physicians, the emergency departments of most hospitals and some community health centres.

Medical Practice. Private practice either on a solo or group basis is the traditional form of medical practice in Toronto. Some solo practitioners deputise for one another during periods when one is not available. A group practice may include primary and secondary care physicians. Also, a considerable amount of primary care in Toronto is provided by medical specialists, such as paediatricians, gynaecologists and internists.

Hospitals. Most Toronto hospitals have emergency departments which also provide less urgent primary care services. In teaching hospitals primary care is provided by house staff backed up by medical teaching staff. Emergency departments in non-teaching hospitals are staffed by physicians, either on a shift rotation or an on-call basis, belonging to the medical staff of the hospital.

Community Health Centres. There are 15 organisations operating in Toronto which are called Community Health Centres, including 11 HSOs. Some are hospital outreach clinics funded by hospitals. Others are local community initiative ventures which the provincial government is supporting as part of their evaluative study of this type of primary care facility. These centres attempt to provide as comprehensive a primary health care service for the family unit as their physical and human resources will allow. Some examples of the type of service being provided are: general medical services, well-baby clinics, birth control advice, geriatric care, immunisation, psychotherapy and counselling and a 24-hour on-call doctor or counsellor service.

Mental Health. Primary care for mental illness may be provided in many different ways depending on the circumstances. The patient's initial medical contact may be with the family physician or hospital emergency department or directly with a psychiatrist in private practice, on the staff of a general public hospital, or provincial psychiatric hospital. Care of mental illness, whether by psychiatrist or family physician, is covered by OHIP. Some hospitals take outpatient psychiatric services into the community to reach people who might not otherwise seek mental health care. These centres provide counselling and general assessment services as well as medication. They also act as crisis centres for potential suicide victims.

Secondary Care Services

Hospital Facilities. Within the boundaries of Metropolitan Toronto, 57 institutions are providing hospital care. There are 40 public hospitals, 6 proprietary hospitals, 3 provincial psychiatric hospitals, 1 hospital operated by the Workmen's Compensation Board, and 7 (out of 45) nursing homes, under proprietary ownership, having temporary approval to provide some chronic care. Eleven of the 40 public hospitals are affiliated with the University of Toronto for undergraduate medical education.

The following categorisations are not mutually exclusive, but indicate the variety of types and the range of ownership and operation of the above facilities:

28	institutions provide active treatment care services;
21	provide short-term, acute psychiatric care services;
3	provide long-term as well as short-term psychiatric care services;
20	provide chronic care services;
3	provide special rehabilitation care services;
7	provide general rehabilitation care services (see Tables 5.10 and 5.11).

A variety of other bed facilities exist in Metro Toronto. These include domiciliary units, detoxification units, respiratory disease units, adult group homes and children's mental health centres. Figure 5.1 shows the relative distribution of most hospital facilities in Metropolitan Toronto. Availability of these facilities is reflected by the patient flow into Metro. Table 5.9 shows that 64.6 per cent of persons from outside the Metro area receive their hospital care in the city of Toronto.

Rehabilitation. Rehabilitation services are funded by the Ministry of Health and the Ministry of Community and Social Services and are classified as physical and social rehabilitation services respectively. The physical rehabilitation that is done in the health service is further divided. General services such as physiotherapy and occupational therapy are provided in most acute care hospitals. Special purpose hospitals provide specific rehabilitation programmes for crippled children, paraplegics, amputees and persons with severe speech or hearing problems.

Table 5.9: Movement of Hospital Patients within Metropolitan Toronto

Locality in which patients are treated	City of Toronto	East York	Place of residence of patients York	Etobicoke	North York	Scar-borough	Patients from outside Metro
City of Toronto	77.7	50.4	50.8	43.8	32.4	20.8	64.6
East York	10.3	41.6	0.3	0.3	2.0	9.5	3.5
York	1.5	0.7	37.0	15.5	11.2	0.5	3.1
Etobicoke	0.8	0.3	4.9	34.0	0.7	0.2	6.3
North York	8.8	1.6	6.6	6.1	50.5	9.4	9.3
Scarborough	0.9	5.4	0.4	0.3	3.2	59.6	13.2
Total	100.0	100.0	100.0	100.0	100.0	100.0	100.0

Source: Ibid., Table 6.

Table 5.10: Resources — Number and Type of Hospital Bed, 1975

	Number	Number per 1,000 population
Active treatment	10,683	5.0
Acute care psychiatry (excl. provincial)	740	0.3
Psychiatric (provincial)	941	0.4
Rehabilitation (special)	177	0.1
Rehabilitation (general)	674	0.3
Chronic	2,632	1.2
Nursing home beds (extended care)	7,182	3.4
Total	23,029	10.7

Table 5.11: Resources — Active Treatment Beds by Type, 1975

Type	Number	Number per 1,000 population
Medical/surgical	7,828	3.7
Acute care paediatrician	1,471	0.7
Obstetrics/maternity	945	0.4
Intensive coronary care	439	0.2
Total	10,683	5.0

Figure 5.1: Hospital Facilities in Metropolitan Toronto

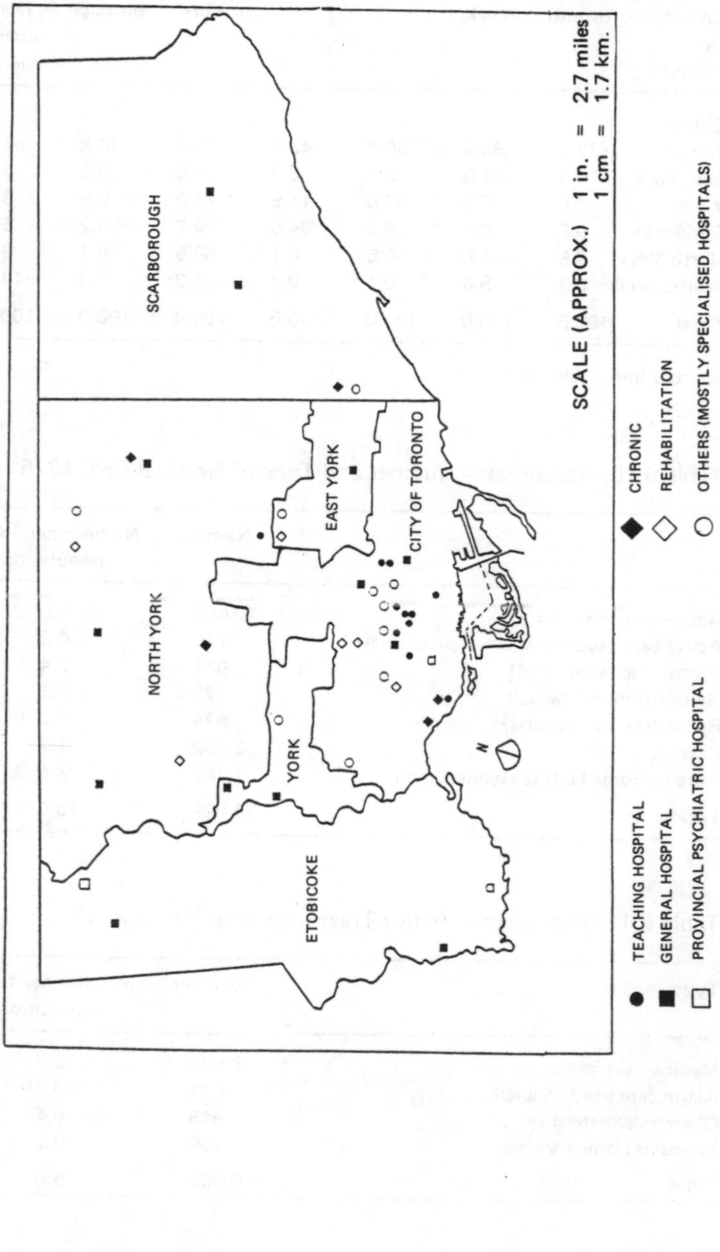

SCALE (APPROX.)   1 in. = 2.7 miles
                  1 cm = 1.7 km.

TEACHING HOSPITAL ●   CHRONIC ◆
GENERAL HOSPITAL ■   REHABILITATION ◇
PROVINCIAL PSYCHIATRIC HOSPITAL □   OTHERS (MOSTLY SPECIALISED HOSPITALS) ○

Chronic Care. A chronically ill person may be cared for under OHIP in a hospital for the chronically ill, a chronic illness unit of a general hospital, or a private hospital. Admission is by medical referral only, usually by transfer from an active treatment hospital. Within Metro Toronto there are 2,632 chronic care beds (see Table 5.10) in 20 institutions, the number of beds in each ranging from 4 to 602. Some of the institutions provide specialised care such as geriatric and child care.

Public Health. The six municipalities within Metro are required by provincial statute to have a department of public health which is controlled by a Board of Health, appointed annually by the local municipal councils. These six boards are autonomous bodies and their composition includes elected representatives, local residents and persons appointed by councils.

The chief function of boards of health is to provide preventive health care services. This is done through such programmes as environmental sanitation, communicable disease control and immunisation under the direction of a salaried physician as Medical Officer of Health (MOH). Public health nursing services include health education, assessment and counselling, pre-natal and post-natal education. The water supply of Metropolitan Toronto has been fluoridated since 1963, following a public referendum approving the measure to combat dental disease.

Home Care. The Home Care Programme of Metropolitan Toronto is operated by a non-profit corporation with a citizens board of directors responsible for policy. Financing is provided by the provincial government on the basis of an approved budget. Admission to the programme is by physician referral. The programme provides home-making services and professional services such as nursing and physiotherapy, in the homes of patients, most of whom have been discharged from hospitals. It also provides some equipment, e.g. wheelchairs and commodes, as well as drugs prescribed by the attending physician.

Nursing Homes. There are 45 nursing homes under proprietary ownership, providing a mix of 'extended care' (partially insured through OHIP) and personal domiciliary or custodial care (fully paid by the patient). There are also 15 Homes for the Aged under municipal, charitable or religious auspices, in which some extended health care services may be provided to ailing residents.

Ambulance Services. The ambulance service in Metropolitan Toronto is the only sector of the health service which is operated directly by the metropolitan level of government. The present system has evolved from a fragmented private operation to a centrally co-ordinated system under which all ambulance vehicles are in radio communication with a central despatch facility. The provincial government covers the major portion of expenditure by Metro for ambulance services. The creation of the Department of Ambulance Services by the Metropolitan Council in February 1975 is expected to result in the implementation of a unified control of ambulance services, improved communication with hospitals and other users and a higher standard of training for ambulance attendants.

Voluntary Organisations and Community Participation. Volunteerism is an integral part of the delivery of health and social services in Canada. Voluntary involvement takes two basic forms. Subject to the over-all legislative authority of the provincial government, voluntary boards of citizens govern the public general hospitals, direct local public health services and lead numerous social agencies. Volunteers also provide a wide range of personal services to the community generally, through organisations such as the Hospital Auxiliary, Meals on Wheels, the Canadian Red Cross, St John Ambulance and the Salvation Army.

The United Community Fund conducts an annual appeal in conjunction with the Red Cross to raise funds for a large number of voluntary service agencies, while others doing voluntary work within Metro prefer to maintain their identity by conducting their fundraising activities independently.

Health Manpower. In the 1971 Census 40,940 persons (9,375 males, 31,565 females) stated that they worked for hospitals in Metropolitan Toronto. The same census identified 4,725 medical doctors (4,095 males, 630 females) working in Metro. A recent study has shown that 64.8 per cent of the physicians in Metro Toronto are specialists, 35.2 per cent are family physicians and that 77.2 per cent are in private practice, with 22.8 per cent in the public sector.

It is estimated that there are 1,250 dentists in Metro, with 19 employed on a full-time basis for the municipal authorities and 70 part-time. The remainder are private practitioners. In 1974 there were

Table 5.12: Resources — Number of Staff and Number of Population
per Health Worker

Staff type	Number	Number of population per health worker
Doctors	4,725	441
Dentists	1,250	1,669
Pharmacists	1,460	1,428

1,460 pharmacists working in hospitals, drug store chains or for themselves in Metropolitan Toronto (see Table 5.12). Other self-employed health practitioners practising in the area include optometrists, podiatrists, chiropractors, physiotherapists, occupational therapists, remedial gymnasts, masseurs and speech therapists.

Information and Communication

There is no single agency in Metropolitan Toronto responsible for collecting and collating epidemiological statistics. The six municipal public health departments are required by law to collect statistics about certain contagious diseases. However, this information is restricted in its value by being based upon arbitrarily defined public health areas which may be widely divergent in their ethnic population and socio-economic mix. Similarly, information regarding the availability and utilisation of health services is available in varying degrees from a number of sources, such as provincial government ministries, public health departments, representative hospital, medical and mental health organisations, the Social Planning Council and the Community Information Centre. Liaison and exchange of data between some of these agencies is reasonably good, particularly where there is a direct financial reporting link to government. In many cases, however, there is no organised means of communication between agencies regarding objectives, future plans and problems. Therefore a recent report of the Ontario Council of Health, the senior advisory body to the Ministry of Health, has recommended the immediate formation of a District Health Council for Metropolitan Toronto. It is anticipated that such an organisation will serve as a central agency for information flow within the health community of Metropolitan Toronto.

B. OPINIONS ON HEALTH CARE SERVICES

The Master Committee invited by the Ontario Hospital Association to guide the Toronto Study encouraged participants in its opinion survey to give particular attention to what they saw as deficiencies and that emphasis is reflected in the following report. To place their specific criticisms in perspective, respondents were asked to state their over-all opinions of the delivery of health services in Metropolitan Toronto. More than 66 per cent personally rated it good to very good; and 77 per cent thought that the general public would give Toronto's health care services the same high rating.

Apart from identifying problems, the survey also asked respondents to list good ideas and practices in Metropolitan Toronto which might be of benefit to other cities, and to suggest changes and studies which might increase the efficiency and effectiveness of health care services in Metropolitan Toronto.

The survey took the form of an open questionnaire. In order to obtain a range of viewpoints, persons able to provide an informed opinion about health care delivery in Metropolitan Toronto were invited to participate as representatives of the following general categories:

(a)   direct patient and community contact;
(b)   administrative or back-up personnel;
(c)   policy formulation and resource allocation;
(d)   informed public;
(e)   influencers;
(f)   academics;
(g)   nominated physicians;
(h)   miscellaneous.

Problem Areas

In this section, general problem areas perceived by respondents in the delivery of health care in Toronto have been identified by the authors of the report from answers to the opinion survey.

Organisation

Opinion expressed in this survey indicated three basic problem areas relating to the organisational structure of health care delivery in Toronto:

(1)   Responsibility for the delivery of services is in the hands of professionals and service organisations but authority rests with

government.

(2)   There is insufficient co-ordination amongst the deliverers of health services in Toronto.

(3)   The health care delivery system does not have a set of objectives.

Finance

Problems with financial arrangements permeate every sector of the health care system and appear to relate chiefly to methods of funding the various segments of the system. It was suggested that present funding mechanisms do not promote the most effective provision and utilisation of available resources.

Primary Care

Lack of co-ordination in the primary care sector is blamed for a proliferation of access routes into the system, resulting in disorganisation, increasing cost, and duplication of effort by a number of health care providers. No organisation is responsible for controlling and co-ordinating the primary care services being provided in Toronto, while the process of entering its health system is not clearly understood by the public.

Active Treatment

Historical emphasis on the hospital as the major component in health care may be hindering attempts at providing a more balanced system. There is seen to be an inappropriate mix of different types of hospital beds available for use in Toronto, and the relationship between the hospitals and the other sectors of Toronto's health care system is not fully developed. It was believed that these defects were particularly evident in the areas of geriatric and psychiatric care.

Socio-Economic

Citizens of Metro Toronto are served by four levels of government, each level having responsibility for the formulation and implementation of different policies which directly or indirectly affect the delivery of health care. Fragmentation of government may be hindering solution to the socio-economic problems being encountered by deliverers of health care within the Metropolis. Furthermore, it was suggested that:

(1)   The heavy influx of immigrants creates particular strains on the health services of Toronto.

(2)   Health and social services are directly affected by problems

in housing and transportation.

(3)   The universal health services being underwritten through the Ontario Hospital Insurance Plan are not equally benefiting all strata of society.

Planning and Information

The absence of a recognised planning agency as an integral part of Metro Toronto's health care delivery system was identified by many as a source of problems for the providers of care. Any planning of health and social services which did occur in Metropolitan Toronto was seen to be unco-ordinated.

Staff Training

The absence of an over-all long-term plan for administering health services appears to prevent the full benefit of the investment in educational programmes from being realised. Thus, in particular: anticipated benefits of educational programmes are not always fully achieved; the fee-for-service method of paying physicians inhibits more effective utilisation of non-physician personnel; health workers have not been educated to adapt to a changing health system.

Good Ideas and Practices; Recommended Changes and Studies

In preparing the following sections it was difficult at times to differentiate between 'practices' and 'good ideas'; and 'changes' and 'studies'. Some respondents were practising what others saw as 'good ideas'. Studies that were recommended by other respondents have already occurred and resulted in some degree of change. This situation indeed suggests a need for a better communication within the health care community in Metro Toronto. It should also be noted that several respondents made essentially similar recommendations. Because of that, and the desire to list as many recommendations as possible in the limited space available, it has not been practical in this section to identify sources.

Good Ideas and Practices

Organisational Structure.

(1)   Hospitals in Metropolitan Toronto benefit from the co-ordination of management services achieved through their own voluntary representative organisations. Joint programmes for purchasing, laboratory and laundry services have been developed from initiatives of the Hospital Council of Metropolitan Toronto and turned over to

independent boards for operation. Examples of province-wide services provided directly by the parent Ontario Hospital Association include employee pension and insurance plans, management statistics and a voluntary mechanism for joint collective bargaining with employee unions.

(2)   Interaction between local boards of health and local school boards has identified areas of health need and led to co-operation and programme development in health education − although much more could be done. Interaction between the local board of health and hospital boards is a growing trend.

(3)   Co-ordination of certain tertiary care services through an organised approach, e.g. chronic renal disease and cardiac surgery.

(4)   The use of role studies to try to determine the 'role' of each institution as part of a total system.

(5)   The universal Health Insurance Programme of the provincial government.

Primary Care.

(1)   A co-ordinated Metro-wide ambulance service.

(2)   Home care on a Metro-wide basis under the aegis of a non-profit corporation has been very effective in Toronto.

(3)   Outreach programmes, particularly the assumption of the responsibility for the complete medical care of residents of extended care facilities.

(4)   Detoxification centres including half-way houses to handle and rehabilitate alcoholics.

(5)   Trained volunteers, working under the direction of an ophthalmologist, are testing junior kindergarten children. This is a great saving of professional time.

(6)   The Addiction Research Foundation Employees Assistance Programme uses the Foundation staff to encourage various organisations in the community to adopt policies which will enable the identification and treatment of employees with alcohol and drug problems.

(7)   The concept of community-run health centres, breaking down the 'big city' notion into many smaller communities.

Acute Hospital Services.

(1)   The achievement of shared services in laundries, purchasing, laboratories, steam plant, computer, printing, bio-medical engineering, management consultant services and public relations.

(2)   Strong medical and nursing committee structure in our

hospitals which provides continuing monitoring and assessment of patient and community needs.

(3)   The establishment of out-patient clinics within the various main hospitals throughout the city.

(4)   A nurse receptionist meets the patient in the emergency department, to direct the most urgent to the appropriate place and to aid relatives.

(5)   Smaller hospitals benefit from contract services in dietary, housekeeping, laundry, radiology, laboratory and grounds maintenance.

Rehabilitation.

(1)   The excellent programme in physical rehabilitation of cardiac patients through running and exercise, operated by the Toronto Rehabilitation Centre as an ongoing collaborative study with the University of Toronto.

Geriatric Care.

(1)   The Baycrest Centre for geriatric care provides an integrated health and social services system.

(2)   Homemaker services contribute to keeping elderly independent and out of institutions.

(3)   Guaranteed holidays for elderly persons living at home with relatives or emergency relief for the family by admission of these persons on a temporary basis to hospitals or homes for the aged.

(4)   Audiometry testing programme for senior citizens enables the client to obtain the most suitable hearing aid and reduces the risk of the equipment not being properly used.

(5)   'Meals on Wheels' programme provides hot meals prepared by hospitals and delivered to homes of senior citizens and 'shut-ins'.

Psychiatric Care.

(1)   The Family Services Association has acted as the central co-ordinating agency between community services projects and local mental health association.

(2)   Community Resource Consultants — an experimental agency to co-ordinate psychiatric rehabilitation, identify gaps in services and help fill the gaps.

(3)   A novel method of treating maladjusted and potentially psychopathic children as out-patients is being effectively used by a small group from the Children's Hours Clinic in North York.

(4)   One of the community colleges in Toronto is establishing a

post-graduate course for nurses that will prepare persons to work in
the area of child and family mental health.

Planning and Information.
(1)   The computerisation of financial and statistical data makes
it possible to retrieve information easily. Comparative information
allows institutions to compare their operations in various departments.
(2)   Medical staff involvement in capital and operating budget
planning and control.
(3)   Departmental operations analysis by specialists in this field
helps to ensure maximum efficiency and productivity of staff and
other resources.

Recommended Changes and Studies
Organisational Structure: Changes.
(1)   Many reports are lying around unused. What is required is a
plan of action and then specific studies on problems encountered.
(2)   The development of a strong epidemiology research and
planning capability in the two universities, which will be available
to the health care community in Toronto.
(3)   More emphasis and better utilisation of home care services.
(4)   District health councils whose decisions are binding.
(5)   There should be some way of informing non-government,
lay organisations about health care matters, so that they can express
their opinions.
(6)   The development of adequate organisational models to
co-ordinate existing services and develop new, relevant services.

Organisational Structure: Studies.
(1)   A study should be made of the appropriate role for public
health in the future.
(2)   Considerable benefit could flow from a study to identify the
impact of combining a number of institutions under one board and
medical staff.
(3)   A study should be made to identify the blurred responsibilities
for policy-making and action amongst the Ministries of Health,
Colleges and Universities, Labour and the Environment.
(4)   The potential role of metropolitan government in health care
services in Metro should be studied.

Financial Arrangements: Changes.

(1)   Many reports have been prepared over the past few years with little action resulting. It is doubtful that any further studies will accomplish a great deal at this extremely difficult financial period.

(2)   Establish some form of mechanism for policing the over-utilisation by the public of physicians' services.

Financial Arrangements: Studies.

(1)   There should be more costing studies to provide a stronger basis for realistic rationalisation.

(2)   Study utilisation of services – by whom they are used and how often, with the aim of reducing cost.

(3)   The role of the community health clinic and the financing of active social services should be examined.

Primary Care: Changes.

(1)   Finding supportive home situations for ex-alcoholics as a step beyond the half-way house.

(2)   The establishment of more family practice clinics that could be operated in conjunction with hospital emergency departments.

(3)   Some mechanism should be devised for preventing, or limiting, the practice of 'doctor shopping', i.e. seeing several doctors in a short time for the same problem.

(4)   The nurse in an expanded role could provide services in the home at night and over weekends.

Primary Care: Studies.

(1)   The number of persons using emergency departments instead of doctors' offices, and the number sent by doctors.

(2)   The available hours that doctors' offices are open in a given area and on weekends.

(3)   The ambulance service should be studied, especially to look at its abuse and also alternatives in a given situation.

(4)   The emergency services in Toronto should be studied. Who is responsible for taking action?

(5)   A study of the health care needs of the community could tell us where we should be allocating our health resources in the future.

Acute Hospital Services: Changes.

(1)   Some procedure should be developed, possibly through use of a computer, for reviewing the daily utilisation of all types of beds in

Toronto.

(2)   Where possible, patients should undergo pre-admission screening in order to avoid hospital delays.

(3)   There should be more inter-hospital communication to avoid duplication of expensive medical services.

(4)   The local hospital council should act as a means of inter-hospital communication and liaison between local and provincial governments.

Acute Hospital Services: Studies.

(1)   A study on patients awaiting placement from active treatment hospitals to next mode of care.

(2)   Someone, other than the government, possibly the voluntary organisations, should conduct a study to identify the criteria for closing hospitals when it is necessary to do so.

Geriatric Care: Changes.

(1)   There should be some form of central agency for placement of patients ready for discharge from acute and secondary care hospitals.

(2)   There should be a wider acceptance and use of alternative service personnel.

(3)   Tax incentives should be provided to families to care for their senior members.

Geriatric Care: Studies.

(1)   There is need for a study on the elderly at home in Toronto to examine services necessary to keep them there.

(2)   There is a need to study alcoholism in subsidised housing for the elderly.

(3)   There should be some assessment of the distribution of nursing home beds around general hospitals.

Psychiatric Care: Changes.

(1)   General dental practitioners should be taught how to treat and care for mentally handicapped people in their offices.

(2)   Allow entry into psychiatric care through other than the medical profession.

(3)   There should be housing for ex-psychiatric patients, more work in the homes of emotionally disturbed children and families, community health and social services centres that relate to the neighbourhoods. All of these are very helpful in the area of early intervention.

Psychiatric Care: Studies.

(1)   A study should be made of ways to improve mental health services by linking general hospitals and provincial psychiatric hospitals.

(2)   Child and family mental health as it relates to housing conditions, and cultural traits should be studied.

Socio-Economic: Changes.

(1)   There should be some means of co-ordinating VD control amongst provinces, municipalities, hospitals and private doctors.

(2)   Public health should be more geared towards mental health and social problems within the community.

(3)   The health status of immigrants (which, it is hoped, is determined before they entered the country) should be made available to the municipality where they take up residence.

(4)   New immigrants should be instructed about our health care delivery system.

(5)   The development of multiple day-care centres with some co-ordination within our urban society would be a worthwhile investment.

Socio-Economic: Studies.

(1)   How new immigrants are oriented to our health service.

(2)   How people who live in subsidised housing gain advice in obtaining a family doctor.

(3)   The socio-economic status of persons using the emergency departments.

Planning and Information: Changes.

(1)   An over-all plan for health care delivery in Metro is the first step.

(2)   What is required is a plan of action and then specific studies on particular problems.

(3)   There should be a channel for ongoing dialogue between all hospitals and related services at a senior level in order to improve patient care before and after the patient moves through a hospital.

Staff Training and Attitudes: Changes.

(1)   The nurse practitioner should be used to provide some defined aspects of primary care in Metro Toronto.

(2)   The amalgamation of closely related health disciplines, so that a limited number of types of 'generalists' could be educated on a full-

time programme. All speciality training could then be post diploma on the appropriate generalist base.

(3)   There is a need for students to experience working in community health care centres.

(4)   Methods should be developed to strengthen the co-ordination of nursing services amongst the Department of Public Health, Victorian Order of Nurses and the hospital.

(5)   Educational programmes should be geared towards competency tests and based on a task analysis of the job function that is expected.

(6)   In order to establish an interdisciplinary approach to health problems, personnel should receive training in group dynamics which involves conflict management.

Staff Training and Attitudes: Studies.

(1)   A study should be conducted of the health manpower needs within the community as well as in health institutions. Educators should be involved so that courses can be developed.

Summary

It is important to record that the survey was undertaken in a period of intensive pressure on health service funds and of consequent uncertainty for the future. The concerns expressed about health services in Metropolitan Toronto raise many points of discussion. However, two main themes predominate: concern that there is no central co-ordination of services and planning, and a related fear that financial constraints imposed by government may adversely affect the present standard of health care.

The province's tax-supported health care system is seen as having many virtues, particularly the accessibility of prepaid primary care around the clock to persons in need. However, Ontario is still wrestling with the problems of reconciling free access to the system with the provincial government's concept of reasonable cost.

In the absence of a planned approach to the supply and financing of balanced hospital facilities in Ontario, the Ministry of Health has resorted to *ad hoc* economy measures designed to lower utilisation by reducing the beds and services available. In Metropolitan Toronto this has included a declared intention to close one 319-bed active treatment hospital altogether. Many respondents in this study have pointed specifically to inappropriate use of high-cost acute care beds as a major reason for unwarranted hospital expense. The apparent shortage of suitable accommodation for patients needing long-term or nursing home care suggests an unbalanced mix of facilities. Similarly, the needs for certain types of specialised medical care, notably in geriatrics and mental health, are seen to be particularly inadequate.

As physicians hold the key to utilisation of both medical and hospital services, the prevailing fee-for-service method of reimbursement is seen by some as a contributory factor in rising utilisation and cost of insured medical care.

On the bright side of the coin, respondents pointed to many commendable innovative programmes and activities, and a substantial majority of them believe that health services deservedly rate very highly with the people of Metropolitan Toronto. There is also a feeling that some of the defects of planning and co-ordination may be resolved if the Ministry of Health proceeds, as expected, to establish a District Health Council to advise it on the development of future services in Metropolitan Toronto.

Appendix: The Committees Responsible for this Report

MASTER COMMITTEE

R. Alan Hay (Chairman), Executive Director, Ontario Hospital
Association.

W.A. Backley, Deputy Minister, Ministry of Health, Province of
Ontario.

J.R. Haslehurst, Associate Executive Director, Ontario Hospital
Association.

Dr J.E. Hastings, Associate Dean, Community Health, Faculty of
Medicine, University of Toronto.

Dr G. Liguori, Executive Director, Metropolitan Toronto, Hospital
Planning Council.

S.W. Martin, Chairman, Ontario Council of Health.

C.A. Wirsig, Executive Director, Hospital Council of Metropolitan
Toronto.

WORKING COMMITTEE

Peter L. Wood (Chairman), Assistant Executive Director, Ontario
Hospital Association.

R. Baker, Professor, University of Toronto.

N. Chenoy, Assistant Executive Director, Hospital Council of
Metropolitan Toronto.

C.B. Halpin, Area Planning Co-ordinator, Ministry of Health,
Province of Ontario.

J.R. Haslehurst, Associate Executive Director, Ontario Hospital
Association.

E. Wiancko, Economist, Ministry of Health, Data Development
and Evaluation Branch.

PROJECT CO-ORDINATOR

Tim Lynch.

Bibliography

de Buda, Dr Yvonne. *Metropolitan Toronto Directory of Family Physicians.* Women's College Hospital, Toronto.

Directory of Community Services in Metropolitan Toronto (1976). Community Information Centre of Metropolitan Toronto.

Health Facilities in Metropolitan Toronto (1975). Metropolitan Toronto Hospital Planning Council (4th edition, June).

Metropolitan Profile (1975). Social Planning Council of Metropolitan Toronto (September).

Social Policy in Metropolitan Toronto (1975). Background study prepared for the Royal Commission on Metropolitan Toronto.

In addition, several of the Boards of Health and public hospitals provide annual reports which give further insight into the delivery of health services in Toronto. A number of background studies prepared for the Royal Commission on Metropolitan Toronto provide broader reading about aspects of Metropolitan Toronto which influence the delivery of health care. Also the Metropolitan Toronto Planning Board, a department of the metropolitan government, has published a number of background papers for its official plan.

6 BOGOTÁ

Jaime Arias

A. EXISTING PATTERN OF SERVICES

Bogotá, Distrito Especial, is the capital city of Colombia. It covers an area of 1,528 square kilometres at a height of 2,630 metres above sea level. The greater part of the territory of Distrito Especial consists of a flat plateau, surrounded by the Cordillera Oriental; approximately 50 per cent is a densely populated urban area. The Distrito Especial of Bogotá includes the city of Bogotá and the municipalities of Bosa, Engativá, Fontibón, Suba, Usaquén and Usme. Administratively, it is divided into 18 minor mayoralties.

Bogotá operates as a Distrito Especial, that is to say, on a par with any department or province; it has a Chief Mayor, nominated directly by the President of the Republic, and 18 Minor Mayors, designated by the Chief Mayor. The organs of the national government, the district governments and the Departmental Government of Cundinamarca operate from the capital city. The greater part of the economic, industrial and commercial activity of the country is concentrated in Bogotá which accounts for about 50 per cent of the national income.

The Health Secretariat constitutes the Health Authority of the city; it is a body directly under the Chief Mayoralty and fused with the Health Service of Bogotá, an administrative body directly under the control of the Ministry of Health. The Secretariat is a body with political-administrative powers and the Health Service of Bogotá (SSB) functions pre-eminently in the technical field (see Figure 6.1).

Demography

Bogotá had a population in 1976 of 3,677,398, of which 46.6 per cent were male and 53.4 per cent female (see Table 6.1). The population is increasing at an annual rate of 6.4 per cent, principally as a result of immigration from other cities into the capital. It is calculated that by the year 2000 the population of Bogotá will be about 14,000,000. The present population density is 2,200 inhabitants per square kilometre and this will rise by the end of the century to some 5,000. At present, 45.2 per cent of the population is under the age of 15, but this proportion is decreasing rapidly and in 25 years is expected to be 30.5 per cent. Meanwhile, the population over 60 years of age, which

161

today represents only 2.3 per cent of the total, is expected to increase to 4.5 per cent by the year 2000. Children under one year of age represent 2.1 per cent of the population, a percentage that has been falling rapidly thanks to the intensity of family planning programmes during the last decade; this age group will probably fall to 1 per cent of the total population over the next ten years.

Economic Distribution

The average income per inhabitant in the city of Bogotá is taken to be US $700, but there is a notorious inequality in the income distribution, more than 70 per cent of the population having an annual income of less than US $250. The rate of unemployment in the city of Bogotá is approximately 7 per cent, despite the fact that the city contains a good proportion of industrial, commercial and banking firms and a very high proportion of the government offices.

Geographical Distribution

In conformity with the regionalisation of Health Services, Bogotá is divided into six regions, with the following populations: North-East 791,282; North-Central 442,180; North-West 387,656; Central 840,955; South-East 943,348; South-West 520,895. In recent years, there has been a tendency for the city to expand to the west, but the government programmes have sought to contain this geographical growth, concentrating it in the so-called urban perimeter that has recently been delimited.

Population under the Care of the Health Service of Bogotá (SSB)

It is thought that the Health Service of Bogotá should concern itself with the poor. It is calculated that about 60 per cent of the population of Bogotá comes within this category, so that the population under the care of the SSB in 1976 was about 2,400,000, situated throughout the city and concentrated in the poorest areas of it, that is the southern and western zones. The remainder of the population, that is some 1,200,000 inhabitants, are served by the private sector or by the existing services of social security.

Health Status

Mortality and Morbidity

The general mortality rate for Bogotá has been calculated at 8.4 per 1,000 and the infant mortality rate at 46.7 per 1,000 live births (see

Table 6.2); the life expectancy in Bogotá is calculated to be 68 years for 1976 and it is expected that it will reach 75 years by the end of the century. The infant mortality rate has been falling rapidly and it is calculated that by the end of the century it will reach the level of 20 per 1,000 live births.

The principal causes of death in children under one year are infectious diseases, bronchopneumonia, anoxic and hypoxic complaints, diarrhoeal illnesses and enteritis caused by other germs and lesions caused at birth (see Table 6.3). For the population in general, the principal causes of death are bronchopneumonia, diarrhoeal illness, anoxic-hypoxic complaints, road accidents and malignant stomach tumours. There is a tendency towards a change in the order of the causes of both, both for children under one year and for the general population, and it is hoped that by the end of the century, the principal causes may only be malignant tumours, ischaemial heart disease, cerebral haemorrhage and other chronic diseases.

As far as causes of morbidity are concerned, the principal causes for children under one year and for the population at large are listed in Table 6.4. As might be expected, there is also a change in the order of these over the last fifteen years, and it is hoped that by the end of the century the principal causes of morbidity will be very similar to those prevalent today in the industrialised countries.

Malnutrition

One of the principal causes of morbidity and mortality among children under five years of age is malnutrition, a condition that is much higher in Bogotá than in other cities in the country, even the rural areas. The figures calculated by the Welfare Institute (Instituto de Bienestar) indicate that about 16 per cent of the children under one year are suffering from severe malnutrition and 18 per cent from some degree of malnutrition. In the one to four age group, 21 per cent suffer severe malnutrition and 18 per cent a degree of malnutrition.

Incapacitating Diseases

Data from the National Enquiry on Morbidity indicate that about 9.4 per 1,000 inhabitants suffer from deafness, 3.7 per 1,000 paralysis, 1.7 per 1,000 are deaf-mutes, 1.6 per 1,000 have suffered the total or partial loss of a limb, and 1 per 1,000 is totally blind. These incapacitating illnesses make demands on the rehabilitation services and those for the chronic sick.

Table 6.1: Population of Bogotá by Age and Sex, 1976

Age	Males		Females		Totals	
	Number	Per cent	Number	Per cent	Number	Per cent
0—4	216,966	5.9	220,643	6.0	437,609	11.9
5—14	478,061	13.0	489,095	13.3	967,156	26.3
15—44	809,028	22.0	1,003,930	27.3	1,812,958	49.3
45—64	161,806	4.4	198,580	5.4	360,386	9.8
65 and over	47,806	1.3	51,483	1.4	99,289	2.7
Total	1,713,667	46.6	1,963,731	53.4	3,677,398	100.0

Table 6.2: Vital Statistics

Infant mortality rate	46.7 per 1,000 live births
Death rate	8.4 per 1,000 population

Table 6.3: Mortality — Principal Causes of Death

	Children under 1 year		General population
Rank	Cause	Rank	Cause
1	Bronchopneumonia	1	Bronchopneumonia
2	Anoxic and hypoxic conditions	2	Diarrhoeal diseases
3	Diarrhoeal diseases	3	Anoxic-hypoxic complaints
4	Enteritis	4	Road accidents
5	Lesions caused at birth	5	Malignant tumours of the stomach

Table 6.4: Principal Causes of Morbidity

	Children under 1 year		General population
Rank	Cause	Rank	Cause
1	Diseases of respiratory system	1	Diseases of respiratory system
2	Intestinal infections	2	Diseases of the sense organs
3	Diseases of the sense organs	3	Ankylostomiasis-helminthiasis
4	Gastro-intestinal tract diseases	4	Genito-urinary diseases
5	Vitamin deficiency and anaemia	5	Intestinal infections
6	Ankylostomiasis-helminthiasis	6	Diseases of gastro-intestinal tract
7	Other infectious diseases	7	Vitamin deficiency — anaemia
8	Accidents — attacks	8	Accidents — attacks
9	Children's diseases	9	Other infectious and parasitic diseases
10	Genlto-urinary diseases	10	Mental disorders

Table 6.5: Resources — Number of Doctors and Number of Population per Doctor

Number of doctors	Number of population per doctor
4,720	779

Table 6.6: Distribution of Doctors by Speciality

Speciality	Per cent
Surgeons	32.3
Gyno-obstetricians	17.6
General practitioners	16.6
Medical interns	14.9
Paediatricians	14.3
Administrators	4.3
All	100.0

Table 6.7: Resources — Hospital Beds

Specialty	Class of institution			Total	Beds/1,000 population
	Assistance	Social security	Private		
General	1,815	2,012	1,108	4,935	1.3
Children	740	165	24	929	0.3
Gyno-obstetrics	479	0	72	551	0.1
Psychiatric	0	0	957	957	0.3
Other specialties	827	0	357	1,184	0.3
Total	3,861	2,177	2,518	8,556	2.3

Table 6.8: Utilisation of Hospital Services

Number of hospital admissions	Average occupancy	Average length of stay
265,000	87 per cent	10 days

Table 6.9: Finance

		Per cent	US $
Estimated total expenditure on health			300,000,000
Contribution of health services of Bogotá			20,000,000
Distributed:	Running of hospitals	40.5	
	Staff salaries	20.8	
	Building and equipment	17.2	
	Repayment of debts	13.7	
	Health centres	3.5	
	Other	4.3	
	Total	100.0	

Figure 6.1: Constitution of the Health Authority in Bogotá, DE

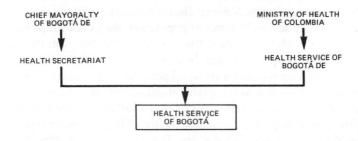

Figure 6.2: Organisation of the Health Service of Bogotá, DE

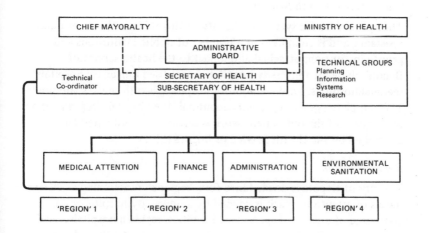

Organisation of the Health System

In Bogotá, the health system operates on a base of three subsystems: public assistance (called National Health System), social security and the private sector. In terms of population, the public assistance system deals with two-thirds of the population and the other two systems about 17 per cent each. In terms of finance, the public assistance system represents about 45 per cent of the money devoted to health, the social security system about 40 per cent and the remainder, the private sector. As was stated earlier, the health authority for the city of Bogotá is the Health Service of Bogotá, which represents the national·system in the city. The functions of the Health Service of Bogotá include not only the provision of primary medical attention in health centres and local hospitals, but also the financing of major hospitals (regional and university) attached and linked to the national health system, and the task of assessing and supervising the network of services provided by itself and the two other subsystems (social security and private). Optimum co-ordination of the health services in Bogotá remains an objective to be achieved, and to date it operates only at the level of the institutions of the national health system, but it is hoped that in the future this co-ordination will include the two other subsystems.

The National Health System

The national health system in the city of Bogotá is in charge of public assistance and is composed of a number of public institutions and private institutions attached and linked to the health service of Bogotá; these are university hospitals, specialised university hospitals, regional hospitals, local community hospitals, health centres and posts. The complete system represents about half the hospital beds, and about 60 per cent of the out-patient work is directed, co-ordinated and controlled by the Health Service of Bogotá (SSB).

Regionalisation

The city of Bogotá is divided into four 'regions', functioning at different 'levels of attention'; each is headed by a university hospital and is composed of a series of specialised hospitals, regional hospitals, local community hospitals and health centres and posts. All the activities of the Health Service of Bogotá (SSB) have been decentralised, and are carried out through this system of regionalisation and levels (see Figure 6.2).

Health Service of Bogotá: Organisation

The Health Service of Bogotá (SSB) comes under four main boards.
One is financial, and is charged with the financial aspects, not only of
its own service but also those of the hospitals attached and linked to
the National Health System. The second is the Environmental Health
Board, whose functions include the checking of the environment
and foodstuffs, zoonosis, and enquiries into the running of public
establishments. The third board is concerned with administration and
deals with all matters relating to personnel and the running of the
service as well as those of the hospitals and health institutions. The
fourth board is that concerned with medical attention and this
directs the activities of the health centres and regional and local
community hospitals and co-ordinates the activities of the university
and specialised hospitals (see Figure 6.2).

Planning, Policies and Development

The city of Bogotá has a health plan that sets out the aims of the
activities of each of the 'regions' into which the health system of the
city is divided, and in addition states the strategies and the use of
resources to achieve these goals. This plan is based on the health
policies that are formulated each year after a series of consultations
with the different organisations and individuals interested in the
problem of the health of the city. The plan is reviewed every three
months and reformulated in relation to the results of this assessment.

Information and Co-ordination

There exists for the city an automated system for information and
assessment that provides the SSB with an instantaneous, comprehensive and trustworthy picture of the development of the different health
activities in the whole city. The assessment includes the quantification
of the resources being employed, the effectiveness of the different
programmes, the standards reached by the actions of the health work
and the quantification of the cost-benefit.

By means of the different boards composing the Health Service of
Bogotá and the Technical Co-ordinator, co-ordination is achieved
between all the health services of the city, including not only those
related to medical attention, but also those concerned with environmental health, health education and special programmes, both in the
realm of the public assistance subsystem and the two other subsystems.

Financing

It is calculated that the total expenditure on health for the city of Bogotá in 1976 was about 300 million dollars, of which the Health Service of Bogotá contributed about 20 million. Of this sum, about 40 per cent is devoted to the running of the hospitals, 20 per cent to staff salaries, 17 per cent to buildings and equipment, 14 per cent to the repayment of debts and 3.5 per cent towards the costs of health centres and local hospitals (see Table 6.9).

Only 20 per cent of the population of Bogotá has any kind of prepayment medical insurance. Most of these belong to the social security system; another 15 per cent pay directly for the services when they use them, and the remainder is considered to be indigent and requires to be covered by the public assistance services. Out of this population only some 40 per cent are covered, almost 30 per cent remaining out of the reach of any kind of service.

From 1977, substantial reforms are planned in the system of social security, with measures that will seek to increase the percentage of persons insured with the system. It is hoped that by the end of the century, more than 80 per cent of the population of Bogotá will be affiliated to some kind of total or partial medical insurance.

Health Resources and Availability

Hospitals and Health Centres

In Bogotá there are 67 hospital units, of which 4 are general university hospitals, 27 are specialised hospitals and 31 are general non-university hospitals, these including the regional and local hospitals. Together the hospitals provide a total of 8,556 beds, of which 3,861 belong to public assistance, 2,177 to social security and 2,518 are private beds. More than half are general beds, 929 are for children, 551 for gyno-obstetric cases and 957 for psychiatric cases; the remaining 1,184 beds are for other specialised cases (see Table 6.7).

In addition, in the city there are 64 health centres and 10 health posts offering primary medical attention to the patients, and together they deal with 3,361 consultations per day. There are approximately 530 private registered surgeries, which attend to 1,424 patients per day and there are also the hospital consultations, dealing with 12,525 patients daily. This represents more than one million consultations in the course of a year. Of these, about 32 per cent are emergency cases.

Support Services

The city of Bogotá has a central blood bank, a general hospitals
laundry, a public health laboratory, and a series of specialised laboratories that support the remaining hospitals. There is also a hospitals
co-operative that supplies drugs and materials to all the network of
hospitals in Bogotá.

The city has approximately 110 ambulances, of which one-third
belong to the Red Cross, another third to the Health Service of
Bogotá and the remainder to private bodies and to social security.
These ambulances are co-ordinated through the Centre for Information
and Co-ordination that provides a round-the-clock service from the
SSB.

Doctors

In Bogotá there is a total of 4,720 registered doctors, of whom one-
third are surgeons, 17.6 per cent gyno-obstetricians, 16.6 per cent
general practitioners, 15 per cent medical interns, 14 per cent medical
paediatricians and the remainder, that is 4.3 per cent, concerned with
administration (see Tables 6.5 and 6.6).

Hospital Admissions

There are approximately 265,000 hospital admissions a year in Bogotá
of which about 50,000 are emergency cases and the remainder are cases
admitted according to schedules. Almost half the admissions are to
hospitals attached and linked to the national health system. The average
rate of occupancy of the hospitals in the city is 87 per cent and the
average duration of stay is ten days.

Students of the Health Sciences

In 1976 there was a total of 8,538 students distributed as follows:
3,547 medical students (213 graduations annually); 1,334 dental
students (109 graduations annually); 669 nursing students (71 graduations annually); 374 students of nutrition (38 graduations annually);
1,914 students of bacteriology (210 graduations annually); 30 students
of public health (30 graduations annually); and 670 auxiliary nursing
trainees (670 graduations annually).

Other Health Programmes

Apart from the medical attention programmes, Bogotá has a series of
programmes aimed at the improvement of health. Among the most
prominent of these are the programmes of attention to the environment,

directed by the Health Service of Bogotá, programmes of health education, conducted by the same institution, programmes of rehabilitation, of mental health and a series of special programmes co-ordinated directly by the Ministry of Health, the most notable being those for the control of venereal diseases and tuberculosis, the vaccination programme, the occupational health programme and mother-child programmes.

B. PROBLEMS, CHANGES AND STUDIES

Problems

(1)   There exists a significant proportion of the population (about one-third) with no, or very limited, access to the health services, either because these do not reach them, they are not an integral part of their life, or are inadequate or not available at the right times.

(2)   Complete or specific malnutrition is highly prevalent in the city, affecting most severely children under the age of five and the mothers of the low-income groups.

(3)   A high proportion of the urban and rural inhabitants are still without water and drainage services compatible with an acceptable level of health.

(4)   The incidence of communicable infectious diseases is very high, resulting in excessive infant mortality rates and rates of morbidity, whether among those in hospital or not.

(5)   The indicators of the contamination of the environment, including noise and undesirable odours, point to a serious problem and the danger of an accelerated increase in the factors causing contamination.

(6)   Accidents within the home and on the roads show high rates of incidence, the former affecting especially children under 5 years of age.

(7)   The prevalence of chronic and degenerative diseases is equivalent to that in the industrialised cities without our being able to combat them with timely and adequate measures.

(8)   The first National Enquiry on Morbidity indicated a high incidence of incapacitating diseases and of pathological conditions such as hypoacusia and defects of vision that seriously affect the productivity of the student and working population.

(9)   The Medical Attention Resources of the city are inadequate to meet current demands; the present organisation, co-ordination and utilisation reduce their efficiency.

(10) There is virtually no check on the quality of the direct services, and this is one of the reasons why the quality is unsatisfactory at all levels and in all sectors, whether public, private, or social security.

(11) There are evident imbalances in the effective utilisation of the primary (basic) resources, the secondary (intermediate) resources and tertiary (super-specialised) resources that are detrimental to the whole system of medical attention. The demands made of the hospitals are very high, especially in the area of emergency cases, while the Centres for Primary Attention are working at 50 per cent below their capacity.

(12) The city does not possess a co-ordinated emergency system and this lack creates a series of problems in medical attention that is becoming ever more acute. Neither does Bogotá have an emergency plan to deal with civil or military catastrophes.

(13) The city lacks adequate provision of medical information allowing for the collection, analysis and use of data in a reliable, timely, comprehensive and simple form. Under the present circumstances, the programming of activities and the measurement of the results is not possible.

(14) The system of selection, buying, storing and distributing the supplies is anachronistic and bears no relation to the size and complexity of the services nor to the requirements of the units of the health services.

(15) The means of communication available to the health system of Bogotá are very poor and are badly utilised.

(16) The units concerned with medical attention (with a few exceptions) do not operate according to the same criteria as business enterprises and their budgets and financial affairs follow no set system. Furthermore, the financial resources of the services are clearly inadequate to meet the demands made on them.

(17) Bogotá has no health plan allowing it to opt for better strategies and tactics conducive to maximising the productivity of the resources.

(18) Basic and applied research is inadequate and allows of no innovation in the health system of the city.

(19) The distribution of the budgeted resources and the control over their management still lack effective rational means to assure the greatest productivity from financial investment in health.

(20) The Health Service of Bogotá still has no infrastructure that would allow it to operate fully as laid down by the legislation.

(21)   The measure of enforcement allowed by the law to the health sectors to see that obligations are met are still incomplete and inefficacious.

Changes

(1)   Increase in the accessibility of the services, especially for those inhabitants without insurance and without the means to pay, those in the marginal and rural zones and those most at risk. To achieve this goal, the following policies need to be followed:

(a)   A search for a balance within the health system, between medical attention and education and prevention, between primary, secondary and tertiary levels of attention, and between geographical zones within the city. This balancing of the system involves a major boost to the health centres and polyclinics in co-ordination with the referral hospitals, the distribution of resources according to needs, and greater emphasis on preventive measures and public health.

(b)   Greater use of the basic staff and an interdisciplinary focusing on problems and solutions will be required. This will involve the development of 'health teams' to get the most out of the work done through the greater use of paramedical staff, auxiliaries and health promoters.

(c)   Development and implementation of an integrated emergency programme with the participation of all the available resources in the city to carry out the programme; the improvement of radio and telephonic communication and the ambulance service; the putting into effect of a referral system for patients; the adoption of new financial methods and the better equipping of the emergency services of the hospitals and polyclinics.

(d)   Better publicity about the services and education of the users so that they may get the best out of them. This will be achieved through greater participation of the community, by means of better health education programmes, and the work of health promotors.

(e)   Comprehensive and continuing attention, which is to be achieved through regionalisation and with information aids, such as telecomputer data bases or similar methods.

(f)   Better contact with the people, from the moment of entry until they leave the institution; for this, promotors or other voluntary workers are to be used.

(2)   Protection of the groups at most risk, which is to be

achieved by means of the following policies:

(a)   Implementation in the city of the National Nutrition Plan
with the maximum collaboration of the Health Service of Bogotá;
nutritional education programmes and massive encouragement of
breast feeding.

(b)   Increase and consolidation of the preventive programmes of
immunisation and epidemiological vigilance.

(c)   Growth of the programmes for pre-natal and infant care
and medical attention at the birth, provided by the polyclinics and
hospitals for all mothers.

(d)   The offering of permanent, or at least frequent and regular,
basic medical services in the marginal areas, whether urban or rural.

(3)   Co-ordination of all the existing health resources, whether
within the official sector or the mixed and private sectors; to be
achieved through the following policies:

(a)   Development of the health 'regions', with the active participation of the attached and linked organisations.

(b)   Creation of solid mechanisms for co-ordination and integration
with the Colombian Institute for Family Welfare (Instituto Colombiano
de Bienestar Familiar) and with the Colombian Institute of Social
Security (Instituto Colombiano de Seguros Sociales), for the benefit
of all institutions and the avoidance of duplication. This will also be
achieved through effective co-ordination with the private sector.

(c)   Close co-ordination with the Ministry of Health for the
implementation in Bogotá of the National Health System and the testing
in the city of the subsystems that compose the National Health System.
Co-operation in all the areas of common interest, such as health
laboratories, environmental checks and detection.

(d)   The active participation of the Faculties of Medicine and
other health sciences in the regional health programmes and the
technical studies promoted by the Health Service of Bogotá.

(e)   Co-ordination of the activities of the Health Service of
Bogotá with those of the other dependencies of the district
administration.

(4)   Strengthening of the infrastructure of the Health Service of
Bogotá, through the following policies:

(a)   The setting up of a medical-epidemiological and financial-administrative information system that will allow for a diagnosis of the situations met by the service and for the planning and evaluation of its activities and programmes.

(b)   The development of a systematised plan for simple assessment, that is decentralised and automated so that it allows for the measurement and evaluation of the programmes, policies and projects in terms of their effort, efficiency, effectiveness, impact and cost-effectiveness.

(c)   The setting up of the national subsystem of costs and financing health in the city and the development of guidelines and standards for the institutions linked and affiliated to the service, with direct auditing of such organisations.

(d)   The setting up of a national health system of supplies, and decentralisation of the provision of supplies to the health 'regions'.

(e)   Development of a plan for human resources in the field of health, in collaboration with the Ministry of Health and the universities and technical schools.

(f)   The drawing up of a health plan for Bogotá with sectional and regional levels and the working out of a budget for programmes, through decentralisation.

(5)   The use of proper techniques for the organisation and management of the services, at the levels of both sectional and regional service and executive bodies.

(a)   The setting up of better mechanisms for administrative control and the assessment of activities.

(b)   Consultancy advice for the health organisations on administrative techniques for organisational development, personnel management, cost systems and budgetary control, internal and external programming and co-ordination.

(c)   Financial advice for executive organs, following the National Health System Financial Subsystem. The setting up of costs studies for hospitals and health centres.

(d)   Indirect help in the running of the health organisations through co-operatives, supplies centres, laundry centres, laboratories, etc., where the size of the operation will make them economical.

(6)   Encouragement of the testing of new types of health attention and organisation of the services, with research evaluation. Quality control of health attention.

(a)   Support for experimental programmes allowing for the development of new models and technologies for health attention, based on the use of basic resources according to the conditions prevailing in the city.

(b)   Testing of the subsystems of the National Health Service in Bogotá, in collaboration with the Ministry of Health.

(c)   Development of measures for the quality control of the health and medical attention services, with the co-operation of the Faculties of Medicine and Health Sciences.

(d)   Co-ordination with the Research Division of the Ministry of Health and 'Colciencias' to support medical research.

(7)   Support for the active participation of the community in the organisation, development and control of the peripheral health services, by means of the following policies:

(a)   Identification, organisation and development of community groups or Communal Action Boards interested in the health services.

(b)   The fostering of the promotors programme (MAC 1) after an evaluation of its effect in the community and on the services.

(c)   Participation of the members of the community in the local and regional services boards.

(8)   Protection of the environment through the following policies:

(a)   The enforcement of the legal requirements on drainage and ecology and support for programmes leading to the protection of the environment.

(b)   Support for the programme to construct a new municipal abattoir and to intensify the checks on milk.

(c)   The re-equipment of the health laboratory in collaboration with the National Institute of Health. Strengthening the zoonosis programmes and the controls on industrial and domestic contamination of air and water.

The foregoing policies will have differing priorities, to be determined in the health plan for the city; the plan will indicate the level of fulfilment expected with regard to each policy and the strategies to be employed to distribute the use of the different resources between the various policies.

Studies or Experiments

(1)   The use of auxiliary personnel for tasks that are today carried out by professional staff but could be delegated.

(2)   Comparative studies on the costs of different types of hospitals (according to size, location, system of financing, specialty).

(3)   Studies on the effectiveness of the local community hospitals, and analysis of the utilisation of the health centres.

(4)   Analysis of the administrative procedures at the central level of the SSB.

(5)   Studies on the participation of the community in the management of the health institutions.

(6)   Testing of 'TRIAGE' systems in the emergency services in the hospitals.

(7)   Feasibility of the setting up of 'prepaid medical practices'.

(8)   Analysis of the effectiveness of 'multiple group practices'.

(9)   Different formulae for the staffing of hospitals and health centres.

(10) Studies on the integration at field level of the services of the social security and medical assistance.

(11) Studies on the extension of services to the elderly and the mentally ill.

(12) Studies on the criteria for the distribution of funds between hospitals and other institutions.

7 MEXICO CITY

Guillermo Fajardo Ortiz

A. PATTERN OF EXISTING SERVICES

Mexico City, known as Distrito Federal (or Federal District), covers
an area of only 1,499 square kilometres, representing 0.1 per cent of
the national territory. It is the smallest unit in Mexico, but nevertheless
is the political, economic and social centre of the country.

Demography

There has been a vast increase in the population of the Federal District
during the last forty years. In 1930, it had 1,229,576 inhabitants;
in 1940, the population rose to 1,757,530; in 1950, it was 3,050,442;
and by 1960 it had reached 5,017,000. The 1970 census recorded a
population of 6,955,004, and in 1976 this number had increased to
slightly more than 9,000,000, representing approximately one-
seventh of the population of the Republic. Distributed between the
1,499 square kilometres of the Federal District, this gives a density
for 1976 of 6,000 inhabitants per square kilometre, compared to a
figure of only 32 inhabitants per square kilometre for the rest of the
country. In 1976, 42 per cent of the inhabitants were under the age of
14, showing that the population of the city is predominantly a young
one, making proportionately greater demands than the rest of the
population on the health services (see Table 7.1).

Health Statistics

In 1940, the birth rate was 43 per thousand inhabitants; in 1950 it
was 38, in 1960 it was 43 and in 1976 it was 41. The rate is stable,
though the level is high. A considerable decrease is observable in the
death rate, for in 1940 it was 24 per thousand inhabitants; in 1950
it dropped to 15; by 1960 it had fallen to 9.9 and in 1976 to 8
(see Table 7.2). The high birth rate level and the marked decrease
in the death rate, combined with increasing immigration into the
Federal District, are the factors responsible for the remarkable rise in
its population, which increases by more than 1,000 daily.

   There were 72,000 deaths in 1976; the ten most frequent causes
of death are listed in order of decreasing frequency in Table 7.3. These
ten causes accounted for 73 per cent of all deaths.

It is worth pointing out that the deaths attributable to influenza and pneumonia and to gastro-enteritis and colitis, which together accounted for 28 per cent of the total, are intimately linked with poor environmental conditions, a lack of timely medical attention, malnutrition and the lack of education in hygiene. Deaths caused by chronic degenerative diseases and by accidents are on the increase. Accidents give rise to a large number of cases of disability and thus economic loss; those occurring in the home are the most numerous, followed by those in the street and those at work and school.

The percentage distribution between age groups of the deaths occurring in 1976 is shown in Table 7.4. Infant mortality is therefore very high, even though there has been a considerable fall in the course of the last forty years. In 1940, the rate was 196 per thousand live births, and in 1976 it was 72. In spite of this, the rate leaves much to be desired, for compared with the rate in industrialised countries it is still excessively high.

More than half of the deaths of infants under the age of one are due to enteritis or other diarrhoeal illnesses, influenza and pneumonia. During the first year of life, the period when the risk is greatest is the first month, 46 per cent of the deaths occurring during this time. The factors that sustain the high level of infant mortality are: lack of medical hygiene attention during pregnancy; poor physical living conditions; feeding deficiencies; culturally motivated behaviour patterns that have an adverse effect on health; and inadequate parental attention given to the child.

Maternal mortality has also fallen significantly, from 5 per thousand live births in 1940, to 1.2 in 1976. Some 46 per cent of the deaths are due to deficient ante-natal care; 33 per cent to inadequate attention at the birth itself; 11 per cent to abortions (generally those that have been induced); and the remaining 10 per cent to other causes. This indicates that the mother-and-child group is one of the most important in the context of health needs.

The significant decrease in mortality levels is due to the fall in deaths from communicable diseases, and this has resulted in an equally significant increase in life expectancy. In 1930 it was 39 years and it is now 63. Nevertheless, entirely new health problems have arisen as a consequence of industrialisation, population growth, increased life expectancy and psycho-social factors.

As far as ill health is concerned, in the public sector of medical care, the conditions met most frequently are listed in Table 7.5. There is evidence that problems of drug addiction and alcoholism are increasing.

Socio-Economic Status

The working population numbers a little over three million, one-third of the total population. Of these, 40 per cent are engaged in providing services, 40 per cent in manufacturing industries, and 20 per cent in commerce and other activities. In 1976, the *per capita* income per annum of 85 per cent of the population was less than 2,500 dollars, the remainder having higher incomes than this. This is very important considered in the light of the relation between income and health, because in general those in the lower-income groups are those with the greatest health problems, particularly problems of infectious diseases.

In 1976, 1,700,000 children attended primary schools. In the same year 800,000 were enrolled in secondary schools and 180,000 in establishments of higher education. Despite the efforts made by the public authorities, the number of illiterates over the age of 10 is 600,000, 7 per cent of the population. No figures are available, but the need to increase programmes of education in hygiene is obvious.

Statistics for housing in 1976 revealed that the number of dwellings was 1,600,000; of these, 28 per cent had only one room, 25 per cent had two, 17 per cent had three rooms and the remainder had four or more. Of the total number of dwellings, 89 per cent had walls of brick or thin partitioning, 6 per cent were of adobe, and the remainder of wood, plaster or other material. In 95 per cent of the dwellings the floors were of cement, tile, mosaic or similar material and only in 5 per cent were they of earth. Seventy per cent have running water indoors; 19 per cent have running water available, but outside; the remainder have access to stand-pipes or public hydrants, or have no piped water at all. As for drainage, 78 per cent of the dwellings have this facility, serving 77 per cent of the population.

The principal supplier of meat for the population of the Federal District is the central slaughterhouse, which has adequate installations and facilities for the killing, storage and distribution of meat to satisfy the greater part of the needs of the capital. There are other slaughterhouses of less importance on the outskirts of the city, where the installations need modernising. As far as markets, supermarkets and self-service shops are concerned, there are sufficient to supply the needs of the population. Nevertheless, the population is nutritionally deficient in its calorific and protein content; 91 per cent eat bread made from wheat three or more days of the week, 73 per cent eat meat, 82 per cent consume milk, 5 per cent eat fish and 0.5 per cent eggs. The deficiencies are most obvious among children that are not yet

Table 7.1: Population by Age Groups, 1973

Age	Number	Per cent
0–4	1,191,617	15.3
5–14	2,030,564	26.2
15–44	3,468,426	44.7
45–64	809,429	10.4
65 and over	267,997	3.4
Total	7,768,033	100.0

Table 7.2: Vital Statistics, 1972

Births	325,768	Birth rate	43.5	per 1,000 population
Infant deaths	22,388	Infant mortality rate	68.7	per 1,000 live births
Deaths	66,804	Death rate	8.9	per 1,000 population

Table 7.3: Mortality — First Ten Causes of Death by Rank

Rank	Cause
1	Influenza and pneumonia
2	Gastro-enteritis and colitis
3	Heart disease
4	Perinatal conditions
5	Cancers
6	Cirrhosis of the liver
7	Diabetes mellitus
8	Cardiovascular diseases
9	Violent and accidental deaths
10	Bronchitis

Table 7.4: Percentage Distribution between Age Groups of Deaths, 1976

Age	Percentage	Age	Percentage
Less than 1 year	35	25–44	11
1–4	7	45–64	17
5–14	2	65–74	12
15–24	4	75 and over	12

Table 7.5: Morbidity — Common Conditions seen in Public Sector
Medical Care

Acute respiratory infections
Enteritis and other diarrhoeal diseases
Accidents caused by animals (mainly dog bites)
Bronchitis
Emphysema and asthma
Other infectious and parasitic diseases
Diseases affecting teeth and bones
Other diseases of digestive tract
Adenoids and tonsils
Malnutrition
Diseases of the urogenital tract

Table 7.6: Resources — Number of Staff and Number of Population
per Health Worker

Staff type	Number	Number of population per health worker
Doctors	19,000	474
Qualified nurses	12,500	720
Nursing auxiliaries	16,000	563
Dentists	3,200	2,813

Table 7.7: Resources — Number of Hospital Beds

Agency	Number
Secretariat of Health and Welfare	5,764
Mexican Institute of Social Security	6,577
Institute of Social Security and Social Services of State Workers	2,711
Department of the Distrito Federal	2,513
Mexican Institute of Child Welfare	370
Others, including private sector	8,074
Total	26,009

(2.8 per 1,000 population)

weaned, those of pre-school age and among pregnant women.

Health Organisations and Resources — Financing

Mexico City has a multiplicity of organisations concerned with medical care, reflecting traditions and priorities of a social, economic and political order.

The medical care organisation can be divided into two groups on the basis of their backing and their financing: the public sector and the private sector, and these in their turn are subdivided. This indicates that these services as a whole correspond to a 'mixed economy', and the characteristics of the principal elements are as follows:

Public Sector

(1)   Governmental:
    (a)   federal;
    (b)   municipal.
(2)   Decentralised: i.e. belonging to decentralised organisations or to firms with state participation:
    (a)   social services;
    (b)   social security;
    (c)   organisations for the production and distribution of goods and services.

Private Sector

(1)   Philanthropic organisations.
(2)   Private organisations.

Governmental Medical Organisations

This group includes the medical services and establishments that are supported by funds from the federal government or from the government of Mexico City; they provide protection for about 3,600,000 inhabitants. Health services of the Secretariat of Health and Welfare (Secretaria de Salubridad y Asistencia) and the Medical Services of the Department of the Federal District Government of the City) belong to this subgroup.

The Secretariat of Health and Welfare is directly responsible to the Federal Executive Authority; its brief being basically to supply medical attention to the poor. It is funded through taxes. This Secretariat includes general hospitals, specialist hospitals, surgeries and health centres. Its units form a co-ordinated network of services. It is also concerned with the following public health functions:

monitoring and prevention of the contamination of the soil, water and atmosphere; sanitary functions concerned with food, drink and drugs; sanitary engineering; industrial hygiene; supervision and authorisation of laboratories for clinical analysis; mortuaries; pest control; international health and other public health programmes.

The capital of the Mexican Federation also has another type of medical benefit – the medical services of the Department of the Federal District, consisting mainly of hospitals for urgent cases, paediatric hospitals and hospitals in institutions for the retired. In all of these medical attention is free, being paid for through taxes. In addition, this department also deals with the removal of rubbish, sewerage, water services and industrial effluents, as well as the provision of drinking water and the administrative supervision of food supplies, especially in slaughterhouses and markets.

Decentralised Medical Organisations

These are establishments administered by employers' associations or by institutions with a certain degree of autonomy despite their official nature. This subgroup comprises:

(a)   social service medical units, such as:
        National Institute of Cardiology;
        Mexico Children's Hospital;
        'General Maximo Avila Camacho';
        Mother and Child Centre;
        Mexican Institution of Child Welfare;
        Infant and Family Units of the Mexican Institute.

To some extent the Secretariat of Health and Welfare has a say in the management and organisation of the above-mentioned establishments, supporting them financially and paying patients' fees.

(b)   Medical units of the Mexican Institute of Social Security,
        of the Institute of Security and Social Services of the State
        Workers and the medical services of the armed forces.

The Mexican Institute of Social Security is a decentralised, national, compulsory body, to which are affiliated, by law, those persons who are bound to others by contract of work and to population nuclei ranging from the very rural outskirts to suburban and urban areas (Social Solidarity). In the current year it provides protection for

1,600,000 inhabitants against accidents at work, sickness, maternity, invalidity, old age, death and retirement at an advanced age; it is supported by contributions from the workers, the employers and the state.

For traditional and politico-social reasons, there are two other organisations with activities very like those of the Mexican Institute of Social Security. These are the Institute of Security and Social Services of the State Workers, which provides protection for just over a million people, supported by workers and the state; and the social security for members of the armed forces, paid for by the government, which covers some 50,000 persons. These social security medical services are graded hierarchically.

(c)   Medical units of organisations for the production and distribution of goods and services for the market.

There are some organisations with medical services for their workers and their families, such as the hospitals and surgeries of the Mexican Oil Corporation, of the Mexican National Railways, etc., and these cover about 100,000 people.

The health organisations of the public sector are under the control and supervision in matters of planning, finance and administration of three State Secretariats: the Secretariat of the Presidency (concerned with planning and supplies); the Secretariat of the Exchequer and Finance (matters of finance); and the Secretariat of the National Heritage (buildings).

Philanthropic Medical Organisations

These are philanthropic trusts administering private funds to provide hospital care. They are non-profit-making and without individual designation of beneficiaries. Examples are the Red Cross Hospital of Mexico City, and the Hospital of Jesus (the oldest still functioning in Latin America).

Private Organisations

These are establishments owned by private individuals or societies and run at their own expense or for profit. Examples include the Surgical Centre of Mexico City, and the Sanatorium of the Union of Workers of the Cinematography Industry. There is little liaison between the two types of private sector services.

In most cases, the different health organisations of the public sector of Mexico City operate independenly of one another in matters of planning and operation. In an attempt to overcome this situation there is a public body, the Joint Co-ordinating Committee for Public Health, Welfare and Social Security Activities which aims to eliminate duplication, multiplication and omissions within the services.

Health Personnel

Within the Federal District there are 250 hospital units, which together provide 26,000 beds. The Secretariat of Health and Welfare has 5,764, the Mexican Institute of Social Security 6,577, the Institute of Security and Social Services of the State Workers 2,711, the Department of the Federal District 2,513, the Mexican Institution of Child Welfare 370; with other institutions including the private sector having 8,074. This provides 2.8 beds per 1,000 inhabitants, a higher figure than for the rest of the country, where the average is 1.6. It must of course be remembered that many of the national resources are concentrated in the hospitals of the Federal District.

Since the doctor is the basic human component in medical care, it is important to give some details about numbers in Mexico City and in the country as a whole. It is estimated that about 19,000 doctors are in practice in the Federal District, representing more than one doctor per 475 inhabitants, a figure that is high compared to that for the remainder of the country, where there is only one doctor per 1,250 inhabitants. This means that 35 per cent of the doctors in the country are found in the Federal District, while its population represents only 15 per cent of the national population. About 14,916 doctors work in the public sector and receive a salary; while some 4,000 are in private practice only. It must be mentioned that an unknown number of doctors work both in public organisations and privately.

Contrasting with the number of doctors, there are 12,500 qualified nurses and 16,000 nursing auxiliaries; the former being less numerous than the doctors, whereas they should perhaps be more numerous. This shortage of nurses is one of the most serious problems of medical care in Mexico City. For other types of medical personnel, there are 3,200 dental surgeons, 1,110 technicians, and 9,131 para-medical staff.

Demands on the medical services constantly increase in all fields, resulting in delays or overburdened services or, worse, a combination of both.

Health Administration

The administration of medical care and its organisations is very frequently hampered by rigid and unworkable structures. In a few cases there has been some effort at planning, organisation and direction and evaluation, but in the majority of cases effective planning and programming are lacking.

In the medical care services, and thus in clinics and hospitals, the head is a doctor who is responsible for clinical and administrative matters. Since in most cases these doctors have had no training in the administration of medical care, it is clear that severe problems can arise.

B. PROBLEMS AND ATTEMPTED SOLUTIONS

Summary of the Problems that Affect the Planning and Operation of Services

(1)   Concentration of inhabitants and the high rate of population increase.

(2)   Prevalence of infectious and parasitic diseases, especially influenza, pneumonia, bronchitis, enteritis and other diarrhoeal illnesses.

(3)   Increasing incidence of chronic and degenerative diseases (heart diseases, malignant tumours, cirrhosis, diabetes and cardio-vascular diseases and accidents).

(4)   Problems of medical care for the mother and child, especially perinatal problems.

(5)   Low *per capita* income.

(6)   Problems of nutrition.

(7)   Inadequate education in hygiene.

(8)   Problems caused by contamination of soil, water and air.

(9)   The multiplicity of organisations concerned with health.

(10)   The shortage and poor distribution of resources.

(11)   Inadequate administration.

Attempted Solutions

The Joint Co-ordinating Committee for Public Health, Welfare and Social Security activities has put in hand various programmes for the improvement of the health of the inhabitants of Mexico City, all based on co-operation and reciprocal help between institutions and private bodies. These programmes are part of the National Health Plan, started in 1975.

The main component of the health plan of the Federal District is a series of actions now being taken that are related to the main health needs and available resources. The following are the most important programmes.

Responsible Parenthood Programme

It is thought that a considerable limitation of demographic growth can be achieved by means that allow a couple to decide freely the number of children they will have and the intervals between them. Abortion facilities are being provided in collaboration with a National Programme for Family Planning. The results so far seem promising.

Programme to Foster Family Unity

This programme is based on the following activities:

(1)   family planning orientated to responsible parenthood;
(2)   organisation of schools for parents and the formation of mothers' clubs;
(3)   support for the Mexican family programme to legalise marriage and legitimise the children;
(4)   fight against alcoholism;
(5)   programmes to prevent drug addiction;
(6)   specific work to combat prostitution and delinquency;
(7)   integration of the family unit to avoid the partial or total abandonment of mothers and children, especially those under 15.

Programme of Mother and Child Medical Care

Activities aimed at the physical, mental and social protection of mothers and children are being intensified in the following fields:

(1)   premarital education of the couple from the point of view of heredity, eugenics, mental health and family organisation;
(2)   orientation of the family to responsible parenthood;
(3)   regular medical and hygiene supervision during pregnancy, encouraging medical attendance at the birth;
(4)   adequate attention for the newly born child and regular medical and hygiene supervision, especially for infants under a year old;
(5)   improvement of nutrition and health attention for the 0-14-year-old age group, with special care for those of pre-school age.

Programme against Communicable Diseases

In order to reduce the incidence of these diseases, the following activities have been stepped up:

(1)   epidemiological surveillance of communicable diseases;

(2)   specific prevention;

(3)   primary and secondary prevention of infectious diseases of the respiratory and digestive tracts; of other common illnesses such as rheumatic fever and skin conditions, as well as of systemic infectious and parasitic problems;

(4)   sanitary controls over food and drink, the suitability of water for drinking, noxious fauna and hygiene education for those who handle food;

(5)   orientation of the public in general towards the prevention, both primary and secondary, of communicable diseases.

Programmes for the Early Diagnosis and Treatment of Chronic Degenerative Diseases

(1)   Timely detection of cervical-uterine and mammary gland cancers.

(2)   Early diagnosis and adequate treatment for persons with diabetic problems, as well as education of their families about this disease.

(3)   Prevention and treatment of other chronic diseases, especially those of the cardiovascular system, through programmes of mass screening and the creation of automated diagnostic services.

Programme against Accidents

The co-ordinated efforts of the various health organisations and other governmental and private bodies are resulting in greater efficiency in the prevention and treatment of accidents, through a better and wider public information service. This deals with the prompt attention needed by accident victims, medico-legal problems arising from accidents and the prevention and specific treatment of accidents at work.

Programme of Medical Care

Attempts are being made to relieve the pressure on the medical services by the measures detailed below:

(1)   technical and administrative restructuring of the hospitals

and clinics;

(2)   integration of medical care and rehabilitation with the preventive health programmes and those encouraging health, in order to avoid duplication of effort and wastage of resources;

(3)   the setting up of procedures for the maintenance and conservation of buildings and supplies;

(4)   training of staff for the services;

(5)   encouragement of academic teaching work and research.

Programme for Health Education

(1)   Intensification of the education message, through the mass media.

(2)   Increasing participation by health personnel in the orientation of the public in matters of hygiene.

(3)   Orientation in matters of hygiene for specific groups, especially those who handle food.

(4)   Encouragement of and collaboration in health orientation for teachers in primary schools.

(5)   Co-ordination of the work of hygiene education with other work carried out by other sectors of the community.

Housing Programme

The problem of housing, one of the chief preoccupations of the government, is receiving attention from various institutions. Because of its close connection with health, health organisations are working to see that buildings meet the minimum requirements from the point of view of hygiene. Of prime importance in this respect is the construction of housing units by the Department of the Federal District and multi-family dwellings by the Mexican Institute of Social Security and the Institute of Security and Social Services of the State Workers and other organisations.

Programme of Nutrition

The health organisations are concerned to improve nutrition through:

(1)   orientation in matters of nutrition, especially concerning the quantity and quality of nutrients;

(2)   distribution of food with high protein value, in particular to nursing mothers and children of pre-school age;

(3)   improvement of co-ordination between organisations concerned with the production, storage, distribution and sale of foods;

(4)   specific consultation for the prevention and treatment of malnutrition.

Programme for Environmental Improvement

(1)   Provision of drinking water and main drainage for the population.

(2)   Increase in the number of units for the collection and removal of rubbish, as well as its processing.

(3)   Legislation to control the release of fumes contaminating the atmosphere.

(4)   Legislation to control soil contamination.

(5)   Elimination of poor conditions connected with the retailing of foods on the public highway, which encourages the spread of gastro-intestinal diseases.

Other Programmes

(1)   Community participation in health activities.

(2)   Social welfare.

(3)   Administration of Public Health and Sanitary Legislation.

These programmes have only been in operation for a year or so, so that it is not possible to attempt an assessment of the achievement of their aims; nevertheless, the results that are emerging are encouraging.

Bibliography

Campillo Sainz, C. (1976). *Co-ordination of the Health Services of the Federal District.* Proceedings of the Fifth Regional Conference of Hospitals and Second National Congress of Hospitals, Mexican Association of Hospitals, A.C. Mexico.

National Health Convention (1974). *Proceedings.* Mexico.

Navarro, G. (1973). *Health Plan of the Federal District.* First National Health Convention. Mexico D.F.

Subsecretariat of Welfare (1974). *Project for the Improvement of the Co-ordination of Health Services in the Federal District.* S.S.A. Mexico.

8 SAO PAULO

Odair P. Pedroso and Associates*

A. AREA CHARACTERISTICS

The county of Sao Paulo is located in the south-east part of the Sao
Paulo state and has eight districts, divided into 48 sub-districts. The
total area of the county is 1,515.5 square kilometres and its altitude
varies between 750 and 820 metres. It has a population of 7,394,823
(see Table 8.2), 39 per cent of whom are engaged in industrial production.

The county's water and sanitation services are maintained by the
state government, only 50 per cent of the population being supplied
with piped water and only 36 per cent with proper sewerage.

In the educational area, there are kindergarten, elementary grades,
high school, technical and university levels. These are maintained by
the federal, state and municipal governments. There are also private
schools. In 1972, there were 87 institutions providing university
teaching and, of these, 13 are concerned with the medical and bio-
logical sciences (1 federal, 7 state and 5 private schools). Sao Paulo
University was founded in 1934. It has 31 units and 4 museums covering
almost all disciplines, and caters for almost 40,000 students and
employs approximately 4,000 teachers (Universidade de Sao Paulo,
1974).

The Metropolitan Area of Sao Paulo was officially created in 1973.
A Metropolitan Area is defined as 'an intensely urbanized, territorial
entity, with a marked demographic density, that constitutes the pole
of economic activity, with its own structure, defined as private
functions and special fluxes, representing a social economic community
in which the specific necessities can be attended in a satisfactory way,
through government functions exercized in a coordinated manner'
(Grau, 1974). The Metropolitan Region of Sao Paulo is made up of 37
counties within 7,951 square kilometres. Its estimated population for
1975 was nearly 10.5 million. It should be noted, however, that the
data presented in this paper refer to the county of Sao Paulo, since
information and studies on the Metropolitan Region, as a whole, are

---

* Dr Pedroso's associates in the production of this chapter and that on
'Determining General Hospital Needs' (Chapter 18) are listed in an appendix at
the end of this chapter.

194

not yet available.

During the last few years there has been intense population growth, due mainly to enhanced employment prospects in new industries, which have attracted migrants to the area. This immigrant population has settled in the county's peripheral areas, where health facilities are almost non-existent. It is exactly this type of socio-economic condition that breeds all types of diseases and presents a major problem for any programme of health provision. It is indeed a general defect of the current health service that existing facilities do not reflect the geographical requirements. As a result of this situation, the occurrence and dissemination of multiple types of communicable diseases are relatively common problems. Infections spread by the faecal-oral mechanism, and then via the respiratory tract, such as tuberculosis, are common. Scabies, pediculosis and venereal diseases constitute severe problems in the population today.

Basic sanitation in the county of Sao Paulo is still far from being satisfactory. Only 36 per cent of the urban population of the metropolitan area is served by sewerage systems, and in only 10 per cent of these systems is the effluent treated before being discharged into creeks and rivers. The rest of the population makes use of cesspools, but the waste again is ultimately discharged into the rivers, which are already polluted by industrial waste from some 40,000 industrial establishments. The quantity of polluted material thrown into the rivers in the Metropolitan Region of Sao Paulo is almost 500,000 tons as estimated in terms of biochemical demand of oxygen (Ministerio de Saude, 1976). This pollution problem is undoubtedly one of the main causes of the high infant mortality rates in Sao Paulo.

The state and municipality governments have been alerted to the problem of air pollution since 1973, especially as respiratory and eye troubles are common complaints today (Ministerio de Saude, 1976). Table 8.1 presents the annual mean and the maximum concentration of sulphur dioxide and particles in suspension for four different locations in the county. It can be seen that the permitted level of 80 ug/m^3 is exceeded in several situations.

B. DEMOGRAPHY

1. Population

The growth of the population of Sao Paulo in the course of this century is shown in Table 8.2. The last census data show that the population of Sao Paulo is predominantly young: data are given in Table 8.3. This

Table 8.1: Annual Mean and Maximum Concentration of SO_2 and Particles in Suspension in Different Parts of the Metropolitan Region of Sao Paulo, 1975 (in ug/m^3)

Pollutant	Annual mean				Maximum concentration			
	A	B	C	D	A	B	C	D
SO_2	189	129	136	115	1,150	466	498	564
Particles in suspension	54	66	130	91	809	558	434	319

A,B,C and D are different locations for collection of data.

Source: 'Companhia Estadual de Tecnologia de Saneamento Basico e de Defesa do Meio Ambiente' (not yet published).

Table 8.2: County of Sao Paulo Population, 1900-75

Year	Number of inhabitants
1900	245,155
1920	588,818
1940	1,326,261
1950	2,198,096
1960	3,788,857
1970	5,924,615
1975*	7,394,823

* Estimated by the Department of Economics and Planning, Sao Paulo State.

Table 8.3: Population of Sao Paulo, 1975

Age	Number	Per cent
0—14	2,395,923	32.4
15—59	4,518,237	61.1
60 and over	480,663	6.5
Total	7,394,823	100.0

population lives in a heavily urbanised area and presents a life expectancy at birth of 60.44 years for males and 68.16 for females (unpublished data).

2. Birth Rate

The changing birth rate in Sao Paulo has been well studied since 1940. Data for the thirty-five-year period, 1940 to 1975, are presented in Table 8.4.

Table 8.4: Number of Live Births, Stillbirths and Rates (per 1,000 inhabitants and 1,000 live births respectively) in the County of Sao Paulo, between 1940 and 1975

Year	Live births		Stillbirths	
	Number	Rate	Number	Rate
1940	33,503	25.48	1,761	52.56
1945	39,404	23.18	2,072	52.58
1950	61,733	28.08	2,382	38.59
1955	93,789	32.61	3,102	33.07
1960	119,775	32.59	3,001	25.06
1965	144,288	30.36	3,910	28.10
1970	152,427	25.70	3,739	25.43
1971	166,175	26.75	3,775	22.72
1972	173,548	26.71	3,859	22.24
1973*	182,765	26.91	4,038	22.09
1974*	197,097	27.78	4,054	20.57
1975*	207,055	28.07	4,076	19.64

* Preliminary estimates (provisional data).

Source: Governo do Estado de Sao Paulo, Secretaria de Economia e Planejamento, Movimento do Registro Civil, 1940/72 (Sao Paulo, 1974).

The birth rate, measured in terms of the number of live births divided by the number of inhabitants, is affected by a number of factors and therefore presents problems of interpretation. The concepts of live birth and stillbirth are frequently the subject of some misunderstanding. The Inter-American Investigation of Mortality in Childhood — a research study made in 15 areas of the Americas, including Sao Paulo, during the period of 1968/70 — revealed the existence of cases in which infants, although having been registered as live births who had died shortly after birth, were, strictly speaking, stillbirths (Puffer and Serrano, 1968). Conversely, a study done on

foetal deaths in the district of Sao Paulo showed that, for the same
period, 2.5 per cent of the infants registered as stillbirths should have
been classified as live children who died shortly after being born
(Silveira, 1974). The picture is further distorted by the revelation by
a similar study that live births were under-registered by about 5 per cent
(Silva, 1970). The percentage of births that took place in the hospital
was approximately 92 per cent for live births and 87 per cent for stillbirths (Silveira, 1974). This number seems high but is accounted for by
the fact that approximately 90 per cent of the population benefits
from some type of social security.

3. Mortality

General Death Rate

The death rate in the county of Sao Paulo has maintained itself around
8.5 per 1,000 inhabitants since the end of the 1950s, although it
increased a little from 1970 onwards (see Table 8.5). An analysis of the
etiological factors involved shows that the distribution has not changed
significantly in the last few years.

Table 8.5: Number of Deaths and Mortality Rate (per 1,000
inhabitants) in the County of Sao Paulo, 1940-75

Year	Number of deaths	Rate
1940	11,116	13.02
1945	19,981	11.75
1950	22,267	10.13
1955	27,819	9.67
1960	31,361	8.53
1965	39,379	8.29
1970	51,299	8.65
1971	54,496	8.79
1972	57,569	8.86
1973*	62,355	9.18
1974*	64,544	9.10
1975*	64,253	8.69

* Preliminary estimates (provisional data).

Source: As for Table 8.4.

Table 8.6: Main Causes of Deaths (per cent) in the County of Sao
Paulo, 1970-3

Causes of death	1970	1971	1972	1973
Infectious diseases	11.56 (2)	12.63 (1)	13.36 (1)	13.30 (1)
Malignant tumours	10.42 (3)	10.28 (3)	9.96 (3)	9.81 (4)
Ischaemic disorders of heart diseases	12.23 (1)	11.74 (2)	11.56 (2)	11.44 (2)
Cerebrovascular diseases	9.58 (4)	9.33 (5)	8.83 (6)	8.74 (6)
Pneumonias	9.17 (5)	9.53 (4)	9.93 (4)	10.58 (3)
Delivery complications and perinatal diseases	6.80 (7)	6.37 (7)	6.11 (7)	6.00 (7)
External causes	9.16 (6)	8.66 (6)	9.28 (5)	9.42 (5)

Note: Number in parentheses represents the rank of the cause.

Table 8.6 shows, for the period 1970-3, the percentages relative
to the first seven causes of death, according to the B List of the
International Classification of Diseases (Laurenti, 1975). Despite the
fact that in some respects Sao Paulo is a well-developed area, this study
of the principal causes of death gives indications to the contrary. The
high incidence of the infectious diseases group during the four years of
the study, is, of course, highly significant. Although ischaemic diseases
of the heart seem now to represent the second most frequent cause
of death, its frequency may well be overrated due to errors in the
preparation of death certificates (Fonseca and Laurenti, 1974; Laurenti,
1973; Milanesi and Laurenti, 1964).

Nevertheless, it is also evident that there is a high incidence of
malignant tumours, of accidents as a whole (external causes) and of
cerebrovascular diseases. These are the very factors that are associated
with mortality in highly developed urban areas. In this sense, therefore,
Sao Paulo shows a similar profile to other well-developed areas.

Infant Mortality

The infant mortality rate, expressed by the relation of the number of
deaths of infants less than one year old divided by the number of
live births, represents, without doubt, one of the most sensitive
indicators of a community health level. Table 8.7 presents the total
numbers of infants who died at less than one year of age and the
corresponding infant mortality rate for the period of 1940 to 1975.
It should be noted that about 82 per cent of the deaths of infants of
less than one year took place in hospital (Puffer and Serrano, 1975).

Table 8.7: Number of Deaths of Infants of less than One Year of Age and Infant Mortality Rate (for 1,000 live births) in the County of Sao Paulo, 1940-75

Year	Number of deaths	Rate
1940	4,154	123.99
1945	3,999	101.49
1950	5,538	89.71
1955	8,114	86.51
1960	7,539	62.94
1965	10,010	69.38
1970	13,636	89.46
1971	15,244	91.73
1972	15,871	91.45
1973*	17,016	93.10
1974*	16,882	85.65
1975*	18,202	87.70

* Preliminary data.

Source: As for Table 8.4.

Table 8.8: Proportional Mortality according to Age Groups in Sao Paulo County, 1970-3

Age	1970	1971	1972	1973
0–1	26.08	27.69	27.68	27.10
1–5	3.18	3.72	3.48	3.52
5–20	3.13	3.27	3.47	3.58
20–50	19.19	18.70	19.20	19.87
50 and over	48.42	46.62	46.17	45.92

Mortality by Age

The proportional mortality according to age groups can be appreciated by the data presented in Table 8.8. It is important to notice in this table that the proportion of deaths of people 50 years of age and over, although having small variations, has diminished in the four years considered.

4. Migration

The data referring to migration demonstrate that Sao Paulo constitutes a pole of attraction not only for foreigners but also for Brazilians from other areas. The foreign population represented a total of approximately 7 per cent of the county's residents in 1970. Of this group, Portugal is the country with the largest representation (34.26 per cent) followed by Italy and Japan (14.52 per cent and 14.32 per cent) and then by Spain with 12.52 per cent.

Internal migration is much more extensive: the census data demonstrate that approximately 30 per cent of the resident population are not native to the state of Sao Paulo. Most of the internal migrants are poorly educated and work as unskilled labourers. They are partly responsible for the high general and infant mortality rates and low life expectancy. From the point of view of health, migration is a highly significant phenomenon since the states whence this population originates are endemic zones of Chagas' disease and schistosomiasis, which in Sao Paulo account for approximately 6 per cent of the death total for infectious diseases (1970 to 1973 data) and were responsible for 3.5 per cent of the hospital deaths due to infectious diseases in 1972 (Goldemberg, 1974).

C. MAIN HEALTH PROBLEMS

1. Infectious Diseases

That infectious diseases are currently responsible for the largest percentage of the county's deaths suggests that the health services of Sao Paulo are underdeveloped. The extremely high infant mortality rate for infectious diseases — 24.3 deaths per 1,000 live births — is higher than the infant mortality rate from all causes in developed countries.

Infectious diarrhoea is currently the most serious disease. It was primarily responsible for infectious diseases of the groups of children less than one year old (81.4 per cent) and infants less than 28 days (81.3 per cent) during the period of 1968 to 1970. It is important to note that even within the neonatal mortality, among infectious diseases, diarrhoea shows up as an important cause of death. In a sample taken by the Inter-American Investigation of Mortality in Childhood, 1,958 neonatal deaths were studied. The causes of death of 438 (22.37 per cent) were due to infectious diseases, and of these 356 (81.28 per cent) were due to diarrhoea. It was also verified that almost half of these deaths occurred in hospitals, where newborn babies, who for several medical or social reasons, had to stay longer in the hospital nurseries, caught infectious diarrhoea.

Prevention of hospital nursery infections would obviously therefore produce an immediate decrease of mortality in infants less than 28 days old. On the other hand, eliminating diarrhoea (in or out of hospitals) would reduce neonatal mortality from 33.7 to 27.5 per 1,000 live births, i.e. an 18.4 per cent decrease.

Other controllable infectious diseases — those preventable by vaccination — were responsible, altogether, for approximately 6 per cent of infant mortality due to all infectious diseases during the period of investigation (Laurenti, 1975). It also emerged from this study that in children of one to four years of age, infectious diseases were the main causes of death, with diarrhoea and measles the most important. It is to be noticed that measles represents the most frequent cause of death in the age groups of 2 to 4, followed closely by tuberculosis. Data for the general distribution of types of infectious diseases as causes of death are given in Table 8.9.

Table 8.9: Main Causes of Death due to Infectious Diseases (per cent) in the County of Sao Paulo, 1970-3

Infectious diseases	1970		1971		1972		1973	
Enteritis and other diarrhoeas	(1)	63.47	(1)	63.24	(1)	62.23	(1)	59.47
Respiratory tuberculosis	(2)	10.19	(2)	8.69	(2)	7.11	(2)	7.25
Other tuberculosis	(2)	1.73	(2)	1.48	(2)	1.36	(2)	1.22
Diphtheria	(10)	0.31	(8)	0.68	(8)	0.46	(9)	0.5
Whooping cough	(6)	0.79	(7)	0.71	(9)	0.42	(10)	0.35
Meningoccocical infections	(8)	0.67	(6)	0.95	(5)	2.19	(5)	3.26
Poliomyelitis	(11)	0.17	(9)	0.66	(11)	0.2	(7)	0.62
Measles	(4)	3.46	(3)	5.17	(4)	4.11	(4)	4.26
Syphilis and sequelae	(7)	0.72	(10)	0.53	(7)	0.59	(8)	0.58
Tetanus	(9)	0.4	(11)	0.31	(10)	0.32	(11)	0.34
Tripanosomiasis	(3)	5.11	(4)	4.59	(3)	4.69	(3)	4.45
Schistosomiasis	(5)	1.44	(5)	0.97	(6)	1.42	(6)	1.37
All others		11.54		12.12		14.9		16.33
Total		100.0		100.0		100.0		100.0

Note: The numbers in parentheses represent the rank order of the cause.

Source: Governo do Estado de Sao Paulo — data not yet published.

Tuberculosis, measured by means of PPD-test positive reactors among municipal elementary schoolchildren, is shown to account for 7 per cent (Certain, 1975), a figure well above the 1 to 2 per cent prevalence in schoolchildren considered acceptable by WHO. Particular mention might also be made of the marked mortality increase caused by meningococcical diseases. The number of cases in the population began to increase in April 1971, and in the second half of the year assumed the characteristics of an epidemic of meningococcus C group. In April 1974 an increasing number of cases due to meningococcus of the A group became evident and a new epidemic appeared in addition to the first one (Iverson, 1975).

2. Maternal and Infant Mortality

Maternal Mortality

Maternal mortality is that group of deaths of women caused by so-called 'maternal causes', which correspond to the complications of pregnancy, labour and puerperium. It is measured by the maternal mortality rate:

$$\frac{\text{Number of deaths by maternal causes}}{\text{Number of live births}}$$

Between 1960 and 1970, the rate decreased from 9.94 to 6.89 per 1,000 live births (Governo do Estado de Sao Paulo, 1975). Analysis of these figures indicates that during the period 1960-1, labour complications accounted for most cases, followed by pregnancy complications and then by puerperal complications and abortion. At the beginning of the present decade, the rates were not only much lower, but also were reversed as far as the main causes were concerned.

The relative incidence of abortion among maternal caises has been growing continuously from 10.48 per cent in 1970 to 15.97 per cent in 1971, and 19.13 per cent in 1972. It is important to note that, during this period, only 1.92 per cent were declared as being induced abortion (and specifically by medical advice). There is no mention of other types of legally admitted abortions or ones induced by other means.* Death due to spontaneous abortion occurred in 19.92 per cent of the cases, the same happening in relation to mole pregnancy. In 94.24 per cent of the cases there was no information as to whether the abortion was spontaneous or induced.

Approximately 60 per cent of the total number of cases were represented by infected abortions and 9.62 per cent had toxaemia

---

* According to Brazilian legislation, abortion is only permitted when no other way of saving the mother's life exists, or in cases where pregnancy was due to rape.

and infection, which suggest that they are probable cases of induced abortion (Silveira, 1976).

Data from a research study conducted in Sao Paulo showed that the reliability of the death certificates, when studying abortion, is quite suspect, since additional information used for the codification of causes of maternal death increased the maternal mortality rates. In this case, mortality due to abortion appeared to account for more than 50 per cent (Laurenti, 1973; Puffer, 1968). This problem was measured by a project undertaken in 1965, which showed that .5.9 per cent of the pregnancies were terminated by an induced abortion; the same study estimated the total number of induced abortions as 250,000 for that year (Milanesi, 1969).

Stillbirth Mortality

The concept of stillbirth employed here is that recommended by the World Health Organization. Thus the natimortality rate is given by the ratio:

Number of stillbirths

Number of live births

The changing pattern of natimortality in Sao Paulo is shown in Table 8.4. Even the recent lower rates (19.64 per 1,000 live births in 1975) are high compared to data for representative developed areas. The study of natimortality causes shows the group of anoxias to be responsible for 65 per cent of cases, infections of the placenta and umbilical cord for 12.27 per cent, with nearly 12 per cent due to unknown causes. The value of this last figure is explained by the small number of autopsies performed on the stillborn (Silveira, 1974).

Perinatal Mortality

Perinatal mortality in well-developed areas, such as Sweden (with a rate of 18.9 per 1,000) and West Germany (25 per 1,000 live births) makes it clear that in spite of low infant mortality rates prevalent in these countries, there is always a certain number of inevitable perinatal deaths in even our most technologically advanced societies.

The rate of perinatal mortality is given by the ratio:

Total late foetal deaths + deaths of infants from 0 to 7 days of life

Total live births

This rate was studied in Sao Paulo during the period 1968 to 1970 (Laurenti *et al.*, 1975), and it produced a figure as high as 42.04 per

1,000 live births. This figure is evidently well in excess of the rates found in developed countries. The particular causes of perinatal mortality are evaluated in Table 8.10. Analysis of this table reveals that the perinatal mortality rate in Sao Paulo could be reduced by treating some specific causes at the prenatal level, or by giving more attention at delivery or to the newborn infant.

Table 8.10: Perinatal Rates by Causes (per 10,000 live births) in the County of Sao Paulo, 1968-70

Causes	Rates
Perinatal causes:	3,858.55
maternal causes associated with pregnancy	67.15
maternal causes specific to pregnancy	96.28
delivery complicated by distocia and trauma	235.85
other pregnancy and delivery complications	140.38
placenta and cord affections	472.10
pregnancy interrupted	17.40
hemolytic diseases of the newborn	31.15
anoxic and hypoxic affections	2,341.91
prematurity	166.67
other foetal and newborn affections	82.53
foetal death of unknown cause	208.34
Congenital causes	167.08
Infectious causes	67.15
Respiratory causes	92.64
Accidents	19.01
Total	4,204.43

Source: R.R. Puffer and C.U. Serrano, *Patterns of mortality in childhood* (OPS/OMS, Washington, DC, 1975. Sc. Pub. 262).

Infant Mortality

Infant mortality can be studied through its sub-categories, neonatal and post-neonatal mortality, the deaths occurring from 7 to 27 days of life and from 28 days to one complete year. In the county of Sao Paulo, data from the Inter-American Investigation of Mortality in Childhood showed that of the 3,788 deaths which occurred in infants under one year of age during the research period, 1,958 (51.69 per cent) occurred in the neonatal period and 1,830 (48.31 per cent) in the late infant period (Puffer and Serrano, 1975). This research was carried out simply by interviewing people in their homes or in hospitals or by interviewing doctors who assisted the children involved, and the

Table 8.11: Neonatal, Post-Neonatal and Infant Mortality, according
to Basic Causes in the County of Sao Paulo, 1968-70

Basic causes	Neonatal mortality rate		Post-neonatal mortality rate		Infant mortality rate	
	Number	Per cent	Number	Per cent	Number	Per cent
Infectious diseases	438	22.37	973	53.17	1,411	37.25
diarrhoea diseases	356	18.18	793	43.34	1,149	30.33
measles	—	—	52	2.84	52	1.37
other	82	4.19	128	6.99	210	5.55
Malnutrition	2	0.10	59	3.22	61	1.61
Respiratory	184	9.40	420	22.95	604	15.94
Congenital trauma	117	5.97	96	5.25	213	5.62
Perinatal cases	1,183	57.87	15	0.82	1,148	30.31
Other diseases	84	4.29	267	14.59	351	9.27
Total	2,008	100.00	1,830	100.00	3,788	100.00

Source: As for Table 8.10.

findings are presented in Table 8.11.

The group of infectious diseases has already been discussed in a
previous section. It is important, however, to point out that the
infectious diseases were often associated with malnutrition. Nutritional
deficiency, as a basic cause, represented only 1.61 per cent, but as a
cause associated with mortality, it was quite high in all the age groups
studied: it was present in 28 per cent of the deaths of one-year-old
infants and in 47.9 per cent of those from one to four years old.
Another factor that contributes largely to the high infant mortality
rate in Sao Paulo is the lack of basic sanitation. Of the children studied
by the Inter-American Investigation, only 51.8 per cent of the homes
of the deceased children had piped water and the proportion of homes
with water closets connected to the sewerage system was also quite
low (Puffer and Serrano, 1975).

3. Chronic and Degenerative Diseases

Cardiovascular Diseases

The analysis of the death rate due to cardiovascular diseases, including
rheumatic diseases of the heart, hypertension, ischaemic diseases of
the heart and cerebrovascular diseases, shows a growing trend. For
example, cardiovascular diseases, which accounted for 16.1 per cent of
the total causes of death in 1940, went up in 1969 to 30.2 per cent.

On the other hand, the risk of dying from cardiovascular disease, measured by the mortality rate, grew from 209.7 to 258.4 per 100,000 inhabitants. The relative growth was greater than the death risk due mainly to the reduction of the death rate due to other factors (Laurenti and Fonseca, 1976). Details of death from cardiovascular disease are presented in Table 8.12.

Table 8.12: Deaths by Cardiovascular Diseases according to Type — Rates in Sao Paulo in 1940, 1950, 1960 and 1969 (rates per 100,000 inhabitants)

	1940		1950		1960		1969	
	Per cent	Rate	Per cent	Rate	Per cent	Rate	Per cent	Rate
Rheumatic disease of the heart	2.6	33.3	1.9	19.7	1.5	13.3	1.3	10.8
Hypertension	—	—	5.1	52.1	5.0	42.6	2.8	24.0
Myocardial ischaemia diseases	12.7	35.6	10.6	108.3	10.5	90.1	11.5	98.5
Other cardiovascular diseases	10.8	140.7	9.8	100.0	12.1	103.4	14.6	125.0
Total	26.1	209.7	27.6	280.1	29.2	249.5	30.2	258.4

Source: D. Certain *et al.*, 'Analise dos resultados da pesquisa de infeccao tuberculosa e do primeiro programa de vacinacao pelo BCG intrademico em escolares de Sao Paulo, Brasil, 1971-4', *Rev. Saude Publ. Sao Paulo*, 9 (1975), pp. 125-36. No data record.

Malignant Tumours

In regard to the malignant tumours, the rates in the period 1962-4 were approximately 102.6 and 95.9 per 100,000 inhabitants, respectively for males and females. The proportional mortality during the same period was around 16.2 per cent for males and 22.5 per cent for females, falling to a mean of 10.42 per cent in 1970, with significant variation in the following years. Table 8.13 shows the distribution of deaths by malignant tumours. These data were obtained in the 'Investigation of Adult Mortality' (Puffer and Griffith, 1968).

4. Accidents

The number of violent deaths, in particular homicides and suicides, is increasing daily. Included here are deaths caused by all types of accidents. Violent deaths have always represented, in the four years studied from 1970 to 1973, one of the six major causes of death. The

Table 8.13: Rates of Death per 100,000 Inhabitants in Five Groups of Malignant Tumours, by Sex in Adults aged 15 to 74 years, in Sao Paulo, 1962-4

	Male	Female
Digestive tract and peritoneum	49.0	35.7
Respiratory tract	20.4	3.6
Breast and genito-urinary	10.9	41.1
Limphomas and leukaemias	8.7	5.6
Other sites	13.6	9.9

Source: R.R. Puffer and G.W. Griffith, *Caracteristicas de la mortalidad urban, OPS/OMS* (Washington, DC, 1968).

high figures are due mainly to the occurrence of a great number of traffic accidents, with a lower, but significant, number of home and occupational accidents (see Table 8.14). There is an evident difference between the respective patterns for males and females.

In a paper published in Sao Paulo (Laurenti, 1975) in which 1,746 deaths due to motor-vehicle accidents in a one-year period were studied, it is stated that 65.41 per cent of the injured received hospital care. The length of stay was not determined. Considering the number of injured during the same period — 21,335 — and considering that 50 per cent of them had to be admitted, the result in terms of hospital demand is evident.

Table 8.14: Mortality Specific Rates, Males and Females according to Subgroups of Causes of Violent Deaths, County of Sao Paulo, 1970-2

	1970		1971		1972	
	Male	Female	Male	Female	Male	Female
Accidents by motor vehicles (BE. 47)	4.61	1.36	4.93	1.38	5.16	1.75
Other accidents (BE. 48)	3.12	0.79	2.96	0.83	3.24	0.77
Suicides (BE. 49)	1.12	0.36	1.08	0.40	0.97	0.47
Homicides (BE. 50-A)	1.70	0.32	1.71	0.23	1.98	0.27
Other causes (BE. 50-B)	0.64	0.15	0.37	0.11	0.37	0.09
Total	11.19	2.98	11.05	2.95	11.72	3.35

Source: M.H. Silveira and S.L.D. Gotlieb, 'Acidentes, envenamentos e violencias como causa de morte dos residentes no municipio de Sao Paulo Brasil', *Rev. Saude Publ. Sao Paulo*, 10 (1976), pp. 45-55.

Another type of accident which deserves consideration is that of 'on-the-job' accidents, increasing because of industrialisation occurring in Sao Paulo. In 1971, the county presented a mean accident frequency of 44 to a million man-working hours, the variations depending on the type of job (Laurenti, 1975). The great majority of the accidents still happen on construction sites, where workers, of whom no special qualification is required, are generally migrants from the rural areas and of low educational level, if not entirely illiterate.

A more detailed study on homicides and suicides (Silveira and Gotlieb, 1976) shows that homicides, whose proportion in the total number of deaths is increasing, are most frequent in men aged 25 to 30 years. As regards suicide, represented by a proportional death rate of 9.29 per cent in the three years studied, the highest risk factor is also for males, increasing with the age group considered. For females, the highest risk occurs in the 20 to 25 years age group, decreasing in the following groups up to 70 years old, when the value rises again.

5. Morbidity

The ten most important diseases, according to the International Classification of Diseases, in a significant group of hospitals, were, for 1975:

(1) dehydration;
(2) gastro-enteritis and colitis;
(3) bronchopneumonia;
(4) malnutrition;
(5) inguinal hernia;
(6) senile cataract;
(7) acute otitis;
(8) acute bronchitis;
(9) gastritis and duodenitis;
(10) chronic amygdalitis.

D. MEDICAL AND HOSPITAL CARE

Medical and hospital care in the county of Sao Paulo, until the beginning of the century, were almost exclusively provided by voluntary institutions. Government participation, which started with isolation hospitals, has been gradually increased, though only significantly after the appearance of social security in the country. The first of such institutions was the Railway Workmen's Pension Fund, providing medical care to its associates. After that, there was the Seamen's Pension

Table 8.15: Number of General Beds and Beds per 1,000 Population
in the County of Sao Paulo, 1935-74

	1935		1953		1974	
	Number of beds	Beds per 1,000 pop.	Number of beds	Beds per 1,000 pop.	Number of beds	Beds per 1,000 pop.
Government	540	0.5	2,345	0.9	6,741	1.0
Voluntary/non-profit	1,990	1.9	5,389	2.1	8,744	1.2
For profit	974	0.9	2,765	1.1	8,167	1.2
Total	3,504	3.3	10,499	4.1	23,652	3.4

Source: C. Guimaraes, 'Evolucao da assistencia hospitalar geral no Estado de Sao
Paulo, Brasil, no periodo de 1935 a 1974', *Rev. Saude Publ. Sao Paulo*, 10
(suppl. 2) (1976).

Fund (1933), the first social security group of workers organised
under federal law. Since then, the provision of welfare and of health
have merged. In 1966, several workers' unions amalgamated to form
the 'Instituto Nacional de Previdencia Social' (INPS). The 'Instituto'
is now subsumed under the 'Ministerio da Previdencia Social', created
in 1974.

A study of the evolution of medical and hospital care in the county
of Sao Paulo from 1935 to 1974 shows that, in spite of an increase in
the number of beds from 3,504 (1935) to 23,652 (1974), rate of
increase of beds per 1,000 population was negligible. In 1935 there
were 3.3 beds per 1,000 population; in 1953, this rose to 4.1, but by
1974 it was back again to 3.3. This was due to the increase in population, primarily a consequence of extensive migration (Guimaraes,
1976). Comparative statistics for the years 1935 and 1974 are given in
Table 8.15.

It should be noted that at the beginning of the period more than
50 per cent of the general beds providing hospital care were in
voluntary institutions. By 1953, however, the governmental share
had increased from 15.41 per cent to 22.34 per cent, and in 1974
reached 28.50 per cent. The for-profit hospitals increased their share
of the number of beds from 27.8 per cent in 1935 to 34.53 per cent
in 1974. This pattern of events corresponded to changes in the
main structure of medical care in the county. Table 8.16 shows the
situation by 1975.

Among the 127 hospitals the bed capacity varied from 6 to 409,

Table 8.16: Number of General Hospitals and Beds according to Ownership, Sao Paulo County, 1975

	Hospitals		Beds	
	Number	Per cent	Number	Per cent
Governmental	20	15.7	6,701	29.2
Voluntary/non-profit	35	27.6	8,857	38.6
For profit	72	56.7	7,401	32.2
Total	127	100.0	22,959	100.0

with 48 hospitals having less than 100 beds. The 1975 ratio of 3.1 beds
per thousand population is lower than the figure for 1974. This rate
could be seen as adequate for the county's needs, but this is unlikely
because, first, the INPS frequently limits routine admissions, giving
emphasis to emergency services, and, second, the turnover of beds in
the commercial hospitals is high, the length of stay in many of them
being less than five days. Furthermore, theoretical estimates suggest
that a figure of 4.5 to 5.5 general beds per 1,000 population is the sort
of level of facility required for big cities such as Sao Paulo (Mountin
et al., 1945; Organizacao Panamericana de Saude/OMS, 1966).
   Of the twenty government hospitals, five are officiated by the
federal agency, nine by the state, and the remaining six by municipal
authorities. Four of the state hospitals are maintained by the
Department of Health, two being paediatric institutions, one for heart
diseases and the other for communicable diseases. The importance of
infectious diseases, especially in childhood, has been emphasised
already. The above-mentioned hospital has a capacity of 400 beds.
Also state-controlled is the 'Hospital das Clinicas', a teaching institution,
operated as a complement to the Sao Paulo University School of
Medicine. Altogether, there are three teaching hospitals in the county,
with a bed capacity of 3,170. Of the six municipal hospitals, two
are for children and one is for maternity. The four hospitals owned
by social security collectively represent the largest number of beds in
the country.
   The 'Instituto Nacional de Previdencia Social' (INPS) has gradually
become the greatest provider of medical and hospital care, either
through its own hospitals, or through agreements with voluntary or
commercial institutions. Actually 6 per cent of the commercial
(i.e. 'for-profit') and voluntary hospitals provide medical and hospital

care for the INPS under such agreements.

The Sao Paulo Municipality is obliged by law to be responsible for emergency services which are offered by teaching hospitals, voluntary and for-profit institutions, through agreement on the cost per patient-day. Unfortunately, the state and county departments do not possess comprehensive statistics concerning hospital utilisation, since there is no law compelling institutions to make data publicly available. The numbers and rates shown in Tables 8.16 and 8.17 were therefore obtained by a direct survey of 112 of the 127 hospitals (which corresponded to 94.8 per cent of the beds).

Table 8.17: Length of Stay, Percentage of Occupancy and Hospital Death Rate, according to Ownership, Sao Paulo County, 1975

Hospitals	Length of stay (days)	Occupancy rate (per cent)	Death rate (per cent)
Government	10.5	68.3	6.7
Voluntary/non-profit	7.5	78.1	3.4
For profit	6.8	87.2	3.5
Total	7.8	78.2	4.0

Although the figures for the total number of hospitals at the base of Table 8.16 might appear satisfactory, there appear to be discrepancies between the various hospital types. These can be explained by a number of factors. Thus the length of stay in government institutions is greater than that in the commercial because the latter depend on a rapid patient turnover for their financial survival. It is also true that the government-controlled university hospital has many long-stay patients to aid teaching demonstrations. The occupancy rate again illustrates the financial motives of the commercial sector and also reflects the larger bed capacity of the government institutions. The death-rate statistics are somewhat deceptive: they are higher in the government hospitals because several of them have to deal with the county emergency casualties, but the low figures for the commercial institutions can be explained by their practice of discharging patients early, when they may be critically ill, subsequently to die at home or in governmental institutions.

The staffing situation in the Sao Paulo health services is far from satisfactory. There are unfortunately no municipal data available on the subject, although statistics do exist for the state as a whole. However it is evident that, with the exception of physicians, additional professional qualified personnel are urgently needed. There is in fact an excess of MDs in Brazil today, there being one doctor per 1,400 inhabitants. But they are concentrated in big cities, Sao Paulo being no exception. The ratio of doctor to registered nurse is 5 to 1, a figure that is exactly the reverse of what would generally be considered reasonable.

Health care is also administered outside the hospitals. There are 202 health centres in the county, 144 belonging to the state and 8 per cent to municipal government. During 1975, the state health centres gave care to 393,846 children and the municipal centres to 264,552 children. Neither type of centre is co-ordinated with the hospital network, a situation that has been known for some time to be unsatisfactory (Pedroso, 1969, 1975). No major move towards integration has been made as yet, however, primarily because of the inscrutability of the barrier between state and private institutions.

Nevertheless, in one area, an integrated Health Unit has been established. This is at Cotia, a city situated some 30 kilometres from Sao Paulo. There is no sewerage in the city and only 23 per cent of its population is provided with piped water. Before the setting up of the unit, the only places where medical care was available were the State Health Centre and a municipal health post. The main activity of the above-mentioned health post was to provide an ambulance service to a hospital in Sao Paulo, although in some cases death would occur during the trip.

Two full professors of the School of Public Health and a group of Cotia citizens decided to raise funds in order to start a campaign for the construction of the integrated Health Unit. This unit would entirely change the traditional roles of hospitals and health centres, with preventive and curative medicine practised side by side. The construction of the hospital health centre started in 1968, with a 150-bed capacity for internal medicine, surgery, maternity and paediatrics. With the help of federal, state and municipal governments and funds from the community, it was possible to start the health centre activities in 1975, and in March 1976 the first in-patients were admitted. At that time 60 beds were operational. Simultaneously an agreement was signed between the hospital and INPS, a valuable source of operating income.

The number of children registered at the health centre in 1975 was over 5,000, with more than 11,000 consultations. More than 2,000 children were vaccinated, equivalent to more than 12,000 vaccine doses applied. From March to August 1976, 87 children were admitted and from May to August 1976, there were 314 obstetric patients admitted, with 287 deliveries, an average of 3 deliveries a day. Health education is transmitted through classes and demonstrations to mothers. Powdered milk is distributed only under medical prescription, since emphasis is placed on breast-feeding, a practice that is carried out by approximately 90 per cent of the mothers in Cotia. The Cotia Hospital/Health Centre is also a teaching and training institution for the School of Public Health and medical schools.

The experience of Cotia has received the encouragement of the federal government, which intends to utilise the unit for training of health personnel and to repeat the project in other areas of Brazil.

Appendix

The following is a list of those who assisted Dr Pedroso in the preparation of this chapter, and of Chapter 18.

Lourdes de Freitas Carvalho, Professor, Hospital Administration, School of Public Health, University of Sao Paulo.

Ruy Laurenti, Associate Professor, Department of Epidemiology, School of Public Health, University of Sao Paulo.

Cid Guimaraes, Assistant Professor, Department of Practice in Public Health, School of Public Health, University of Sao Paulo.

Jose Maria Pacheco de Souza, Assistant Professor, Department of Epidemiology, School of Public Health, University of Sao Paulo.

Maria Helena de Mello Jorge Silveira, Assistant Professor, Department of Epidemiology, School of Public Health, University of Sao Paulo.

Sabina Lea Davidson Gotlieb, Assistant Professor, Department of Epidemiology, School of Public Health, University of Sao Paulo.

Jose Gabriel Borba, Associate Professor, Department of Practice in Public Health, School of Public Health, University of Sao Paulo.

Bibliography

Certain, D. *et al.* (1975). 'Analise dos resultados da pesquisa de infeccao tuberculosa e do primeiro programa de vacinacao pelo BCG intrademico em escolares de Sao Paulo, Brasil, 1971-1974.' *Rev. Saude Publ. Sao Paulo*, 9, pp. 125-36.

Fonseca, L.A.M. and Laurenti, R. (1974). 'A qualidade da certificacao medica da causa de morte em Sao Paulo, Brasil.' *Rev. Saude Publ. Sao Paulo*, 8, pp. 21-9.

Fundacao, Ibge (1973). *Censo Demografico de Sao Paulo*. Rio de Janeiro: Recenseamento Geral do Brasil, 1970.

Goldemberg, P. *et al.* (1974). 'Coeficiente de positividade das reacoes de Machado Guerreiro em convocados para o Servico Militar no Estado de Sao Paulo de 1968 a 1971.' *Rev. Ass. med. bras.*, 20, pp. 307-8.

Governo do Estado de Sao Paulo (1974). Secretaria de Economia e Planejamento. 'Movimento do Registro Civil, 1940/1972.' Sao Paulo.

Governo do Estado de Sao Paulo (1975). Secretaria de Estado da Sauda. 'C.S.T. Mortalidade matema e na infancia no Estado de Sao Paulo de 1960 a 1970.' Sao Paulo.

Grau, E.R. (1974). *Regioes metropolitanas*. Sao Paulo: Bushatsky.

Guimaraes, C. (1976), 'Evolucao da assistencia hospitalar geral no Estado de Sao Paulo, Brasil, no periodo de 1935 a 1974.' *Rev. Saude Publ. Sao Paulo*, 10 (suppl. 2).

Iverson, L.B. (1975). 'Meningite meningococica no Municipio de Sao Paulo no periodo – 1968-1974. Aspectos epidemiologicas.' Faculdade de Saude Publica USP, Sao Paulo (Monografia de Mestrado).

Laurenti, R. (1973). 'Causas multiplas de morte.' Faculdade de Saude Publica USP, Sao Paulo (Tese de Livre-Docencia).

Laurenti, R. (1973). 'O atestado de obito: a importancia de seu preenchimento de maneira correta.' *Residencia Medica*. Sao Paulo, 2 (6 marco).

Laurenti, R. (1975). 'Alguns aspectos particulares referentes aos resultados da Investigacao Interamericana de Mortalidade na Infancia na area do projeto de Sao Paulo, Brasil.' *Bol. Of. Sanit. Panam.* Washington, DC, 79 (1), pp. 1-14 (julho).

Laurenti, R. (1975). 'O problema das doencas cronicas e

degenerativas e dos acidentes nas areas urbanizadas da America Latina.' *Rev. Saude Publ. Sao Paulo*, 9, pp. 239-48.

Laurenti, R. and Fonseca, L.A.M. (1976). 'A mortalidade por doencas cardiovasculares no Municipio de Sao Paulo em um periodo de 30 anos (1940-1969).' *Arq. bras. Cardiol.*, 29 (2), pp. 85-8.

Laurenti, R. *et al.* (1975). 'Mortalidade perinatal em Sao Paulo.' *Rev. Saude Publ. Sao Paulo*, 9, pp. 115-24.

Milanesi, M.L. (1969). *O aborto provocado.* Sao Paulo: Pioneira.

Milanesi, M.L. and Laurenti, R. (1964). 'O Estudo Interamericano de Mortalidade. Estado atual da certificocao medica da causa de obito no distrito da Capital.' *Rev. Ass. med. Brasil.*, 10, pp. 111-16.

Ministerio da Saude (1976). 'Anais do Seminario Situacao de Saude nas Areas Metropolitanas Brasileiras.' Faculdade de Saude Publico USP, Sao Paulo.

Mountin, J.W. *et al.* (1945). 'Health service areas: requirement for general hospitals and health centres.' *Publ. Health Serv. Bull.*, 292.

Organizacao Panamericana da Saude/OMS (1966). 'Administracion de servicios de Atencion Medica.' Washington (Publ. cientifica no. 129).

Organizacao Panamericana da Saude/OMS (1969). 'Classificacao Internacional de Doencas, Lesoes e Causas de Morte, 81.' Revisao, 195 (1965). Washington, DC.

Pedroso, O.P. (1969). 'Assistencia hospitalar e Saude Publica.' *Rev. Paul. Hospitals*, Sao Paulo, 17 (9), pp. 3-8 (setembro).

Pedroso, O.P. (1975). 'Hospital e Saude Publica.' *Rev. Paul. Hospitals.* Sao Paulo, 23 (4), pp. 137-9, abr. 1975.

Puffer, R.R. and Griffith, G.W. (1968). 'Caracteristicas de la mortalidad urban.' OPS/OMS, Washington, DC.

Puffer, R.R. and Serrano, C.U. (1975). 'Patterns of mortality in child-hood.' OPS/OMS, Washington, DC (Sc. Pub. 262).

Silva, E.P.C. (1970). 'Estimativas de coeficientes e indices vitais e de sub-registro de nascimenios no distrito de Sao Paulo, baseados em amostra probabilistica de domicilios.' Sao Paulo (Monografia de Mestrado. Faculdade de Saude Publica da USP).

Silveira, M.H. (1976). 'Abortamento espontaneo e provocado. Estudo epidemiologico.' *Rev. da Feder. bras. da Soc. Ginec. Obstetr. Rio de Janeiro*, 4, pp. 215-22 (Abril).

Silveira, M.H. (1974). 'Perdas fetais do distrito de Sao Paulo.' Faculdade de Saude Publica USP, Sao Paulo (Mongrafia de Mestrado).

Silveira, M.H. and Gotlieb, S.L.D. (1976). 'Acidentes, envenenamentos e violencias como causa de morte dos residentes no municipio de Sao Paulo, Brasil.' *Rev. Saude Publ. Sao Paulo*, 10, pp. 45-55.

Universidade de Sao Paulo (1974). 'Esboco do Catologo Geral dos
Cursos de Graduacao.' USP, Sao Paulo.

9 HONG KONG

Arthur E. Starling

A. THE PATTERN OF EXISTING SERVICES

Demography

The Crown Colony of Hong Kong consists of the island of Hong Kong, a small area on the mainland of China and a number of small islands, many of which to this day remain sparsely populated and undeveloped. Its total area is some 400 square miles into which are crowded about 4,300,000 people — 10,000 per square mile: three-quarters of the population live in the twin cities of Victoria in Hong Kong and Kowloon on the mainland which together constitute an area of approximately 33 square miles. It is estimated that 1,000,000 are resident in Hong Kong and 3,300,000 in Kowloon and the New Territories. The two cities are therefore among the most densely populated in the world.

The territory was occupied by the Japanese in December 1941 and was liberated in August 1945. At the time of occupation the total population was roughly 1,000,000 people. From the moment of liberation, Hong Kong began a spectacular recovery. The Chinese returned at a rate approaching 100,000 a month and the population, which by August 1945 had been reduced to about 600,000, rose by the end of 1947 to an estimated 1,800,000. Then, in the period 1948-9, as the forces of the Chinese Nationalist Government began to face defeat in civil war at the hands of the Communists, Hong Kong received an influx of people unparalleled in its history. About three-quarters of a million, mainly from Kwangtung province, Shanghai and other commercial centres, entered Hong Kong during 1949 and the spring of 1950. By the end of 1950 the population was estimated to be 2,360,000. Since then, it has continued to rise and the 1971 census put the population at 3,948,179. The immigrants formed a huge reservoir of labour and Hong Kong, which up to this point had earned a living as an entrepot, found herself entering an era of rapid industrialisation.

Constitution and Administration

The office of governor is the central position in the government of Hong Kong. The governor presides at meetings of the Executive

Council, whose advice he must seek on important policy matters. He is also the President of the Legislative Council, where he possesses both an original and a casting vote. All bills passed by the Legislative Council must have his assent before they become law. With strictly defined exceptions, he is responsible for every executive act of the government. A large number of advisory bodies and committees are also appointed, and constitute an effective consultative and advisory machinery which enables public opinion to be brought to bear on policy formation.

The administrative functions of the government are discharged by about 40 departments, most of which are organised on a functional basis and have responsibilities covering the whole of Hong Kong. This form of organisation, rather than one based on authorities with responsibilities in a limited geographical area only, is suitable for this small compact area and enables the government to provide services without regard to the capacity of residents of various districts to pay taxes.

Health Services

Statutory responsibility for administering the services which safeguard public health in Hong Kong rests with the Director of Medical and Health Services, the Urban Council, the Director of Urban Services, the Commissioner of Labour and the Secretary for the New Territories. The Medical and Health Department provides hospital and clinic facilities throughout both urban and rural areas, maintains family health, which includes maternity and child health and family planning, school health and port health services, and is responsible for measures to control epidemic and endemic disease. In addition, doctors are seconded to the Urban Services Department, the Industrial Health Division of the Labour Department, the Criminal Investigation Department of the Police and to the Prisons Department.

A White Paper on the development of medical services in Hong Kong was published in 1964 and established what it then described as minimal ratios of provision necessary for augmented clinics and hospital services to meet the most urgent medical needs. It stated that by 1972 the standards should be:

4.25 hospital beds per 1,000 population;
1   standard urban clinic per 100,000 urban population;
1   standard rural clinic per 50,000 rural population;
1   polyclinic per 500,000 population.

By 1973 the standards laid down had more or less been achieved, but there was heavy demand on general hospital beds, particularly those maintained directly by the government. Furthermore, the distribution of clinics was uneven, contributing to the heavy overcrowding of some general out-patients' clinics and long waiting periods for appointments in specialist clinics.

In 1973, the Medical Development Advisory Committee was appointed with the following terms of reference:

To keep under continuous review and to advise on the development and phased implementation of medical and health services in Hong Kong. Having regard to all factors which would determine the progress of expansion including finance, rate of building construction and the availability of qualified staff, and on the principles of subvention.

The Committee reported in July 1973 and a White Paper entitled *The Further Development of Medical and Health Services in Hong Kong* was tabled in the Legislative Council in July 1974. The principal proposals contained in the White Paper are as follows:

(a) Medical and health services will be organised on a regional basis. Each region to be served with all appropriate general and specialist facilities.
(b) A ratio of 5.5 hospital beds per thousand population should be regarded as a desirable standard for long-term planning.
(c) The building of 3 additional general hospitals and the provision of further psychiatric facilities.
(d) The introduction of day-beds in selected clinics.
(e) The provision of a number of additional polyclinics and clinics in order to serve the developing needs of the community and the movement into planned new towns.

Hospital Beds

At the end of 1975, 18,561 hospital beds were available in Hong Kong. Of these, 16,382 are in government hospitals or hospitals subvented by government and 2,179 are provided by private agencies. Government maintains a total of 51 clinics for general out-patients with specialist facilities being available in the major centres of the urban areas. A number of private clinics operate which are required to be registered under the Medical Clinics Ordinance. There are also low-cost clinics in operation in the housing estates, and a School Medical Service is operated by the School Medical Service Board. Notwithstanding these non-government services, any member of the population can attend one of the government general out-patients' clinics for treatment and can if necessary be referred from there to a government consultant or to one of the government hospitals for treatment. There is no compulsory health service insurance scheme or the equivalent in Hong Kong. Fees for both in-patient and out-patient treatment by government agencies and by the government-subsidised agencies are nominal and can be waived, if necessary, through the medical social service so that, in effect, the population enjoys a nearly free health service which is financed almost entirely by the central government, except for that small section of the community who can afford to and do pay the economic costs for treatment through private practitioners or through one of the private hospitals. It is estimated that the latter would be about 10 per cent of the population.

The distribution of hospital beds is shown in the statistical data included in Table 9.4 in the appendix to this chapter. A new hospital known as the Princess Margaret Hospital is at present partly commissioned. This hospital will be fully functional during the year 1976 and a further 344 general hospital beds will be added to the total available number of beds shown in Table 9.4.

Primary Care

The Medical and Health Department provides primary care facilities and preventive services in the general clinics referred to in the preceding section. These clinics are strategically located throughout the urban and rural areas to serve population centres and a typical clinic will comprise a general out-patients' department on the ground floor with a family health service centre and maternity ward above. Some clinics have a full-time chest clinic and most of those that do not do provide chest clinic services on a sessional basis. Primary care services for venereal diseases are located in separate social hygiene clinics. In addition to primary care of expectant mothers at antenatal clinics, the family health service provides infant and toddler welfare sessions and has recently initiated a child developmental screening programme (see Table 9.7). In addition to the chest clinic sessions held in the general OPDs, the Chest Service operates a number of full-time chest clinics separately located for primary and follow-up out-patient care, and the chest service also has a prominent preventive role, providing BCG vaccination to the newborn. Family planning was pioneered in Hong

Kong by the Family Planning Association and in recent years the Medical and Health Department has taken over from the association much of the routine work in family planning clinics. The Family Planning Association, however, continues to be very active in the field of education and in assessing the needs for additional family planning clinics. Other active areas of health education are in the fields of tuberculosis, social hygiene and the dental service. Health education has tended to be organised on a fragmented basis in the past but will shortly be co-ordinated under a centralised Health Education Unit which will formulate policy and generally direct the work of health education through centres organised on a regional basis.

Staffing

All staff, including doctors, working in the government hospitals and other government agencies are employed by the government on a full-time basis and paid as such. Doctors on these conditions are not permitted to indulge in private practice. In the government-subsidised institutions, doctors are employed on varying terms of service and some may be permitted private practice whilst working on a part-time basis for the subsidised organisations. Doctors in private practice charge the economic fee for their services and are not controlled by the government or their professional body. There are, in addition, a number of voluntary agencies which assist in the health services, e.g. HK Anti-Cancer Society, HK Anti-Tuberculosis and Thoracic Diseases Association.

Ambulance Services

The Ambulance Service is operated by the Fire Services Department. It falls into two categories — the emergency service and the non-urgent service which conveys patients to and from hospitals and clinics as required.

Training

The Medical Faculty of the University of Hong Kong was established in 1911 and the annual intake is now 150 pre-clinical students per year. The Queen Mary Hospital on Hong Kong Island also serves as the University Teaching Hospital. In addition, it is planned to establish a second medical school at the Chinese University of Hong Kong in order to ensure the availability of a sufficient number of doctors in 1985. There are no local facilities for training in dentistry, but it is proposed to set up a dental school shortly in the University of Hong Kong.

Facilities exist for the training of nurses, health visitors and the professions supplementary to medicine except occupational therapists and dietitians.

B. THE MAIN PROBLEMS

In the immediate post-war years, priority was given to the establishment of services concerned with the prevention and control of diseases and particularly of the epidemic diseases of smallpox and cholera. High priority was also given to the development of quarantine and epidemiological services, maternity and child health services and measures to control the major menace of tuberculosis.

The biggest problems have arisen from the very dense overcrowding, inadequate housing and environmental sanitation, all of which have been due to the staggering increase in the population over a period of little more than 25 years. Tuberculosis remains a health problem in Hong Kong and the policy for control of the disease has been to protect, by vaccination with BCG, the newborn, who are particularly vulnerable, and primary school entrants, who may develop active disease later in life. This measure has markedly reduced the incidence of tuberculosis in children under 15 in recent years. For actual cases of the disease, it has been shown that often out-patient therapy is at least as good as institutional treatment. There has been a high degree of co-operation between the government and the voluntary agencies in the treatment of tuberculosis, particularly the Hong Kong Anti-Tuberculosis and Thoracic Diseases Association. Other than tuberculosis and the endemic gastro-intestinal group of diseases, infectious diseases are no longer a problem in Hong Kong and it has been possible to reallocate hospital beds intended for the hospitalisation of infectious diseases to other specialties.

Although training is available in Hong Kong for medical, nursing and most paramedical personnel, there is a large shortfall in most areas. A significant factor is wastage due to emigration, as Hong Kong is in no position to compete with larger developed countries in terms of opportunity and political stability and because travel has generally become easier and cheaper. Additional training facilities are being planned to cope with the large demand for all grades, which is expected to arise as the development programme gains momentum.

Overcrowding in the urban areas has long been recognised as a problem and the government has plans to develop three new towns in the New Territories, where land is more readily available for housing and for industry. It is expected that by 1985 one-third of the population will be settled in these new towns.

Finance

Hong Kong has a relatively young population (see Table 9.1) and the
pressing needs for education and work opportunities must be
considered along with the requirement for improved social services.
Conversely the demand for subsidised health services, despite the
young population, is still great owing to the relatively low socio-
economic capacity of the majority of the population. In most countries
it is claimed that the development of health services is impeded by
inadequate funds. Whilst to some extent this is true, the development
of health services is also dependent on many other environmental
factors and in Hong Kong it is doubtful whether the availability of
additional finance could have speeded up development to any marked
extent.

There is an annual cycle of estimating and budgeting to meet the
cost of the health services. The estimates are prepared by the Medical
and Health Department and submitted to the government, which then
decides on the final allocations between the various service departments.

Rehabilitation

Rapid industrialisation has caused large numbers of accidents and
resultant disabilities, and rehabilitation services both in government
and the voluntary agencies have developed in a fragmented, piecemeal
manner. The maintenance of a large productive working force depends
on an efficient rehabilitation service, and a comprehensive ten-year
development programme for rehabilitation is now being established
to ensure that all such services will in future be properly co-ordinated.

Drug Addiction

Drug addiction is a serious problem in Hong Kong and there is an
estimated addict population of 80,000 or more, mostly on heroin and
morphine. Every effort is made to stamp out the trafficking of drugs
into and through Hong Kong, but the geographical situation renders it
extremely difficult for the law enforcement agencies to do this
effectively. Large seizures of illicit drugs are frequently made, as a
result of which the prices of heroin and morphine fluctuate, and this
in turn affects the numbers of addicts who come forward to take
advantage of the various forms of treatment available. At present the
Medical and Health Department operates 4 Methadone Maintenance
Centres and 12 Methadone Detoxification Centres. The Society for the

Aid and Rehabilitation of Drug Addicts runs a treatment centre on a small island, which houses 500 addicts who stay on the island for about 6 months before returning to their own homes. The Prisons Department also runs a number of treatment centres and rehabilitation services.

Hospital Development

In Hong Kong's overcrowded conditions land suitable for building is both difficult to find and very valuable so that medical projects compete with other agencies for land allocations. As a result, hospitals of 1,300 beds and more have been developed. The first of these was completed in 1963 at a time when the accepted view was that 600-700 beds was the optimum size of a hospital. However, these large medical centres have proved to have advantages which compensate in some measure for the disadvantages which are inherent in any large organisation.

Reference has been made to the assistance rendered by voluntary organisations in the development of health care facilities. Financial assistance, mainly by means of annual subvention, is given to certain voluntary organisations, which maintain hospitals. These range from small hospitals to large general hospitals containing 1,500 beds. They are well equipped and efficiently operated and by reason of the government's financial interest the Medical Department is able to maintain some indirect control over their activities and future development. Additionally, the Department is usually represented on the Executive Board. However, problems do arise which attract a degree of justifiable criticism, and which have not been entirely resolved. There is a tendency for the government hospitals to be overcrowded and for the subvented organisation to be relatively under-occupied. This involves an uneconomic use of expensive resources. There are many reasons for this – whilst the subvented organisations are well run and adequately equipped, the population as a whole tends to move towards the government hospital in preference to the non-government, partly because access to government consultants is easier and perhaps because there is a natural reaction to anything which may be described as charity and it was as charitable organisations that the majority of these hospitals started. A system of regionalisation is being planned for the health services and when this is in operation it is hoped that it will be possible to achieve a more even distribution of patients so that the hospitals will operate more as a unified service than they do now.

Mental Health

Another area for concern is that of mental health. At present Hong
Kong has one psychiatric hospital which was designed for 1,242
patients and now houses well over 2,000 and a relatively small number
of psychiatric beds in general hospitals, plus a number of psychiatric
clinics, some of which contain day beds. That the Mental Health
Service is not adequately developed is perhaps understandable and
the following quotation from a report written by the Colonial Surgeon
in 1875 is of interest:

> At the end of 1874 a European Female Lunatic was sent into the
> Gaol. This young person was very noisy and slept little. Day and
> night her singing, laughter and shouting were to be heard if she was
> in a good temper, which she usually was; but if she was not, her
> howling and screaming was something appalling. This kept most of
> the prisoners awake who had to work hard all day, an additional
> punishment to which they were not sentenced. Not only this, but it
> annoyed the whole neighbourhood among others two unofficial
> members of Council who lived close by and who very forcibly in
> Council backed up my representations that the Gaol was not a fit
> place for the detention of Lunatics. So the half of a building consist-
> ing of two semi-detached houses was fitted up as a Lunatic Asylum
> . . . This was opened the first day of 1875.

The existing psychiatric hospital was completed in 1961 and is
situated in the New Territories, some 22 miles north of Kowloon. It
consists of a number of two-storeyed buildings set in spacious grounds
so that the patients can be permitted the maximum freedom consistent
with their medical condition. It is set in rural surroundings, well away
from the main centres of population and is in many ways ideally sited
for a mental hospital, although access is sometimes difficult due to
limited public transport. This replaced the former mental hospital on
Hong Kong Island which had space for only about 400 patients in
very unsatisfactory accommodation and which was erected in 1919.
An additional psychiatric hospital is now under construction in North
Kowloon. This will have about 1,300 beds and will provide much-
needed relief for this service.

An associated problem is the lack of any domiciliary mental health
service. This is due principally to the conditions under which people
live rather than any conscious decision not to provide it, but it does
mean that patients may have to remain hospitalised for long periods

when in different conditions they could be cared for at home.

Dental Care

No comprehensive dental service has yet been established. Government operates a dental service for its employees and their dependants but, except for dealing with a number of dental emergencies, this is not available to the public who have to use private dental practitioners.

A dental nurses' training school is being established and a school dental service will then be developed. The proposed establishment of a dental school in the University of Hong Kong has already been noted.

Housing

It is impossible to discuss the development of Hong Kong's health services without mention of the housing programme. The congested conditions in which a large proportion of the population live influence the manner in which the health services have developed, in that they inhibit and even preclude the development of domiciliary and community health services.

The present housing target is to give every inhabitant of Hong Kong self-contained accommodation in a reasonable environment within ten years. In hard figures this means that the government plans to build new housing for 1.8 million people at a cost of HK $3,340 million. It also means new towns, new roads to link them with the old urban areas, and a full ration of the essentials of modern life: schools, medical facilities, parks, playgrounds, services and markets. There is no field in which Hong Kong's overcrowding has produced more acute problems, or one in which the government has responded more vigorously, than housing.

Since the first resettlement blocks were built following the great squatter fire of 1953, which made 53,000 homeless, more than 1.6 million people have been housed in government-built low-rent estates. The early resettlement blocks were rudimentary, but they offered security and a real home to people who until then had lived in cardboard or corrugated iron shacks, with no protection from flood and fire.

The new estates are fine examples of how Hong Kong has coped with housing people at densities higher than anywhere else on earth and today the rash of squatter huts that used to disfigure the hillsides has diminished. Many of the ageing and dilapidated pre-war tenement houses have also been replaced by private development.

But in spite of all this, problems remain. There are still more than a quarter of a million squatters and many rooms in the earlier resettlement estates are badly crowded and, in the private sector, over 300,000 people are living in unsatisfactory conditions in shared flats or tenements.

C. SOME GOOD IDEAS

The following extracts from the White Paper tabled in the Legislative Council in July 1974 entitled *The Further Development of Hospital Services in Hong Kong* describe in some detail the present approach to the administration of medical and health services:

A Regional Approach

Since 1949 there has been an increasing concentration of population in the urban areas, particularly Kowloon. With the development of Kwun Tong and Tsuen Wan a new pattern of population distribution has occurred, which will be further accentuated by the development of the new towns at Sha Tin and Tuen Mun. Medical and health planning must take this into account with a view to ensuring that medical services are available within reasonable access of the new centres of population. It is accordingly proposed to introduce a fresh approach to the administration of medical and health services which will ensure a better appreciation of the medical and health needs of each of these main population centres.

Some parts of the health services are already administered on a regional basis; the administration of medical services (concerned particularly with the hospitals) remains centralised at Medical and Health Departments.

To provide a soundly based regional service and to enable the best use to be made of resources, planning will be based on the need for each region to be served by:

(a)   a regional hospital: this would be a major acute hospital, equipped to treat patients requiring the highest level of specialist care; some highly specialised facilities may be concentrated in a particular hospital but otherwise a regional acute hospital should be capable of providing the region which it serves with all major general specialist services to an appropriate degree of sophistication;
(b)   one or more district hospitals: these hospitals will provide the basic hospital services in the region and will receive patients whose condition is not such as to warrant referral directly to the regional

hospital; a district hospital will perform a dual role: a patient whose condition so warrants will be referred to the regional hospital for the more specialised levels of treatment; a district hospital will also receive patients from the regional hospital for the later stages of their treatment, when it is medically appropriate for them to be transferred;

(c)   one or more specialist clinics or polyclinics: these will provide the necessary support and out-patient specialist services, including those for patients before and after any hospital treatment; and

(d)   a number of general clinics based on the needs of the population of the area providing both out-patient and general public health services.

Such a regional organisation can be built around the major hospitals (Queen Mary, Kwong Wah, Queen Elizabeth and Princess Margaret). There will therefore initially be four regions served by these hospitals respectively:

(a)   Hong Kong Island;
(b)   West Kowloon;
(c)   East Kowloon and East New Territories;
(d)   West New Territories.

However, with the anticipated movement of population it will be necessary at a later stage to establish a fifth region to serve East New Territories separately. The need to establish another region for the Tuen Mun area will be kept under review but for the present it is considered likely that the needs of the latter area can be effectively combined in the same region as Tsuen Wan and Kwai Chung.

The Economic Use of Hospital Beds

The introduction of a regional approach to medical and health services and the establishment of regional administrative offices will make it possible to secure a more even use of the general beds available in government and government-assisted hospitals.

A patient is in need of the more specialised facilities for only part of his stay in hospital. Depending on the course of treatment required, therefore, he should continue the remainder of his in-patient treatment in a bed with appropriate but simpler services.

The maximum use of beds would mean that a patient should usually first attend a general out-patient clinic, or hospital casualty department in the case of an emergency. Where treatment can be continued on an out-patient basis, but specialist attention is required, the patient would normally be referred to a specialist clinic serving the region and within reasonable travelling distance of his home. If the doctor at a general or specialist clinic considers that in-patient treatment is necessary, the patient will be referred to a district hospital serving the region or to the regional hospital, depending on the treatment required. Subsequently when his condition permits, he would be transferred to a non-acute bed for convalescence in a district hospital. Thus a patient not considered to require highly specialised treatment would not normally be referred to a regional hospital; one whose treatment requires a stay in an acute hospital bed would be transferred to a non-acute bed for convalescence.

Accident and Casualty Services

With the establishment of this integrated structure it will be possible to undertake a detailed investigation of the accident and casualty services. Before the Medical Development Advisory Committee report was submitted, advice had been received on a number of improvements to these services. It may be that these services should be reorganised into a two-tier system of Designated Accident Centres and Accident Centres. A reorganisation on these lines could be effected on a regional basis. When the establishment of the new regional structure permits, proposals will be worked out in detail.

The introduction of the regional approach should:

(a)   ensure that patients are treated with facilities more appropriate to their ailments;

(b)   ensure at a time when there is increasing pressure on hospital beds, that the maximum use is made of them; and

(c)   improve the accident service.   *[End of White Paper extracts.]*

Day Beds

The provision of day beds is being pursued as a means of reducing the shortfall in in-patient facilities and, it is hoped, as a further means of ensuring a more economic use of hospital facilities. The present proposals envisage approximately 60 day beds being provided in certain general clinics. A day bed is far cheaper to maintain than a hospital bed; it enables the patient to remain in his home environment and at the same time to receive the benefit of medical care and rehabilitation. The success or otherwise of day beds has yet to be proved, but present indications are that they will help to ensure the maximum use of hospital beds, and at the same time compensate in some way for the present lack of domiciliary services.

Maternity Homes

For some years, maternity homes have been incorporated into a number of the general out-patient clinics for uncomplicated deliveries. Patients go into these homes which contain 25 beds, have their babies in clean and modern conditions with skilled staff in attendance, remain for about 2 days after delivery and are then discharged. These units are cheaper to operate than hospital beds and enable the patient to remain near her home.

Hospital Design

In order to keep abreast of the expanding population, hospital development in Hong Kong over the last 30 years has been impressive. Both government and the voluntary agencies have played their part, and a number of the voluntary agencies have been granted capital subventions for building new hospitals and upgrading existing facilities. As has been noted, this has resulted in an uneconomic use of hospital beds, but a number of new ideas on hospital design have emerged and deserve comment. Reference has been made to size: 1,300-bedded hospitals or over have been developed rather as a matter of necessity than of choice, but apart from being perhaps more impersonal than is desirable size alone has presented no real problem, and has in fact proved to have advantages. It is very much easier to ensure that the full range of specialist services is available throughout the 24 hours. The casualty services can function more efficiently under these conditions and there is no doubt, certainly in Hong Kong, that operating costs of large hospitals are comparatively less. Nursing units of 66 beds have developed: these are divided into two sections with a centre span which houses a service area shared by both. Each section is divided into cubicles of 8 with 2 single rooms for isolation or special care. These units seem to suit the needs of Hong Kong well and avoid under-utilisation or duplication of treatment rooms, utility rooms, etc.

The New Medical School

A project which is now in the preliminary stages of planning and which will create a degree of interest in the future is the establishment of a second medical school in the Chinese University of Hong Kong. This is being designed for an annual intake of about 100 medical students and will be associated with the Sha Tin hospital, which is being developed as part of the new town and will be about three miles away from the university. The complex will house the hospital, specially designed with the teaching element in view, a polyclinic which will be connected to the hospital by a covered passage-way, and the teaching or professorial suites which will each be adjacent to the appropriate patient area. It will include day centres for geriatric and psychiatric cases and adequate lecture theatres, seminar rooms, library facilities, reading rooms and hostels for the students. The project presents an almost unique opportunity to develop both a medical school and teaching hospital simultaneously, but will require a lot of detailed planning and organisation to ensure that the hospital can be used for teaching when the first intake of students finish their pre-clinical studies.

The Auxiliary Medical Service

The purpose of the Auxiliary Medical Service, which was formed in 1950, is to reinforce the regular medical services and ambulance services in any type of emergency by providing additional medical and paramedical services as necessary.

Its function is that of a civil defence medical unit and in an emergency, covering part or the whole of the territory, members would be required also to work closely with the Civil Aid Services and other rescue services. All members of the Service are volunteers and included in the membership are doctors, nurses and others who are anxious and willing to help their fellow-citizens in times of need. Unqualified members are given training in first aid, home nursing and search and rescue operations. They have assisted at the scenes of disasters wrought by typhoons, landslides, fires and bombs, have helped in epidemics and more recently are giving assistance in drug addiction treatment centres. Members enjoy the respect of the community for their voluntary service and have helped various branches of the regular health service on many occasions in the past.

SUMMARY

Hong Kong has long been described as a 'Problem of People'. The rapid increase in the population over recent years has impelled the expansion and development of the social services, and that it has not always been even is understandable. Primary health care, health education, specialist services and hospitalisation are available on a nearly free basis for that portion of the community which cannot afford the services of a private practitioner. It is perhaps a matter for future policy as to whether the population should be or will be required to pay more for these services.

The deficiencies in health care are recognised and every attempt is being made to identify these and clarify some of the issues involved. They stem from a shortage of space, an overcrowded community and difficulties in the recruitment, training and retention of skilled staff. None the less Hong Kong has enjoyed many years of prosperity and continued improvement in the standard of living of its people. Although still subject to a form of colonial administration, the government maintains a large number of advisory bodies and committees. Through these it is able to assess public opinion and the needs of the community and can react quickly to criticism and changing conditions.

Appendix: Health Statistics of Hong Kong

Table 9.1: Population of Hong Kong by Age and Sex, 1975

Age	Males		Females		Totals	
	Number	Per cent	Number	Per cent	Number	Per cent
0—4	207,800	4.8	194,900	4.4	402,700	9.2
5—14	495,500	11.4	473,500	10.8	969,000	22.2
15—44	1,057,100	24.2	914,300	21.0	1,971,400	45.2
45—64	405,600	9.2	379,900	8.7	785,500	17.9
65 and over	85,200	2.0	152,800	3.5	238,000	5.5
Total	2,251,200	51.6	2,115,400	48.4	4,366,600	100.0

Table 9.2: Vital Statistics, 1975

Birth rate	18	per 1,000 population
Infant mortality rate	15	per 1,000 live births
Death rate	5	per 1,000 population
Deaths registered	21,191	

Table 9.3: Mortality — First 10 Causes of Death by Rank, 1975

Rank	Cause
1	Malignant neoplasms
2	Heart diseases including hypertensive diseases
3	Cerebrovascular diseases
4	Pneumonia
5	Bronchitis, emphysema and asthma
6	All accidents
7	Tuberculosis
8	Certain causes of perinatal mortality
9	Suicide and self-inflicted injuries
10	Congenital anomalies

Table 9.4: Resources — Number of Hospital Beds by Specialty and
Total per 1,000 Population

	Government hospital	Government-assisted	Private	Total	Beds per 1,000 population
Med.	875	1,722	649	3,246	0.7
Surg.	1,107	1,006	487	2,600	0.6
Orth.	684	369	42	1,095	0.3
Gynae.	244	403	85	732	0.2
Mat'y	1,135	678	432	2,245	0.5
Paed.	628	649	129	1,406	0.3
Psych.	2,111	28	6	2,145	0.5
Mental retard.	200	44	0	244	0.06
TB	108	1,429	33	1,570	0.4
Others	1,441	1,521	316	3,278	0.7
Total	8,533	7,849	2,179	18,561	4.3

Table 9.5: Utilisation — Number of Patients Treated in All Institutions,
1975

Speciality	Number
General	340,725
Infectious (excluding tuberculosis)	11,866
Tuberculosis	9,919
Maternity	102,073
Psychiatric	9,045
Total	473,628

Table 9.6: Resources — Work of Family Health Service, 1974-5

	Number of centres
Full-time	22
Part-time	15

Table 9.7: Work of Family Health Service, 1974-5

Work of centres	Number of sessions	Number of new attendances	Number of total attendances
Antenatal	3,112	26,334	178,486
Postnatal	1,458	13,748	14,390
Infant welfare	7,582	78,189	1,070,167
Toddler welfare	1,508	35,743	140,087
Family planning*	5,871	31,436	243,318

* Government Family Planning Clinics only; the FPA of Hong Kong also provides a family planning service.

10 MANILA

Gabriel G. Carreon

A. THE PATTERN OF EXISTING SERVICES

Demographic and Other Data

Health services for the 4,953,643 people living in 635.98 square miles of Metro Manila Area (Bureau of Census and Statistics, 1970) are provided as part of the Philippine Health Care Delivery System, envisioned in the National Health Plan 1975-8 (formulated by the Department of Health (DoH) and the National Economic Development Authority, 1975). Broadly, the Philippine health care delivery system may be divided into the government, private and mixed sectors. It consists of a network of facilities dispersed all over the country (see Figure 10.1), loosely linked together but without a formal referral system.

From a national government standpoint, the Department of Health is the primary government agency in the field of health and it runs the bulk of the government health facilities. The DoH co-ordinates its services in the twelve regions of the Philippines, one of which is the Metropolitan Manila Area (for details of the 12 regions see Table 10.8). Under the DoH, various facilities are provided to constitute the health care delivery system. At one end of the spectrum is the medical centre providing highly sophisticated tertiary care while at the other is the unsophisticated barrio health station (Rural Health Unit) providing primary care. Secondary care level facilities (non-departmentalised hospitals) occupy an intermediate position.

Organisation

Being one of the regions of the Philippines, a fair amount of autonomy is given to the Metropolitan Manila Commission to govern Metro Manila Area. From the Commission's viewpoint, the over-all co-ordination of planning, organising and integrating Metro Manila's health and sanitation services is vested in its Action Officer for Health and Sanitation Services. Final decisions (unless explicitly delegated to the action officer) are made by the Governor of the Commission.

The health and sanitation services in Metro Manila are essentially organised along the same pattern as that envisioned in the National

238

Health Plan. It is organised according to the concept of a three-layered structure rendering primary, secondary and tertiary care services. Primary care is delivered by the health centre, secondary care by 'regional hospitals' and tertiary care by 'medical centres' (see Figure 10.3).

The aforementioned services are delivered according to six health zones in Metro Manila. Each health zone is headed by a team composed of the city and municipal health officers of the zone. The designated leader reports directly to the Action Officer for Health and Sanitation Services (see Figure 10.2). The town/city health officers are responsible for the over-all manpower planning and distribution in their respective areas. The action officer, however, reserves the right to transfer people and other resources between areas when it is so merited by the health situation in a particular locality.

In order to ensure co-ordination between the different layers of health care delivery and the general population, it was decided that:

(a)   The primary care unit, i.e. the health centre, should be assigned its own 'territory' of barangays. (A barangay is a political unit composed of 10 puroks, one purok being composed of 10 families.) As such, the health centre shall be responsible for the delivery of primary care needs to the population of the barangay.

(b)   Secondary hospitals have their own 'territories'.

(c)   As a general policy, patients seeking secondary and tertiary care in government hospitals have to be referred by the health centre physician before they are entertained.

Other Main Government Agencies

Apart from the Metro Manila Commission, the Philippine Medical Care Commission, a national agency, makes available medical care through a health insurance scheme with a coverage that currently includes employees but eventually will include the whole population. Moreover, the Office of the President, through the University of the Philippines System, Philippine General Hospital, UP-Infirmary, and other agencies, provides medical care to the general population. In addition, some government agencies provide health services covering specific sectors of the population: Department of National Defence, Bureau of Prisons, Department of Education and Culture and Department of Social Welfare. There are also government agencies which are charged with the responsibility of undertaking specific health activities such as environmental sanitation (partly performed by the National Pollution

Figure 10.1: Philippine Health System

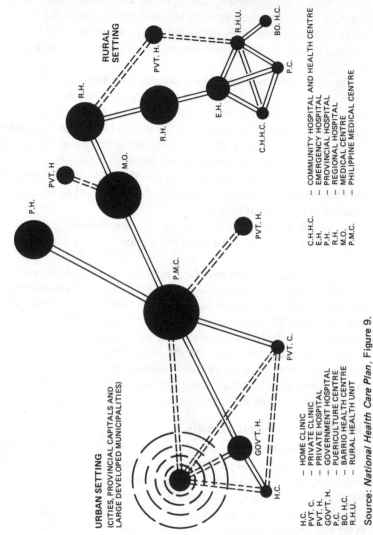

RURAL SETTING

URBAN SETTING
(CITIES, PROVINCIAL CAPITALS AND
LARGE DEVELOPED MUNICIPALITIES)

H.C.	— HOME CLINIC		C.H.H.C.	— COMMUNITY HOSPITAL AND HEALTH CENTRE
PVT. C.	— PRIVATE CLINIC		E.H.	— EMERGENCY HOSPITAL
PVT. H.	— PRIVATE HOSPITAL		P.H.	— PROVINCIAL HOSPITAL
GOV'T. H.	— GOVERNMENT HOSPITAL		R.H.	— REGIONAL HOSPITAL
P.C.	— PUERICULTURE CENTRE		M.O.	— MEDICAL CENTRE
BO. H.C.	— BARRIO HEALTH CENTRE		P.M.C.	— PHILIPPINE MEDICAL CENTRE
R.H.U.	— RURAL HEALTH UNIT			

Source: *National Health Care Plan*, Figure 9.

Figure 10.2: Structure of Health Officers in Metro Manila

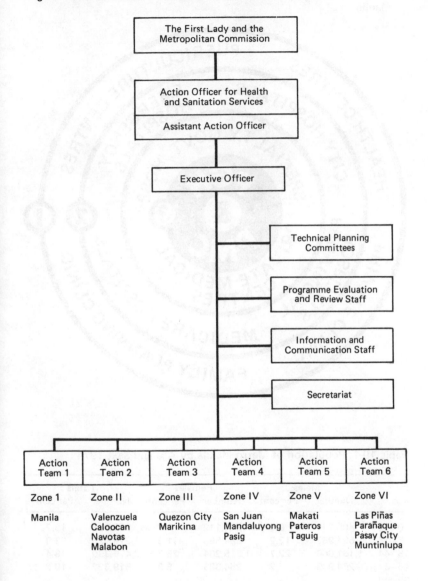

Figure 10.3: Three-Layered Health Care Delivery System in Metro Manila

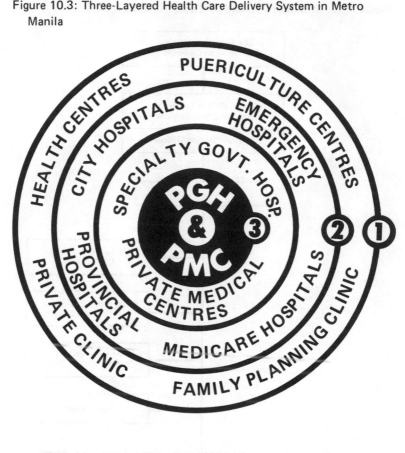

Table 10.1: Population of Metro Manila by Age and Sex, 1974

Age	Males		Females		Totals	
	Number	Per cent	Number	Per cent	Number	Per cent
0–14	408,241	8.0	394,112	7.7	802,353	15.7
5–14	624,957	12.2	594,568	11.6	1,219,525	23.8
15–44	1,161,066	22.7	1,315,264	25.7	2,476,330	48.4
45–64	264,939	5.2	254,383	5.0	519,322	10.2
65 and over	47,348	1.0	46,977	0.9	94,325	1.9
Total	2,506,551	49.1	2,605,304	50.9	5,111,855	100.0

Table 10.2: Vital Statistics, 1974

Birth rate	35.0	per 1,000 population
Infant mortality rate	52.8	per 1,000 live births
Death rate	7.2	per 1,000 population

Table 10.3: Mortality — First 10 Causes of Death by Rank, 1974

Rank	Cause	Rate per 100,000
1	Pneumonia	325
2	Tuberculosis	152
3	Diseases of the heart	84
4	Gastro-enteritis and colitis	72
5	Certain diseases of early infancy	62
6	Vascular lesions of central nervous system	52
7	Malignant neoplasms	44
8	Accidents	41
9	Senility	20
10	Malnutrition	9

Table 10.4: Morbidity — Common Conditions Seen in the Public Sector
Medical Care

Gastro-enteritis and colitis
Tuberculosis (all forms)
Pneumonia
Influenza
Measles
Diphtheria
Gonorrhoea
Cancer
Infectious hepatitis
Typhoid fever

Table 10.5: Resources — Staff Employed by Metro Manila Commission, 1975-6, Number and Number of Population per Health Worker

Staff type	Number*	Number of population per health worker
Physicians	410	12,468
Nursing personnel	675	7,573
Other health workers	1,766	2,895

* Does not include those employed in private sector.

Table 10.6: Resources — Health Centres, Puericulture Centres and Family Planning Centres, by Health Zone

	Zone						
	I	II	III	IV	V	VI	Total
Health centres	40	41	33	20	15	32	181
Puericulture centres		10		3	18		31
Combined HC and PC	1	16	4	35	4	7	67
Total	41	67	37	58	37	39	279
Family planning clinics	91	46	70	37	39	32	315
Other clinics	155	2	17	0	0	6	180

Table 10.7: Finance — Aggregated Expenditures of the Four Cities and Thirteen Municipalities in Metro Manila, 1975-6

		Pesos
(A)	Budget	
	Personal services	16,294,001
	Maintenance and other operating expenses	6,647,708
	Equipment outlay	171,700
	Capital outlay	1,609,279
(B)	Others	
	Salaries and other privileges	15,000
	Mechanics and other supplies	10,000
	Popcom	110,476
	Charity sweepstakes	123,000
Total		24,981,164

Table 10.8: Regions of the Philippines

Region I	—	Ilocos		
Region II	—	Cagayan Valley		
Region III	—	Central Luzon		
Region IV-A	—	Metro Manila		
		1. Caloocan City	10.	Pasig
		2. Manila	11.	Marikina
		3. Quezon City	12.	Malabon
		4. Pasay	13.	Navotas
		5. Las Piñas	14.	Pateros
		6. San Juan	15.	Muntinlupa
		7. Makati	16.	Valenzuela
		8. Parañaque	17.	Taguig
		9. Mandaluyong		
Region IV-B	—	Southern Tagalog		
Region V	—	Bicol		
Region VI	—	Western Visayas		
Region VII	—	Central Visayas		
Region VIII	—	Eastern Visayas		
Region IX	—	Western Mindanao		
Region X	—	Northern Mindanao		
Region XI	—	Southern Mindanao		

Control Commission). Finally, nutrition, population control, the control of drug abuse and other activities are jointly undertaken by a number of multi-sectoral government agencies.

Patients' Access to Health Care Facilities

(a)   As mentioned earlier, health centres run by the Commission are the basic government units that deliver primary care. The delivery of primary care is effected in two ways: either the patient goes to the health centre to seek health care or, as part of the promotive health services programme of the health centre, the centre's personnel goes to the homes of patients.

(b)   Alternatively, individual patients may go to private clinics/doctors who render services for a fee.

(c)   A system, where access to secondary and tertiary government hospitals and medical centres is through a referral system coming from the primary care unit, is at present being developed. Pending the implementation of this system, individual patients go directly to tertiary care centres.

Voluntary Organisations

For the purposes of planning Metropolitan Health Services, the Commission disregards the contribution of voluntary organisations, since for the most part the services they offer are short-term services. This is true except for the Philippine League of Puericulture Centres, which has already been integrated into the over-all organisation of Health and Sanitation Services in Metro Manila. The Commission, however, provides for points of entry for voluntary organisations into the delivery of health care within the over-all context of its plan. Points of entry for voluntary organisations are especially encouraged at the health zone, city, town, individual health centre, hospital and medical centre. Encouragement is given to voluntary organisations through press and other media coverage.

Community Participation

The health centre/barangay link mentioned earlier is the critical point at which community participation is effective. In each barangay, a health and sanitation assembly is organised under the barangay leader. This assembly, which is usually composed of unpaid members, is encouraged to participate actively in the over-all planning and execution of primary care services in the barangay. Also through these assemblies, members of the barangay are encouraged to become aides of the health centre's workers in delivering primary health and sanitation services. (See Chapter 20 for a more detailed exposition.)

Finance

The Metropolitan's health services which are under the Commission are financed through local taxation in each town and city. Those that are directly run by the DoH are financed through the national government subsidy. Others, such as those run by other government agencies, are supported by the agency's budgetary allocation coming from either the national government or other sources. In general, the services offered by the Commission, DoH and other government agencies are not directly paid for by the patients, except those drugs, medicines, laboratory procedures, etc., which cannot be provided by the agency. If the patient, however, wishes to avail himself of paid services (both in government and private hospitals) he can either use his Medicare privileges or, if he is not so entitled, he may pay for the services out of his own funds.

The national government follows an annual cycle of estimating and budgeting. Following this cycle, the Metro Manila Commission prepares two kinds of budget. One is the operational budget of each town and city. For this purpose, each of the towns and cities of Metro Manila prepares its own budget, and this is acted upon by the respective local chief executive. Part of the budget is for the delivery of health care and sanitation services, while the remainder is for the integrated projects of the commission. The health and sanitation services' portion of this integrated budget is prepared by the action officer concerned.

The other national agencies operating in Metro Manila prepare and submit their budgets to their corresponding national offices. Among those agencies which prepare their own estimates and submit them to their national offices without having to pass through the Commission are the Philippine General Hospital, the hospitals run by the Department of Health, and the Armed Forces. These are collated by the Budget Commission in co-ordination with the National Economic Development Authority.

It is basically through these fund allocation schemes that the national government and the commission are able to check, control and direct health and sanitation services according to national perspectives.

Payment of Doctors and Other Health Workers

Doctors and other health workers employed by the Commission, and by the DoH and other government entities, whether on a full-time or part-time basis, are paid salaries either according to the official government WAPCO (Wage Administration and Position Classification Office) rates or according to other duly approved salary schemes. Examples of other salary rates outside of the WAPCO are those paid by individual towns and cities and those in the University of the Philippines System. These agencies and towns pay their doctors according to schemes (due primarily to their budget constraints) approved by the national government.

At present, a study team has been created to recommend ways and means of standardising salary scales of health workers (doctors included) in Metropolitan Manila. This is being done primarily because of evident disparities in salaries of health workers among towns and between cities and towns.

Private Medical Practice

Doctors and other health professionals employed by the government may have their own private practices. The services they render are paid on a fee-for-service basis. The consumers may take advantage of their Medicare and private insurance privileges, or they may pay for the services out of their private funds.

Planning and Information

The entire governmental machinery follows the planning, programming and budgeting system in any given year. In the health services sector, a year is divided into three phases starting with the planning phase and ending in the budgeting phase. In all phases the flow of information starts from the smallest significant unit, namely the town or city; it then passes to the regional level, to the DoH and then to the National Economic Development Authority. The planning phase is basically concerned with setting objectives, goals and strategies, which upon being approved by the DoH and NEDA, are relayed back to the smallest operating unit. The plans and programmes translated into hard cash are then finally approved by specific authorities delegated with such powers. Through the control system infused into the approval of these budgets, a close supervision and control of operations is wielded by the DoH, the national government and the Commission.

The Commission also organises a central information system that generates and maintains relevant statistical and other information regarding its services. Moreover, the Action Officer for Health and Sanitation Services has a separate information system more specifically for managing the health and sanitation services of the metropolis. On a national scale, the DoH and NEDA have their own information systems. Furthermore, universities, especially the University of the Philippines System and other medical schools, generate and maintain their separate information services. These systems and data banks, however, still need to be improved to facilitate the efficient generation, collation, analysis and transmittal of information for planning, general management and other purposes.

The National Economic Development Authority (NEDA) is the highest planning and policy-making body of the Philippine government. The NEDA, together with the DoH, and in consultation with other agencies involved, have evolved a four-year National Health Plan which serves as the basis for all other plans/standards in the delivery of health and sanitation services.

B. THE MAIN PROBLEMS OF THE HEALTH SERVICES

1. Planning

(a)   The present systems for generating concise, up-to-date, relevant information on health and sanitation are inadequate. Although at present there are, as mentioned earlier, several information systems currently in use, these systems have still not proven adequate to satisfy requirements. The central management information team of the Metro Manila Commission, recently installed, has met plenty of hardships in generating the information necessary for planning purposes.

(b)   Health and sanitation services, as one of the basic government services, have not been given financial priority. It is worth noting that in the national budget, only 3.4 per cent was allocated to health and sanitation services in the fiscal year 1973-4.

The expenditure on health has grown at a moderate pace during the last decade from P112 million in 1963 to P477 million in 1974. This growth, however, is due to general increase in total government expenditure and not to the allocation of a larger share of such expenditure to health. Thus, the share of health expenditures in the total government outlay has declined from 6 per cent in 1970 to 3.4 per cent in 1975.

2. Provision of Health Services

(a)   There are at present only 181 health centres and 28 government hospitals in Metropolitan Manila. These facilities yield an average ratio of 1 : 28,038 health centres to population and 1 : 329 government hospital beds to population. (The relatively low ratio of government hospital beds to population is somewhat misleading because 7,000 beds belong to the National Mental Hospital. The effective average government hospital beds to population ratio therefore is only 1 : 603.) The health centre ratio is far below the Philippine standard of 1 centre to 10,000 people.

Private hospital beds, though numerous, are not easily accessible to the general population because of the high cost of hospitalisation, despite the Medicare privileges of the population.

(b)   The continuing drain of skilled manpower (doctors and nurses especially) is another problem of providing effective health care to the general population in Metropolitan Manila.

(c)   The continuing inflation in the Philippine economy aggravates the difficulty of providing effective services in as much as prices of drugs, medicines and other supplies continually increase.

(d)   The underdevelopment of the inter-agency referral system (following the concept of primary, secondary and tertiary layers of health care delivery) contributes to the congestion of hospitals in Metro Manila since the majority of the population would rather go to a hospital than frequent their health centres. (The Philippine

General Hospital alone served an average of 1,200 to 1,400 out-patients daily in 1975.)

(e)   The lack of professional managers in the over-all system of health care delivery has taxed the professional medical personnel in as much as they have had to manage the systems themselves, instead of concentrating on the delivery of professional health services.

(f)   Public education in health and sanitation is another main problem. The ignorance of the general population regarding basic hygiene has aggravated the congestion in hospitals.

C. SOME GOOD IDEAS IN PLANNING AND PROVISION OF HEALTH CARE

(a)   The formulation of the three layers of health care delivery in the Metro Manila area, and the gradual development of an effective inter-agency referral system, are important innovations in the planning of health care in the Metro Manila area and indeed for the entire country. This idea envisages the integration of all existing health care centres into a comprehensive network of graduated levels of delivery of health care; the simplest (represented by the rural health centres) graduating into the more sophisticated regional and emergency hospitals, with the most sophisticated being the tertiary referral medical centres. In 1976 only 900 out-patients were seen daily in the Philippine General Hospital.

(b)   Encouragement of community participation in the barangays through the creation of health councils and committees is also an important step in effectively educating and delivering health services to the general population.

(c)   The integration of all programmes in health and sanitation services (such as nutrition, family planning and environmental sanitation) in the basic infrastructure (health centre) should also prove to be an important step in bringing comprehensive health and sanitation services to the people.

(d)   One hundred and twenty family planning clinics and pueri-culture centres were integrated with the 181 health centres.

(e)   The consolidation of all health and sanitation programmes and services in the Metro Manila Area, under a central authority (action officer) remains as the single most important change and experiment in delivering health and sanitation services to the general population of the Metro Manila Area. If this experiment proves successful, then the health and sanitation condition in the Metro Manila Area will certainly be improved.

(f)   Reallocation of specialised hospital services to general secondary health care.

(g)   Centralisation of authority over health facilities and hospitals in Metro Manila under the Commission (to include other government hospitals such as Departments of National Defence, Health, Justice, Social Welfare, etc.).

11 TOKYO

Kenzo Kiikuni

A. THE PATTERN OF EXISTING SERVICES

Tokyo Metropolis, consisting of 23 wards and satellite regions, covers a total area of 2,143 square kilometres (about 827 square miles). The satellite regions are the Tama Area and the Islands Area which are made up of various cities and townships. The 23 wards, or 'Special Wards' as they are officially known in English, correspond to the area of the pre-war city of Tokyo. It has a radius of 15 kilometres (9.3 miles) and covers 580 square kilometres (224 square miles). The population of the wards today is about 9 million. The 23 wards are roughly equivalent to the city of New York. Each ward is somewhat like a New York borough but is perhaps closer to a London borough.

The Tama Area can be compared to a county of New York. It covers 1,161 square kilometres (about 450 square miles) and has a population of 3 million. It is made up of 26 cities, five towns and one village. The Islands Area is located in the Pacific Ocean some 100 to 1,000 kilometres to the south and includes the Ogasawara Islands. It covers a total of 403 square kilometres (about 155 square miles). Its population is 34,000. When speaking of Tokyo in a narrow sense, however, the Islands Area is not included.

Demographic and Other Data

Tokyo had a population of 11,669,167, according to a census in October 1975. Censuses are taken every five years and have shown that Tokyo's population increased by only 2.3 per cent in the years between 1970 and 1975; this represented a sharp fall compared with the 5 per cent, 12 per cent and 20 per cent increases in the previous censuses. This fall is due to the fact that a considerable number of people in Tokyo have been moving to the neighbouring prefectures such as Saitama, Chiba and Kanagawa because of housing problems. Another tendency over the past five years has been the decrease in the number of people living in central Tokyo, although 8,642,000 (74.1 per cent) do still live there. This may be called decentralisation of the population, but has not led to such a grave problem as in some other big cities.

The distribution of population between various age groups is given

252

Table 11.1: Population of Tokyo (Special Wards) by Age, 1975

Age	Numbers
0–14	555,000
15–64	8,120,000
65 and over	740,000
Total	9,415,000

Table 11.2: Health Indices in Tokyo, 1975

		Tokyo (A)	Japan (B)	A/B (per cent)
Average life expectancy		(years)		
Male		71.30	69.84	102.1
Female		75.96	75.23	101.0
		(per 1,000)		
Death rates		4.7	6.3	74.6
		(per 100,000)		
Apoplexy		113.1	156.7	72.2
Cancer		105.7	122.5	86.3
Heart disease		66.4	89.1	74.5
Suicide		15.7	17.9	87.7
		(per 1,000)		
Infant death rates		8.9	10.0	89.0
Neonatal death rates		14.6	16.1	90.7
Physical measurement		(14 years, male)		
Height	(cm)	162.7	161.9	100.4
Weight	(kg)	51.8	50.7	102.2
Chest	(cm)	79.3	79.1	100.3
Sitting height	(cm)	86.6	86.3	100.3

in Table 11.1. While a relative population reduction of the age group from 0 to 14 years and slight reduction of immediate work group are observed, the older age group tends to increase year by year, its rate of increase being 4.42 per cent. This latter group comprised 5.96 per cent of the whole population in 1974, 6.22 per cent in 1975, and 6.49 per cent in 1976.

Health Status

In 1975, the average life expectancy at birth for males throughout Japan was 69.84 years and for females 75.23 years, one of the highest levels in the world, the result of general advances in medicine and improvements in social and economic conditions. In the same year, the average life expectancy for males in Tokyo was 71.30 years (the highest level in Japan) and 75.96 for females (the third-highest level in Japan). Tokyo has the lowest death rate of Japanese cities, a rate of 4.7 per 1,000 population, while the national average is 6.3. Its infant mortality rate is also the lowest, being 8.9 per 1,000 live births, the Japanese average being 10.0. The principal causes of death are cerebrovascular disease, cancer, heart disease, pneumonia and bronchitis, a pattern consistent with the national statistics; suicide is the fifth most significant cause. However, the Tokyo rate for cerebrovascular disease is below the national average, while the rates for breast cancer and ischaemic heart disease are above the national average. For these and other personal health statistics, see Table 11.2.

Organisation of Health Care

Health care administration in Japan may be broadly divided into the three areas of general public health, school health and industrial health. In the area of general public health administration, the service is rendered by a nation-wide organisation consisting of central government (Ministry of Health and Welfare, Koseisho), prefectural government (public health departments), health centres and municipalities (public health sections). Health centres are established in all prefectural governments and larger cities designated by the Cabinet Order, and are bases of the nation's public health programmes.

Functions of the Ministry of Health and Welfare were defined by law in 1949. The Ministry is composed of the Minister's Secretariat, nine bureaus and agencies which include the Social Security Agency and several institutes including the Institute of Public Health, National Institute of Hospital Administration and National Institute of Population Studies and their local subdivisions. Of these nine Ministerial bureaus, the Bureaus of Public Health, Environmental Health, Medical Affairs and Pharmaceutical Affairs play a central role in the nation's health care administration. To cope with environmental pollution an Environment Agency was established in July 1971. Organisation of the 47 prefectural governments is established by the Local Autonomy Law, under which a department charged with health care administration was established in each prefectural government with elected governors.

The health services in Tokyo Metropolitan Government are conducted by the Bureau of Public Health. It consists of eight divisions: General Affairs, Public Health, Environmental Health, Medical Affairs,

Health and Welfare, Pharmaceutical Affairs, Hospital Administration
and Hospital Building. The major activities of the General Affairs
Division are policy planning, administration of health centres,
statistics and surveys; the last being carried out through 66 health
centres in Tokyo. Within the Public Health Division there are sections
for geriatric disorders, epidemics of communicable diseases, tuberculosis,
maternal and child health and nutrition. In the Environmental
Health Division are units for waterworks, food health, dairy products
and meat health, and food supervision. In the Medical Affairs Division
there are sections which are responsible for medical licensing, mental
health and nursing services; in the Health and Welfare Division are
sections for special diseases. The Hospital Administration Division and
Hospital Installations Division are mainly engaged in the management
of seventeen hospitals which are run by the Tokyo Metropolitan
Government.

Planning
Following the Second World War, a strategy for the provision of equal
opportunities for all citizens to obtain decent medical care was
initiated. To this end, two major problems needed to be solved. One
was the question of financing medical care and the other was the
planning of adequate facilities. The former was rapidly attained by an
arrangement of nation-wide health insurance or by providing medical
care under public financial assistance. However, resolution to the
latter problem was slow in coming.

In 1948, a New Medical Service Law was passed, by which a Medical
Care Council was established for the purpose of discussing various
approaches to the planning of medical care facilities. The Council
released a draft programme for the planning of national medical care
facilities, on the basis of which the Ministry of Health and Welfare in
1959 proposed a long-term medical plan. It was in fact a copy-version
of hospital planning based on WHO's ideas on regionalisation of
hospitals. However, the proposal was not accepted because it was
considered inappropriate to the particular situation in Japan. It failed
to realise the fact that there are some 24 different ownerships of
hospitals in Japan; and each hospital is operating in a competitive
situation. Thus the proposal suggesting the creation of regional, intermediate and local hospitals, assuming that patients, doctors, medical
equipment and supplies would flow freely between them, was
completely unrealistic. Given the rivalry among the hospitals, it is
obvious that such a relationship could not exist.

Meanwhile, many rural areas remained in a situation where their people could not enjoy the benefits of modern medical care at a time when excessive medical facilities were concentrated in urban areas. Nearly 70 per cent of the nation's hospitals are privately owned, and even those public hospitals established by local governments, the Japan Red Cross and social insurance-related organisations, are concentrated in urban centres, contributing to the intensity of the already keen competition existing among these hospitals. In order to encourage a more satisfactory distribution of public hospitals, the Medical Service Law was amended in 1962 to restrict the construction of new public hospitals or the increase of beds in an existing hospital in areas where bed population ratios had reached a certain level.

Despite the advancement of medical science and technology, the medical care system was left in a fragmented form without the guidance of a clear plan, until it finally reached a stage of 'medical crisis'. The chief reasons for this crisis were the growing popular demand for medical care, coupled with rising costs and a shortage of physicians and nurses. The government came up with various measures to deal with the situation, one of which was the promotion of a community health planning programme.

This, however, is not to suggest that there were no voluntary efforts on the part of medical professionals. In fact, local medical associations themselves undertook to establish medical association hospitals where practitioners could care for their own patients. They were also actively involved in various public health activities, developing a system linking the primary and secondary levels of health care. They also established clinical laboratory centres to promote the community health activities of practitioners.

Community Health Planning Programme

Total health care delivery to the Japanese people has so far been unsystematic. It is the basic philosophy of the community health planning programme to remedy this situation. The term 'community', as used in this context, means the range of people's day-to-day activities; this does not necessarily coincide with the administrative divisions such as villages, towns or prefectures. The programme aims to provide systematised health care at the primary and secondary levels within a community. Fortunately, some administrative areas made up of several cities, towns and villages already exist and these can usefully be taken into consideration when implementing the community programme.

In many areas, an emergency medical service system designed to meet the special needs of a given area is already in operation, and in 1975, the Ministry of Health and Welfare launched a Community Health Planning Programme Study Group to formulate, as soon as possible, general guidelines for the decentralisation of health administration.

Hospital Planning

The idea of hospital regionalisation, with integration into local administration, is certainly acceptable in theory. In practice, however, the provision of a system of co-ordinated hospital care facilities is far from being realised. Hospital planning is, of course, a part of the community health planning programme and cannot be discussed separately. Considering the idiosyncratic medical needs of different communities, there can be no such thing as a universal programme. In this sense, the hospital planning of Japan is still in an experimental stage. However, the following points can be mentioned at this stage.

In Japan, the term 'hospital' is used for a medical institution equipped with 20 beds or more, so that in hospital planning it was only these facilities that were considered. However, it must be noted that there are many clinics with 19 beds or less, and the total number of beds in this type of institution in Japan is more than 260,000. In addition, there are other facilities related to the social welfare service such as special nursing homes that maintain in-patient facilities. When considering hospital planning, therefore, the availability of these beds should also be taken into account.

The next question relates to the necessity of clearly grasping the medical functions that each hospital performs. At present, hospitals can be classified according to the types of ownership, number of beds and the types of departments they have, but this gives no indication of their medical function. For instance, there is no way for a patient to know whether a given hospital with a surgery department or urinary department is capable of conducting a special operation. In such a situation, the community health planning programme which is intended to cover the primary- and secondary-level medical service cannot function effectively. Therefore, for hospital planning, it is essential to grasp the medical functions of each hospital. It would perhaps also be worth while to introduce into this situation some of the data-processing techniques which have been brought into the medical service at large in recent years.

Financing

In the fiscal year of 1974, the Japanese people spent a sum of 5,378.6 billion yen which represented 3.95 per cent of GNP, or an average expenditure of 48,375 yen per person. This covers the costs for the care and treatment of diseases and injuries but does not include the cost of normal pregnancy, childbirth, maternity care, health examination, vaccination, corrective eye-glasses, artificial limbs and the like. Nor does it include the additional cost of a private room at the time of hospitalisation, which is not a part of the health insurance benefits, nor the cost of private duty attendants or differences in dental charges. Furthermore, the costs of over-the-counter medicines and treatment for traffic accident cases were estimated somewhat modestly.

Payment of health expenses can be divided into categories as shown in Table 11.3.

Table 11.3: Payment of Health Expenses (billion yen)

		Yen	%
(1)	Government	727.6	13.5
(2)	Employee health insurance	2,508.1	46.7
(3)	National health insurance	1,307.7	24.3
(4)	Other medical insurance	114.3	2.1
(5)	Patients themselves	720.9	13.4
Total		5,378.6	100.0

Japan was the first Asian country to introduce health insurance and now almost all of the population is covered in some form or other. This reflects the constitutional idea that: '. . . all people shall have the right to maintain the minimum standards of wholesome and cultured living. In all spheres of life, the state shall use its endeavours for the promotion and extension of social welfare and security and of public health.' There are two basic programmes of health insurance in Japan. One is employee health insurance which covers 67 million employees and their dependants. The other is 'national health insurance', covering 44 million self-employed people, such as farmers and fishermen, and their dependants.

When the insured person wants to receive medical care, he is free to go to any hospital or clinic upon presentation of a membership card. Nearly all medical care facilities are under a health insurance programme. In the case of injuries or illness while at work, they are covered by the workmen's compensation insurance and premiums must be borne for the full amount by the employer.

Method of Payment

At the end of each month, each participating hospital or clinic prepares a bill for the services rendered, based on a flat fee schedule determined by the Minister of Health and Welfare. The Minister requests the recommendation of the Central Social Insurance Medical Council which consists of eight representatives of insurers, eight of providers (physicians, dentists and pharmacists), and four from the public sector. The fee scale is called the 'point system': and each act of medical care is given a point and the fee is computed by multiplying the point score by the unit costs (at present unit cost is 10 yen). It is determined by consideration of the degree of technical difficulty as well as the economy involved. In paying for drugs used, consideration is given to the standard purchase cost which covers 90 per cent of the price of drugs actually paid by hospitals and clinics, and is usually 20-50 per cent higher than the actual cost.

The 'points' are intended to be revised on the basis of the actual cost survey of participating hospitals and clinics. Lately, however, it has proved difficult to conduct regular financial surveys and, as a result, the previous data were updated in accordance with age and price increases and revision is usually subject to political control. For instance, fees for nursing and hospital food services are revised on the basis of straight cost increase, while technical fees such as those for examination and operation are adjusted through political consideration. The bill then is submitted to the Social Insurance Medical Care Fee Payment Fund which pools the money from each programme and is checked by a medical consultant before payment of the bills. Unnecessary treatment is sometimes deleted; this often causes complaints by participating hospitals and clinics.

The 1976 budget for Tokyo Metropolitan Government for health administration was 41,234 million yen which was subdivided as shown in Table 11.4.

In the financing of 17 metropolitan hospitals, the government spent 21,457 million yen for hospital operation and 4,841 million yen for capital expenses.

Table 11.4: Tokyo Metropolitan Government Health Expenditure

	(million yen)
Public health	10,853
Environmental health	2,540
Medical administration	10,697
Medical welfare work	990
Pharmaceutical administration	776
Child health	3,988
Research	4,395
Capital expenses	2,639

Health Facilities

An Overview of Medical Facilities

Of the 739 hospitals in Tokyo at the end of 1975, mental hospitals accounted for 57, TB hospitals 8, leprosy 1, and infectious diseases 4, the remaining 669 being general hospitals (see Table 11.5). Five hundred and forty-seven hospitals are located in the Tokyo metropolis and 191 are in the suburbs (all except one in the Tama area). There is a tendency towards an increase in the suburbs at the expense of the centre. Thus, between 1970 and 1975, the number of hospitals in the metropolitan area decreased from 559 to 547, while that in the suburbs increased from 183 to 191: changes which reflect the movement of the population.

The total number of hospital beds in Tokyo in 1975 was 116,924. The distribution of this figure among various facilities is shown in Table 11.6, which also records the changing profile over the last twenty-five years. In comparing the 1975 figures with those of 1965, a general increase of 25.7 per cent is seen. There are increases of 50.2 per cent in the number of beds for patients with mental diseases and of 50.6 per cent in beds for general patients, while there are decreases of 47.3 per cent in the number of beds for tuberculosis sufferers and of 31 per cent for patients with communicable diseases. The Tokyo hospital bed/population ratio (see Table 11.7) is slightly lower than the average national figure. Tokyo has also a total of 10,659 clinics, with 18,171 beds. The occupancy rate of hospital beds is 71.3, compared to the national average of 75.9. Groupings of hospitals by size are indicated in Table 11.8.

Table 11.5: Health Care Facilities in Tokyo

	Number of hospitals						Clinics	Dental clinics
	Total	Mental	TB	Leprosy	Infectious diseases	General		
1950	276	12	37	1	10	216	5,191	3,246
1955	464	15	63	1	8	377	7,070	3,983
1960	608	25	54	1	8	520	9,120	4,846
1965	681	39	27	1	5	609	10,010	5,323
1970	743	53	12	1	4	673	10,507	5,697
1971	744	54	10	1	4	675	10,535	5,740
1972	747	57	10	1	4	675	10,697	5,811
1973	744	58	10	1	4	671	10,852	5,965
1974	744	58	8	1	4	673	11,004	6,127
1975	739	57	8	1	4	669	10,659	6,132

Table 11.6: Health Care Facility Beds in Tokyo

	Total	In hospitals					In clinics	In dental clinics
		Mental	TB	Leprosy	Infectious diseases	General		
1950	31,770	3,541	12,582	1,200	1,000	13,447	4,816	9
1955	56,824	5,610	26,247	1,570	2,111	21,286	9,270	21
1960	77,215	10,567	27,101	1,570	2,180	35,797	15,576	3
1965	92,983	15,886	21,110	1,470	2,031	52,486	18,223	43
1970	109,719	22,330	15,970	1,470	1,246	68,703	19,316	20
1971	112,410	22,949	15,008	1,470	1,224	71,759	19,247	28
1972	113,234	22,797	13,475	1,470	1,160	74,332	18,952	2
1973	114,817	22,102	14,135	1,470	1,160	75,950	–	–
1974	115,460	23,471	11,837	1,470	1,167	77,515	–	–
1975	116,924	23,865	11,127	1,470	1,402	79,060	18,171	2

Table 11.7: Beds per 10,000 Persons in Tokyo, 1975

Bed type	Number
Mental	20.4
TB	9.5
Leprosy	1.2
Infectious diseases	1.2
General	67.8
Total	100.1

Table 11.8: Hospitals by Size in Tokyo, 1975

Size (Number of beds)	Number of hospitals	Per cent of total
20—49	231	31.2
50—99	191	25.8
100—199	132	17.9
200—299	78	10.6
300—399	48	6.5
400—499	16	2.2
500 +	43	5.8
Total	739	100.0

B. PROBLEMS, SOLUTIONS AND SUGGESTIONS FOR CHANGE

Although superficially similar to those in some large Western cities, health problems in Tokyo are to some extent unique because of social circumstances. The basic problems peculiar to Tokyo may be summarised as follows.

(1)   Within recent history, the tempo of social change has been extremely high. This was shown in the modernisation process of the Meiji era, and even more acutely after the Second World War — particularly during the 1960s. The process of urbanisation, which in Western cities occupied about one hundred years, took place in Tokyo within a period of only fifty years.

(2)   Under these social circumstances, long-standing problems exist side by side with new ones. This has caused heavy pressure on financial and administrative resources as well as posing socio-political

problems.

Important problems in relation to the health service can be enumerated as follows.

(3)   The major concentration of effort of the health services of this country has been directed toward the spreading of Western medical science. This emphasis has led to priority being given to the Western practice of medicine in health services, to the detriment of consideration of the patient's broad needs which other health personnel could effectively meet. This approach has had an adverse effect on the organisational strength of health services.

(4)   The wide variety of ownership of Japanese hospitals (see Table 11.9), with a majority of private hospitals, is characteristic of the Japanese hospital scene. Most of the privately-owned institutions are medium- or small-sized accounting for 49,027 beds out of Tokyo's total of 116,924.

Table 11.9: Hospitals by Ownership in Tokyo, 1975

	Mental	TB	General	Total
National	—	—	29	30
Local government	3	—	18	22
Municipal	—	—	8	11
Other public	3	2	44	49
Social insurance	—	—	22	22
Private	51	6	548	605
Total	57	8	669	739

(5)   Due to the national efforts of the government after the war to build up the welfare state, medical care has become available to almost all of the people. The social security system has been financed by contributions from social insurance schemes and this has led to the result that the funding of medical care, particularly since the total coverage of health insurance was achieved in 1961, has been controlled by the financial positions of the social insurance schemes rather than by the actual cost of operating hospitals or clinics. A characteristic of Japanese medical care is the fact that a large part of its funds is used for out-patient care, rather than for the specialised

services of hospitals and specialists.

(6)   A high priority for the Japanese health care system is the need to strengthen the functions of hospitals according to the needs of the community, and this calls for a substantial increase in the number of professional personnel.

(7)   There is no established system for continuing the education and training of physicians, nurses and other health workers. Few hospitals are prepared to take an active part in training such personnel. There is an urgent need to provide adequate systems of graduate and further training and to improve the facilities of hospitals for training them.

(8)   The Ministry of Health and Welfare, the Tokyo Metropolitan Government and private organisations are actively involved in the promotion of health planning programmes — and with some success. However, these are still at an infant stage and constitute far from an effective system; this poses the greatest challenge to all concerned.

Other new problems which must be solved during the development of the health services in the coming years are as follows.

(9)   Social adaptation to developments in information science. The intelligent use of information science is an indispensable component in the improvement of the health service. At present, however, social conditioning for this purpose is lacking. Instruction in information science should figure in all education schemes for medical and other health personnel.

(10)   Control of environmental pollution. Environmental pollution has been an extremely serious problem in Japan since the 1960s; and various national counter-measures have been developed. The Fundamental Law for Environmental Pollution Control was enacted in 1967, and the Environment Agency was created in 1971. Related legislation has been enacted and various administrative and voluntary efforts concentrated in an intensive nation-wide campaign. However, prediction of environmental pollution in the coming years is extremely difficult, and, in view of constantly developing technology, optimistic forecasts are not warranted.

There are still many unsolved problems concerning the impact of pollutants on health. For this reason, the Metropolitan Government is carrying out continuous medical examinations, investigations and researches, while trying to preserve the people's health by promoting environmental protection measures. Through health centres, the

Metropolitan Government is, at suitable intervals, monitoring the profile of respiratory diseases of the general public, examining the effect of lead on the health of residents living near major traffic intersections, and assessing local environmental pollution. Researches and surveys conducted by the Metropolitan Government include the following: a survey of photochemical smog, studies on the accumulation of various heavy metals in the human body, and the toxicity of non-ionic detergents, an atmospheric survey intended to grasp the present state of local air pollution, and a survey of PCB. A scheme has already been adopted by the government whereby the cost of medical treatment to persons under 18 who contract diseases attributable to atmospheric pollution (chronic bronchitis, bronchial asthma, asthmatic bronchitis, pulmonary emphysema and secondary diseases of the above) is subsidised.

(11)   Adaptation to an ageing society. It has been of great advantage to the country in the 1960s and 1970s that the productive age groups form a major part of society, with only a small number of aged in the population. However, it seems certain that, because of the sharply lowered death and birth rates, the tempo of ageing of the population will accelerate in the coming decades. Some other countries have already reached this stage, and now face the difficulties. In Tokyo it is necessary to prepare for adaptation and to learn from the experiences of other countries.

The following indicate some of Tokyo's experiences in tackling these difficult problems.

A Basic Survey of Old People's Welfare, conducted by the Tokyo Metropolitan Government in July 1971, disclosed that 39.4 per cent of those surveyed became aware of their old age around the age of 70, and 23 per cent felt old at the age of 65 or so. In reality, the working energies of many persons persist until about 65. Welfare service for the aged is therefore provided for persons of 65 years or more. In Tokyo, there were 620,089 such persons on 1 January 1972 and 740,000 in 1975 (see Table 11.1).

Decline of Patriarchy

For centuries, old people in Japan have been supported by their families under a patriarchal system. With the decline of that system after the Second World War, families have become less considerate of the older generations.

Nevertheless, about 80 per cent of the old people in Japan still live with the families of their children. In Tokyo the percentage is lower,

77.4, as reported in the above-mentioned survey. Of those living with their families, 48.9 per cent appeared anxious about their future health and survival. Provision must therefore be made to meet their needs for stable livelihood, residential security, treatment of diseases and rehabilitation.

From Home Accommodation to Residential Welfare

Many old people desire to remain with their families, being deeply attached to the communities they have always lived in, even if their families do not provide good care for them. In the past, major welfare services for the aged tended to provide homes for the elderly which were unlike those to which they were used. From now on, however, the service must be extended to the old people within the communities themselves so that they may receive essential services at their homes and lead fruitful lives as accepted members of society.

Helping Bedridden Old People

Old people presenting the most serious problems are those long confined to bed. Their number, 60 years old and over, in Tokyo, is estimated at 27,000. It is believed that about half would be able to leave their beds if they could receive rehabilitation training. The Tokyo Metropolitan Old People's Hospital, opened on 1 April 1972, provides general medical services as well as rehabilitation services. The Tokyo Metropolitan Government's medium-term plan aims to construct many nursing homes equipped to offer rehabilitation training as well as proper medical treatment and care.

Physical Check-ups

According to the July 1971 survey on the welfare of the aged in Tokyo, 75.3 per cent indicated that their health conditions were either very good or normal, 19.7 per cent reported that their conditions were poor, and 4.3 per cent were bedridden. Nevertheless, for many, mental and physical problems are arising, yet they are unconscious of them. So it is necessary for the wards, cities, towns and villages of Tokyo to investigate annually the conditions of all its senior citizens in order to discover their problems promptly and offer timely treatment.

Physical check-ups were given to 28.7 per cent of Tokyo's old people in 1971. At that time, 19.2 per cent were found to be in normal health, 6.4 per cent were advised to return for a further examination, and 74.4 per cent required medical treatment. The variety of medical problems found was quite considerable, ranging from total tuberculosis and malignant neoplasms to diabetes and vascular lesions affecting the central nervous system. All those aged 65 years and older who were bedridden were offered physical check-ups in their own homes.

Aid for Treatment Costs

Little value can be obtained from offering medical check-ups if those who are diagnosed as requiring treatment are lacking funds to undergo that treatment. Thus, besides offering free physical check-ups, the Tokyo Metropolitan Government (TMG) offers to pay at least part of the expenses for needed medication. In the case of the aged of limited income, the TMG pays the individual's share of medical expenses under the insurance systems. Thus, by showing both the health insurance certificate and the TMG medical certificate, the patient need pay no hospital bills, with the TMG bearing his portion of the burden. In 1971, a total of 159,881 old persons took advantage of such assistance, requiring 1,193,005 separate treatments. The TMG paid 3,612,989,000 yen for the cost of these.

Aid was offered automatically to all persons of 70 years and more. As for those between 65 and 69 years, if the physical condition of their normal functions was impaired, they too received such assistance. A fairly rigid family income restriction was in effect in 1971. However, this was dropped in July 1972, making eligible all those whose annual incomes were below the level where income tax and inhabitants tax are imposed, without regard to the income level of the other members of their families.

The Old People's Hospital

When aged persons begin to fail in their physical well-being, their mental health invariably suffers as well. As a result, treatment is required from all types of medical specialist. Unfortunately, there are very few hospitals where both medical care and rehabilitation therapy and training are available under the existing health insurance system. For that reason, the TMG opened an Old People's Hospital in June 1972. It has 753 beds, including 119 for those undergoing rehabilitation training. A research unit, the Institute of Gerontology, is now attached to the hospital.

The Problems of the Bedridden Aged at their Homes

Without question, the most unfortunate of all old people are those permanently confined to bed in their homes. Their number is currently estimated at 40,100. This is 4.3 per cent of all the people in Tokyo over 60 years of age who are confined to their homes, and of them 26,600 are confined to bed for periods longer than six months. Still, the number is significant, and 1.2 per cent of them are utterly without someone to care for them at home. Another 82.2 per cent are cared for by spouses or children, and the rest by other relatives.

These people require a great deal of care, both in terms of treatment and rehabilitation training. The TMG is making an effort to assist them. An example of such service has been the construction of nursing homes for the bedridden aged. As for those of limited income who are at home alone and confined to bed, caretakers are sent to their homes twice a week to prepare meals, wash clothes, and offer consultation and sympathetic advice. The TMG subsidises individual wards, cities, towns, and villages for their services in this programme.

PART TWO:
ASPECTS OF CITY SERVICES

12 COMMUNITY INVOLVEMENT IN MENTAL HEALTH

(with special reference to London)

Edith Morgan

London: The Social Problems

London is the ninth biggest city in the world with an area of 610 square miles and a population of 7.2 million. It has many advantages — good sanitation, pure water supply, moderately clean air, and health services that are free at time of use. Its extensive range of open spaces, a comprehensive public transport system, and many pleasant residential areas add to its attractions for people with a reasonable income to live on. London's problems, however, resemble those of big cities all over the world: overcrowding, slums and bad housing, traffic congestion, a high road accident rate and great travel frustration. There is in addition the decay in post-war years of the inner city fabric, social disintegration and increased homelessness, and for many people desperate loneliness and mental stress.

Britain has legislated for a comprehensive welfare system, but the provision of social services in London is complicated by several factors. One is that the city has to serve a population far greater than its own. Over 18 million tourists spent one or more nights in London in 1976, and two million workers travel into London every day by train, bus and private car. The composition of London's population also contributes to its social problems. Many young and middle-aged skilled men and their families have moved away, leaving behind a high proportion of unemployed, handicapped and old people who depend heavily on the social services. London is also still a magnet for people with social problems from other parts of Britain. In addition, 15 per cent of its population are immigrants from other countries, and many of these have pressing needs, particularly in connection with housing and employment.

As a result, London has some of the worst social statistics in Britain, and the figures for mental illness indicate much stress and distress. In some London boroughs, mental hospital admission rates are as high as 654 per 100,000 population, 50 per cent higher than the national average. Not surprisingly, the position is worst in inner London where the over-all admission rate is 512 per 100,000, compared with 381 for outer London.

I shall assume that readers have already studied Chapter 1, describing London's health services, so I will not discuss these now. I will only underline that the separation of the health from the social services creates particular problems for mentally ill people, since the social consequences of mental illness can be as devastating as the illness itself.

The provision of mental health services in Britain has always lagged behind that of most of the other health services and London also has special problems of its own. For instance, the four Thames Health Authorities have to cater for large rural populations outside London, with their particular problems, as well as for inner London with its pockets of acute deprivation. In addition, the isolation of London's 22 mental illness hospitals — nearly all built during the last century in what was then the surrounding countryside — tends to cut patients off from their old neighbourhoods, and often from their families too. Staffing these large hospitals away from natural communities is not easy, and a substantial proportion of their nursing staff come from overseas and may have problems of language and of cultural understanding. Linking London's health services with the 32 separate boroughs — that is, the local authorities — which provide its social services presents yet another problem.

It is in the context of this complicated structure that we find a vital strand of community involvement that runs right through every level of social organisation in the country. It starts with the election by communities of their representatives to Parliament and continues in roughly the same way with local government. In the health services, members are appointed from community groups to both the regional and area health authorities, the bodies responsible for planning and managing the services. But one of the strongest impacts on health provision by the community is now made through the Community Health Councils that were set up in 1974 to represent consumers. The chain of community involvement is further extended by numerous voluntary organisations and a sizeable army of individual voluntary helpers.

Nowadays British people, like those of many other countries, have much higher expectations, not only of normal living standards, but of the care and health provision they have a right to when they need it. These expectations cannot be met from state sources alone. Communities have to look to their own resources as well, and a growing number are responding by offering their voluntary services. That is to say, they are prepared to work without payment for a cause that they find worth while, where the requirements are for common sense and the right personal qualities, rather than for professional training. A recent study indicated that five million people in Britain now work as volunteers — mainly in the field of social welfare — and that their contribution is the equivalent of 400,000 full-time staff each year.

As a rule, these volunteers are ordinary working people who are prepared to give up some of their leisure time. But they also include women who are not in paid employment for a few years while bringing up young children, retired people who want to go on being useful and active, and students and schoolchildren who are learning to be good citizens in a practical way.

Not all voluntary help needs to be organised, of course, and many people are spontaneously aided all over the world without anyone being aware of it except the persons involved. But not everyone can rely on getting the help they need when they need it, and some kinds of problems produce behaviour which repels rather than attracts help. Their problems do need an organised response and one way in which it is made in Britain is through the development of an extensive network of voluntary organisations.

These organisations are voluntary in the sense that they are independent of state control and they nearly always depend on unpaid voluntary helpers. They do, however, have a highly professional approach and the larger bodies employ a nucleus of full-time paid staff to co-ordinate and develop their activities. Their aims vary: some merely raise money and distribute it for special purposes; others put their main emphasis on campaigning about specific issues, or on pressing for improvements in the statutory services. Some, like MIND, use a combination of methods, campaigning for improved services and at the same time providing services themselves, both at national level and through their local groups. They often work on a massive scale and cover the whole country. Many thousands of individual volunteers are involved in the work of MIND through its 150 local associations in England and Wales, while MIND has a paid professional staff of 70 people to facilitate its huge work programme.

The statutory health and welfare bodies sometimes use voluntary helpers directly. In 156 mental illness and mental handicap hospitals and 139 other hospitals, voluntary help co-ordinators have been appointed. Government ministers and official bodies give full approval to the volunteer movement and since 1973 we have had a national Volunteer Centre. Both national and local government give financial assistance, as well as other forms of support, to encourage particular voluntary causes. The present Secretary of State for Health spent many years himself working for voluntary organisations, including MIND. As a result, he has exceptional knowledge and understanding of their work. He expressed this in a recent speech when he said: 'Voluntary bodies can take risks, experiment with new methods and try out innovations which may after a time be accepted wisdom . . . they should be the Minister's conscience, constantly reminding him of his responsibilities in the field in which they are operating.' This kind of acceptance is immensely encouraging to people working in the voluntary sector.

In recent years I have seen mutual respect grow steadily, not only between voluntary organisations and statutory bodies, but also between voluntary helpers and professional workers. It has been strengthened, I believe, by a clarification of the role of volunteers. It is not their job to provide the basic services where these exist. What voluntary helpers rightly do is to bring an extra element of understanding and compassion that can extend the skilled help of professional workers, and improve the quality of life for people in need.

I want now to illustrate the general points I have been making about community effort in London by focusing on the part I know best, the borough of Camden.

The Situation in Camden

Camden, one of the fourteen boroughs of inner London, is an area of strong contrasts, of much wealth and deep squalor, of depressing problems and imaginative solutions. The borough has some of London's most densely built-up areas, with decaying nineteenth-century housing partially replaced by tower blocks, and some of the city's most pleasant residential areas in Hampstead and Highgate. Within its boundaries there are three main railway termini, three important teaching hospitals, the main parts of London University, 200 hotels, the Post Office Tower, the headquarters of the Trades Union Congress, the new head-quarters of the King's Fund Centre and the International Hospital Federation, the house where Freud found refuge for some happy months at the end of his life — and Karl Marx's grave.

Most of London's social trends and problems are to be found in Camden where the population, now 193,000, has declined by half during this century, and currently has a turnover of 10 per cent a year. Camden contains large numbers of immigrant settlers from every part of the world. There is an inward drift of young people — sometimes as

students, sometimes bringing their problems to the city — a daily
flood of commuters, an ever-growing use of private cars, a high
illegitimacy rate, and very poor housing conditions in certain parts
of the borough.

In terms of health provision, Camden forms part of an area health
authority in the north-east Thames region and shares the complicated
health services structure I referred to earlier. People suffering from
mental illness have access to services provided through the National
Health Service in the same way as for any other illness. Most of them
are treated by their own general practitioners and do not need any
kind of hospital care. Others attend out-patient clinics in hospital
psychiatric departments.

For those who do have to be admitted as in-patients to hospital for
treatment there are a limited number of places in the big general teaching hospitals. The majority, however, go to Friern Hospital. This is a
large psychiatric hospital coming under the same administration as the
other health services. It was built over 100 years ago and is situated
outside the borough. The number of patients living there has been
halved in the last 15 years but it still has 1,200 beds. The service that
can be provided in these conditions is far from ideal.

I shall spend the rest of this chapter on the voluntary services in
Camden, but in the context that the health and social services
authorities are the main providers of services. The work I am describing
is complementary to these.

Camden is fortunate in having one of the liveliest Councils for
Voluntary Service in the country, supporting over a hundred local
voluntary welfare agencies. The CVS also has a volunteer bureau,
which is a kind of employment agency, matching voluntary jobs to
voluntary helpers, and this has stimulated voluntary involvement
greatly. Some of the voluntary helpers fill gaps in services that will
eventually be provided by the appropriate authorities, but they
mostly add the extra dimension of ordinary human feeling that I
mentioned earlier. Their work is very varied. Here are a few of the
things they do:

help in children's homes and adventure playgrounds;
visit old people's homes and help in day hospitals;
shop for the housebound;
take old, ill and frail people to hospitals, to clubs and on outings;
work with families in critical situations and provide a valuable
    link between school and home;

visit people in prison, help their families and assist them when they
   leave prison;
teach English to immigrants;
decorate the homes of elderly and handicapped people.

Camden's hospitals welcome voluntary help. University College
Hospital has about 300 volunteers, who help in the small psychiatric
in-patient unit, as well as on the medical and surgical wards. Friern
psychiatric hospital also has about 300 volunteers, including groups of
schoolchildren and other young people. The voluntary help
organisers at both hospitals say that they do not find recruiting
volunteers difficult. It is maintaining their enthusiasm and winning the
goodwill and confidence of hospital staff that present the real challenges
to them. Both staff and patients benefit from their undoubted success.
   Interest in work for mentally ill people outside hospital is also
firmly rooted in Camden through a number of voluntary organisations.
Apart from the Camden MIND group there is:

the British Red Cross Society which runs clubs for mentally frail
   elderly people;
the London Simon Community which runs two hostels for people
   who have become itinerants as a result of psychiatric problems;
a branch of the National Schizophrenia Fellowship, one of many
   self-help organisations, which brings together the relatives of
   schizophrenic patients for mutual comfort and support;
the Samaritans, who help people who are in despair or suicidal,
   often because of clinical depression;
the Richmond Fellowship which has a house for emotionally
   disturbed young people;
the Peter Bedford Project which, by providing a combination of
   work and accommodation, tries to rehabilitate homeless and
   rootless people, many of them former mental hospital patients.

But the organisation most active in mental health work is the
Camden Association for Mental Health, which is affiliated to MIND.
After ten years of life the volume of its work has reached such propor-
tions that it has to employ a part-time paid officer to co-ordinate its
many activities.
   The mention of a paid officer immediately introduces the matter of
finance. The local authority gives the association a grant to cover the
cost of renting an office, which is essential to good administration.

But it has to raise the rest of its income itself. It tries the usual ways of fund-raising — flag days, local appeals, benefit performances and jumble sales. Its steady source of funds, however, is from a shop which sells partly used clothing.

This shop is one of a chain of nearly 50 highly successful Nearly New Shops that have been set up through MIND's own trading company. They are organised and staffed by volunteers, and contain a very high standard of merchandise. The shops do not rely on gifts but sell clothes on commission, giving half the selling price back to the owner of the clothes and keeping half as a donation to mental health work. This is attractive to people disposing of good clothing that they have grown tired of, and invaluable to the local association.

The value of the shops is not merely financial. The volunteers enjoy the work and, since they include people who are regaining confidence after a mental breakdown, the scheme has a therapeutic aspect. The shop premises, moreover, can sometimes house one of the association's social services, a day centre, a counselling scheme, or, as in Camden, living accommodation.

CAMH also adopts several other community roles:

it helps people in the day centre that was started a few years ago by the association for mentally ill people and was later handed over to the local authority;

it runs a variety of clubs and groups during day time and evenings;

it runs a befriending scheme for people who are lonely and isolated;

it runs a Sunday lunch club for people who would otherwise be alone at weekends;

it has a wide-ranging educational programme — as well as public meetings and study meetings, the association does a lot of work in schools in Camden;

its garden allotment scheme gives occupation, enjoyment and companionship to people who have been ill for years and are just beginning to re-learn the pleasures of growing things and of taking physical exercise.

The final project is one that highlights the association's special skills in working in co-operation with all the statutory bodies — health, social services and housing — as well as with MIND nationally. I am referring to the group homes that it runs for people who were living in mental hospitals, and who seemed likely to stay there though they no longer needed specialised hospital treatment. Disabled by illness and long years of institutional living, it was clear that these people could not survive outside hospital without continuing community support as well as suitable accommodation. To meet this kind of need MIND's local associations have pioneered group homes, which now give homes to hundreds of people who would otherwise have ended their days in mental hospitals.

Camden followed MIND's usual pattern of renting houses from the local housing authority, and then organised them as group homes in co-operation with the staff of both the local mental hospital and the social services department. Professional workers were essential in helping to select and prepare the prospective residents, since they had become very dependent on institutional living and had forgotten how to look after themselves. It is amazing to see how well they can adjust to normal living, after twenty, thirty, or even more years in hospital. The essence of these group homes is that they are small, family-style houses of not more than four or five people with no resident staff. They are not to be confused with hostels or half-way houses from which people are expected to move on eventually. Group home residents can leave if they wish, but what many of them need and want is a permanent home of their own.

Selected members of the local association help the tenants to settle in. The main subsequent contact is usually through a volunteer rent collector who when calling for the rent every week looks out for any problems. Social workers keep in touch where necessary but the right to privacy of the residents – not patients, I must emphasise – is insisted on. These are people's homes, not hospitals or hostels to be visited without invitation.

Group homes are not suitable for every patient in a mental hospital, of course, but the thirteen years' experience of MIND has shown that they do answer the needs of many people, especially the kind of long-stay hospital inmates who may need prolonged medication and support, but not intensive psychiatric treatment.

From the community's standpoint one of the bonuses of these group homes, in addition to the new lease of life they give to their occupants, is their very low cost. After initial expenditure on furniture and equipment the rent and running costs can be paid by the residents themselves – from earnings if they go out to work, or from the state allowances to which they are entitled like everyone else if unemployed or over working age. This is dramatically different from the costs of keeping people in hospital.

For the residents the benefits are hard to quantify, but one such resident, who has now spent three happy years in a group home after twenty years in a mental hospital, wrote very movingly about her own experience:

> We cannot remember much about our reactions on the first morning except that it was overwhelmingly wonderful to wake and find ourselves in a bedroom of our own. As the days went by we discovered many delights. The pleasure in little ordinary things to which other people would not give a second thought. The privacy of a bath on your own, the possession of a latch key, the real beauty of a soft-boiled egg or a cup of coffee on your own at midnight if you feel like it. It is simply the joys of ordinary living that were not available in the institutionalised life we had led.

This writer, like other group home residents, has become an ordinary member of her community and is now herself a voluntary helper.

The prolonged discussion and disagreement as to whether modern societies produce more mental illness, or whether the apparent higher incidence is due to improved diagnosis and the increased provision of services, will no doubt continue. What is quite certain, however, is that the conditions that produce mental and emotional strains and stresses do increase with the growth of urbanisation, and that many of these problems are better solved, and sometimes prevented, by the involvement of the community.

13 HEALTH CARE IN A BIG CITY IN A TIME OF FISCAL CRISIS

S. David Pomrinse, George B. Allen and
John C. Rossman

Background

New York City, with 7.6 million residents, is the largest municipality
in the United States and has 42 per cent of the population of the state
of New York, the next level of government. The city and state are
currently in the throes of a fiscal crisis, necessitating cutbacks in many
services. The crisis is the result of a multitude of factors, not least
among them a decline in industrial activity and rapid increases in the
cost of governmental services, particularly those pertaining to health,
welfare and education.

The structure of the city's health care system is multipartite and
diverse. In addition to the government, there are numerous voluntary
and proprietary organisations, as well as tens of thousands of individual
providers of health care. The financing involves all three levels of
government, federal, state and local, as well as private insurers and
direct payment (see Chapter 2). Much of the governmental authority
and responsibility with respect to health care is at the state and local
levels. However, over-all control of New York City's expenditures,
including those for health care, has been vested in an Emergency
Control Board dominated by state appointees. This is a result of the
near bankruptcy of the municipality.

The New York City 1975 *per capita* expenditure for personal health
care services was $ 885, constituting over 13 per cent of *per capita*
income, compared with a US *per capita* expenditure of 9 per cent.
Personal health care expenditures in New York City are more than 2.8
times higher than nine years ago, while *per capita* expenditures for
hospital care are more than 3.3 times higher. Over 23 per cent of the
municipality's budget and over 20 per cent of the state's budget are
devoted to health care. Hospital care accounts for over 63 per cent
of public expenditures for health care in New York City, although it
accounts for only 53 per cent of total personal health care expenditure, public and private. This is due to a comparatively larger
proportion of hospital care being financed through the public sector.
Health care expenditures, in particular hospital services, are thus an

282

obvious major target for cutbacks in this time of fiscal crisis.

History of Rate Controls

There has been a continuing and accelerating pressure to control the increases of health care costs, particularly institutional costs, since, in 1969, the full fiscal effects of the health care programme became evident. The main response has been to implement a system of prospective reimbursement whereby hospitals receive a fixed pre-determined sum per patient-day for Medicaid (medically indigent) and Blue Cross (private non-profit insurance) patients. These sources account for over half of hospital operating revenues. The rate is based on the hospital's past costs, with a factor added to compensate for price inflation.

The effect of this programme through the early 1970s has been to curtail reimbursement to hospitals. This curtailment has resulted in institutional operating deficits funded through the use of unrestricted endowment funds, delays in payments to vendors, bank loans, and the expenditure of funds earmarked for the replacement of plant and equipment.

An evaluation of New York prospective reimbursement rate controls conducted for the US Department of Health, Education and Welfare showed that the rate controls impacted substantially on *per diem* costs and somewhat less substantially on case cost. Comparison with a control group of hospitals also showed that negative incentives built into the rate control system resulted in a differential increase in the length of stay, thus explaining the less significant impact upon case cost. Another negative effect was a differential increase in the admission rate. No significant effect was found upon the offering of new services by hospitals. An analysis of these findings indicates that there is no evidence that any net saving, on a *per capita* basis, has been achieved. Any saving to payers has basically been financed through disinvestment by hospitals rather than a reduction in system expenditures for hospital services.

The financial crisis of both New York State and New York City governments had become so great by 1975 that the limited measures previously implemented through the reimbursement system were seen to be no longer adequate. This resulted in a series of drastic cutbacks in payments to institutions. This approach was taken despite the questionable results of earlier rate reductions. However, these efforts were in part delayed, and to some extent blocked, by litigation initiated by the hospitals.

Basic System Changes

There is a growing awareness by all concerned that meaningful answers to controlling health care costs on a long-term basis lie in areas other than rate control *per se*. These areas include: system planning; the role of teaching programmes in hospitals; utilisation review; the impact of new technology; the efficiency of the individual institutions composing the system; and, possibly most important, a re-evaluation of the role of curative care.

Planning

A very basic question, in respect to both the direct necessities of the fiscal crisis and the basic long-term dynamics of the system, relates to the appropriate size and structure of the hospital system. Mandatory planning controls were implemented in New York State in 1966. The philosophy in the 1960s and early 1970s was to permit system expansion on a controlled basis. Indeed, the number of general hospital beds in NYC increased from 4.67 to 5.02 per 1,000 population between 1966 and 1974. The strategy for hospital planning and construction then changed to one of limiting new construction, but allowing replacement of plant and substantial introduction of new services by present facilities. The climate has now changed to a policy of cutting back facilities, beds, and to some extent services. This is consistent with a new national policy approach as promulgated by the prestigious National Academy of Sciences.

A new planning body, the Health Systems Agency (HSA) created by federal law, in 1976 assumed responsibility for the regional planning process. The final decisions, however, remain under the control of the state government. The pragmatic approach has led to the conclusion that a shrinkage of the system is a necessity. Planning projections, revised within the last three years, show a current surplus of over 5,000 general care hospital beds which by 1980 will exceed 7,000 or over 20 per cent of the total beds, presuming there is *no* new construction in addition to that already approved. This sets the framework for a sharp immediate curtailment in the number of facilities and beds.

It is interesting to examine how this huge 'surplus' of beds has developed. Two years ago planning projections showed a comparatively small bed surplus, and going several years further back, the planning data indicated a bed deficit. The radically changed situation today is partly the result of new estimates for population changes, but more particularly the result of a re-evaluation of such basics as the appropriate percentage of occupancy and the anticipated length of stay.

Comparisons of the admission rate and the length of stay of New York City with pertinent national averages may be useful. The average length of stay of acute general hospitals in New York City is 131 per cent of the average of the 100 largest cities in the US. The admission rate, however, is 66 per cent of the average of these 100 cities. The reasons for the longer length of stay and the lower admission rate are not understood, although many hypotheses, most centring upon differences in medical practice, have been proposed.

State authorities decided to utilise a length of stay figure based on the current norms for all of New York State. This is despite the fact that the demographic, social and economic factors in New York City differ markedly from those in the rest of the state. This is rationalised by comparisons of New York City with other US urban areas which have shorter lengths of stay. There is no consideration given to the fact that the admission rate in New York City is much lower than in these other US urban areas. The low admission rate and the high length of stay, however, may well be interrelated.

Medical Teaching Programmes in Hospitals

One of the constant problems which has concerned many in the health care field has been the source of financing the cost of teaching programmes in hospitals. This educational cost has been, by and large, included in the costs attributable to patient care and paid through the same financing mechanisms. This creates a substantial problem since the community does not necessarily derive the future benefit of having trained the physicians, while the costs of doing so are paid for, in large part, by the community.

There are no adequate studies to date clearly demonstrating the cost of teaching in large teaching centres. The immediate and direct costs are readily identified and include those of House Officers and their supervising physicians. A case can be made that these direct costs may not exceed the costs of the same services rendered by practising physicians. There is a consensus among knowledgeable people in the field that a teaching programme substantially increases the costs of ancillary services (e.g. radiology, laboratory) through an increased quantity and diversity of tests being performed. The hard evidence is scarce, however, because of the difficulty of quantifying the differential impact.

The accepted view in the US is that care at teaching hospitals is distinctly better than at non-teaching hospitals. There is, however, some evidence that the teaching hospitals may hold special dangers to patients. The classic study of Schimmel, supported by the later study of McLamb *et al.*, shows 20 per cent of the patients admitted to the medical service of a university teaching hospital as suffering hospital-induced complications. No comparative study is currently available for non-teaching hospitals.

The state authorities have instituted fund reductions specifically for the medical teaching programmes of hospitals. There have been, however, no meaningful moves made to relate the number and type of teaching facilities to community needs.

Utilisation: Control of Admissions and Length of Stay

Excessive admissions and excessive length of stay are considered, by government, a major problem at the national as well as at the local level. In a country where care is paid for on a *per diem* basis, reductions in admissions and in length of stay are direct attacks on the amount of money which governments must spend on behalf of their clients. The federal government has instituted a peer review system, Professional Standards Review Organization (PSRO), applicable to federally funded programmes. Groups of practising physicians review the appropriateness of admissions and determine appropriate lengths of stay by diagnosis. Nurses responsible to the designated PSRO review body evaluate all patients covered under the programme. Those patients whose stays are growing longer than seems appropriate are brought to the attention of the PSRO physician consultants. The case is then reviewed with the attending physician and either an extension is awarded or the physician and patient are advised that the programme will not pay for the extended stay.

New York State also, because of fiscal pressures, has a New York State Hospital Utilization Review System (NYSHUR) affecting a key government programme for the medically indigent (Medicaid), under which payment may be denied if certain length-of-stay norms and procedural rules are not complied with. New York State has also implemented an 'on-site' programme which parallels that of the PSRO except that the evaluators and reviewers are state employees. The admission and length of stay standards applied also may differ from those applied by the PSRO.

Representatives of PSROs, as well as many hospital administrators, view the federal and state programmes as inappropriately duplicative. Early data indicate that the cumulative effect, however achieved, has been a significant reduction in the length of stay. There is no evidence that these programmes have resulted in any significant reduction in admissions.

Technological Change

The United States, and particularly those areas under financial pressures, such as New York, are faced with a conflict of values. Our history has encouraged the application of new technology with little regard for the cost-benefit ratios involved. Often this meant that very complex care was made available to a small number of patients whose lives might, or might not, be extended for a relatively short time. Thus the received policy was unlimited investment for any extension of life (even when that entailed continued pain or disability). Within the past two or three years in this country we have seen a recognition of this dilemma and a willingness to accept, in a moral context, the fact that not all patients should have their lives extended irrespective of the costs. A rationing of medical services is beginning to evolve by limiting the available supply.

In an era of reduced availability of funds, for capital as well as operating purposes, the decision to invest in expensive new technology is a difficult one. With the pressure on leading teaching hospitals to maintain their technological superiority, the balance between the economic and the clinical priorities becomes extraordinarily difficult. One example is the recent development of computerised tomographic devices. These machines have given a new dimension to diagnostic radiology. The cost, however, is nearly half a million dollars for each piece of equipment, with a per annum cost of operation approximating $150,000. A specific example may be of interest. At Mount Sinai Hospital the computerised scanner has been in operation for some 18 months, resulting in an 87 per cent reduction in the number of air studies and a 21 per cent reduction in the number of arteriograms. The savings which have resulted from finding that the scan was normal and that hospital admission would not be necessary are unknown. It is impossible to determine definitively the number of patient-days which are saved in this manner, but it seems clear from anecdotal reports that the number is significant. A detailed study of this is planned.

There is an evident need for an organised and systematic evaluation of the benefits and costs of new technology. Such evaluations often present major methodological difficulties and can also involve difficult ethical and philosophical issues. It seems much more appropriate, however, to attempt such an evaluation rather than have such control result as an implicit by-product of a general curtailment in payments to health care institutions.

Measures to Improve Efficiency

Great emphasis has been placed by New York State government on attempting to increase the efficiency of operation of individual institutions. The approach used, however, has been, through the use of formulae based on group averages, to penalise institutions considered inefficient. There are no positive incentives to the hospitals nor any effective help provided to improve hospital management. There is no convincing evidence that the systems used by the state have either identified inefficient hospitals or directly assisted institutions to increase efficiency.

The over-all pressures of fiscal constraints imposed on hospitals have, nevertheless, resulted in a greater effort by hospitals generally to improve efficiency. An example of such efforts is the services provided by the Management and Planning Services Programme (MAPS) of the Hospital Association of New York State. The MAPS Resources Monitoring System (RMS) develops labour productivity standards tailored to the unique characteristics of each hospital. It is currently in use in 30 states in the US, and is being applied by hospitals in Canada and Australia.

The Role of Curative Care

A more basic view of the alignment of health care costs with community resources relates to the role that curative health care services can and should play. Are we trying to solve problems through curative health care that can effectively be solved only through social, economic and environmental changes? What price treatment for respiratory disease in a city where the air is heavily polluted? Can the problems of drug addiction and alcoholism be effectively dealt with through curative care?

Curative care can and often does reflect failures in the social, economic and environmental arenas. Prevention in the broad sense may be a more effective way of dealing with health problems of a modern industrial society than any corresponding expenditure on curative care could possibly be. The attitude and expectations of the members of our society for health care may also reflect a lack of realism. Many of the major disease problems relate to poor individual health habits, e.g. over-eating, smoking, lack of exercise and, more acutely, alcoholism and drug addiction. It is a fact of our society that a person, no matter what the disease or condition, is expected to die

in a health care institution. Does this necessarily result in greater
comfort to either the patient or his family? Is the maintenance of life
in the absence of any reasonable chance of recovery a goal worth
the expenditure of very considerable health care resources? The fiscal
crisis is forcing a re-examination of these basic and sometimes
uncomfortable questions.

New Approaches

There is evidence of the growing acknowledgement that new approaches
are needed to address these basic system issues. Mr A.Y. Webb,
Executive Director of the NYS Health Planning Commission, recently
stated:

> Our present system is based almost entirely upon the notion of
> curing or arresting disease, and is essentially organized around
> the hospital as provider of health care. This approach is extremely
> costly. A redirection of some of our resources toward such areas
> as preventive medicine, environmental research and control, and
> health education programs could result not only in reduction of
> cost, but also in elimination of some unnecessary suffering.

The state has acknowledged that the present rate control approaches
require re-examination. Study is being given within and outside of
New York State to various new ways of rate setting. These include
systems which reduce case cost or give other positive incentives to
hospitals to reduce length of stay, and the development of regional
aggregate limits on hospital expenditures.

Legislation has recently been introduced in Congress to establish
a Center for the Evaluation of Medical Practice to stimulate and fund
research in various areas of medical practice, including: (1) the
appropriate use of facilities, equipment and technology, including
indications for hospitalisation and length of stay; (2) the relationship
between educational and training requirements for providers and the
quality of care provided by them; (3) diagnostic and case-finding
techniques including assessment of their specificity, sensitivity,
frequency of application, safety and cost; and (4) therapeutic
procedures, including assessment of their benefits, costs, risks and
indications for use.

Effective action based on these basic system concerns is
unfortunately, at present, too slow to deflect short-term, drastic
and often unproductive measures to curtail health care costs.

The question is whether knowledge as to the system dynamics will be acquired and acted upon quickly enough to limit damage to the system infrastructure.

Bibliography

American Hospital Association (1974, 1975, 1976 edition). *Hospital Statistics*. Chicago.

Carey, Hugh L., Governor of the State of New York (1977). *State of the Health Message*. Albany, New York (17 February).

Dowling, William L., Ph.D. (1976). *The Impact of the Blue Cross and Medicaid Prospective Reimbursement Systems in Downstate New York (Final Report)*. University of Washington, Department of Health Services, School of Public Health and Community Medicine. Washington (June).

Evans, R.G. (1971). ' "Behavioural" Cost Functions for Hospitals', *Canadian Journal of Economics*, vol. 4 (May).

_____ and Walker, Hugh D. (1972). 'Information Theory and the Analysis of Hospital Cost Structure', *Canadian Journal of Economics*, vol. 5, no. 3 (August).

Feldstein, Martin S. (1971). *The Rising Cost of Hospital Care*. Published for the National Center for Health Services Research and Development. Information Resources Press. Washington, DC.

_____ and Schuttinga, James (1975). *Hospital Costs in Massachusetts: A Methodological Study*. Discussion Paper No. 449, Harvard Institute of Economic Research. Cambridge (December).

Fryman, John, MD and Springer, John (1973). 'Cost of Hospital Based Education', *Hospitals, JAHA*, vol. 47 (1 March).

Health and Hospital Planning Council of Southern New York, Inc. (1974). *Hospital Statistics of Southern New York, 1974*. New York.

Health Systems Agency of New York City. *Grant Application for Conditional Designation*. New York (8 January).

Illich, Ivan (1976). *Medical Nemesis*. New York: Pantheon Books.

McLamb, J.T. and Huntley, R.R., MD (1967). 'The Hazards of Hospitalization', *Southern Medical Journal*, vol. 60, pp. 469-72 (May).

Mross, Charles Dennis (1973). *Diagnostic Mix and Cost Variation*. An essay presented to the Department of Epidemiology and Public Health of Yale University in candidacy for the degree of Master of Public Health.

National Academy of Sciences, Institute of Medicine (1976). *Controlling the Supply of Hospital Beds*. Washington, DC (October).

New Jersey State Department of Health (1976). *The Development of a Prospective Reimbursement System for New Jersey Hospitals*

291

(5 August).

New York State Department of Health, Division of Health Facilities Development, Bureau of Facility Planning (1976). *Monthly Inpatient Need Satisfaction, Profiles by County*. Albany, New York (1 August).

New York State Health Planning Commission (1976). *Acute Care Need Estimates*. Albany, New York (9 November).

––––––– Health Advisory Council, Ad Hoc Committee on Hospital Reimbursement (1977). *Executive Health Care Policy Making, Planning, and Regulation in New York State* (18 March).

New York State Legislature, Legislative Commission on Expenditure Review (1977). *Health Planning in New York State*. Program Audit 1.1.77. Albany, New York (3 January).

Piore, Nora, Lieberman, Purlaine and Linnanne, James (1976). *Health Expenditures in New York City: A Decade of Change*. Columbia University Faculty of Medicine, Center for Community Health Systems. New York.

Rossman, John, Dr P.H. and Pomrinse, S. David, MD (1977). 'Health Care in Big Cities: New York', *World Hospitals*, vol. XIII, nos. 1 and 2, pp. 19-31 (January-April).

Schimmel, Elihu M., MD (1964). 'The Hazards of Hospitalization', *Annals of Internal Medicine*, vol. 60, no. 1, pp. 100-10 (January).

United States Bureau of the Census (1975). *Statistical Abstract of the United States, 1975*. Library of Congress No. 4-18089, Washington, DC.

United States Congress (1975). *New York City's Fiscal Problem: Its Origins, Potential Repercussions, and Some Alternate Policy Responses*. Background Paper No. 1, Congressional Budget Office. Washington, DC (10 October).

United States House of Representatives (1977). 95th Congress, 1st Session. Bill H.R. 4869. *To Amend the Public Health Service Act* (10 March).

United States Department of Health, Education, and Welfare (1976). Public Health Service, Health Resources Administration. *Baselines for Setting Health Goals and Standards*. Government Printing Office, DHEW Publication No. (HRA) 76-640. Washington, DC (September).

Waldman, Saul (1972). 'The Effect of Changing Technology on Hospital Costs', *Research and Statistics Note*. US Department of Health, Education, and Welfare, Social Security Administration, Publication No. (SSA), 72-11701, Washington, DC (28 February).

14 REGIONALISATION OF METROPOLITAN HEALTH SERVICES

Anthony I. Adams

Attempts to regionalise health services in large metropolitan areas are by no means new, and perhaps the most publicised example of successful regionalisation has been the development of the hospital services organisation in Stockholm, Sweden. The concept is directed towards the provision of services, whether they be hospital- or community-based, to defined populations in metropolitan areas so as to give all citizens equal accessibility to those services.

The inherent advantage of this is that the needs of the defined population groups can, by means of surveys and data collections, be identified on a continuous basis and services can be adjusted, modified or introduced to meet the changing needs of these populations. It is argued that looking at a city as a whole does not permit the ready identification of local health needs, as smaller subgroups of the population always tend to get overlooked in any macro-view. Hand in hand with the provision of more appropriate services to smaller population groups goes the need for the development of more effective and flexible funding mechanisms with perhaps the allocation of global budgets to regional health administrations to enable them to have more autonomy in allocating funds across the whole range of health services.

In times of rapid escalation of health service costs it could, however, be argued that regionalisation lessens the control of the central authority, arouses unnecessary or unreal expectations on the part of the regional and subregional local populations, and leads to the over-provision of services of all types (plus a proliferation of health administrators) as each region struggles to attain absolute self-sufficiency. It can also be argued that regionalisation of any service in a metropolis runs counter to the very notion of a modern city as a single 'living' indivisible unit or organism which permits of no artificial subdivision into regions or districts.

The city of Sydney, which has a population of approximately 3 million people, has been regionalised since mid-1973 at a time when a new administrative organisation, the Health Commission of New South Wales, was formed from the former departments dealing with public health and hospitals. The four regions were originally designated in such a way as to give each region approximately the same size of population. However, the rapid growth of one region in particular, which occurred as the city expanded away from the coast, meant that within a short period of time we have already had to consider the reallocation of regional boundaries. The inner region, which is really the heart of the metropolitan area, has historically been the centre of the city's hospital services, and the largest amount of money has had to be spent in that region in maintaining traditional hospital services which have been built up around the two major universities and the larger teaching hospitals. In 1974-5 alone, this region spent $130 million on hospital operating costs, the equivalent of 15 per cent of the state health budget. Of the 16 major hospitals in the region the teaching hospitals accounted for 77 per cent and the non-teaching hospitals 23 per cent of total expenditure (see Chapter 4).

When the regions of Sydney were first designated, regional planning teams were built up within each regional health administration. The main task of these planning teams, in the first instance, was to develop a descriptive profile of the population within the region, of the services that existed, and of those that were in the planning stage, in an attempt to develop indicators of the most urgent needs of the population. This approach has been rather revolutionary for Australia, as very few attempts had been made in the past to look at services provided in any area whether rural or urban, from a total viewpoint. Thus, in the last two years the Health Commission, through the Division of Health Services Research and the regional planning teams, has been assisting regional administrations in the development of regional plans.

In two urban regions, namely the Western and Inner (see Figure 4.4, Chapter 4) this has led to some very exciting work with regard to the planning of future hospital services. In the Western Metropolitan Region, where the population had far outstripped the provision of hospital services and where earlier studies had demonstrated the very high rates of leakage from that region to hospitals in older parts of the city, a study was undertaken to assess the propensity of the population to use hospital services both in the immediate and distant future. Using a computer programme which took into account travel costs as well as the propensity for use of hospital services, plus the detailed analysis of existing hospitals, a forward hospital building programme has been devised which will, if funds continue to become available, provide hospital services by the end of this century adequate for most, if not all, the needs of that population. In the Inner

Metropolitan Region the reverse situation applied as the hospitals which had traditionally served most of the city now had a great deal of excess capacity. In addition to having excess capacity they were in many instances in very poor physical shape and they had, over a period of several decades, developed a number of specialist services, largely in a spirit of competition with each other, which had led to a considerable duplication of expensive super-speciality services in the region. We attempted to look at the use of all services in the hospitals in the Inner Region by using a two-week sample of all discharges from all wards and units in the region and to identify the origin of patients to both super-speciality and generalist services, thus calculating propensities of the population to use (or rather be admitted to) a total of 23 identified specialist medical services.

From this study it has thus been possible to start rationalising the services in the Inner Region and to consider closing some of the larger hospitals or changing the role of hospitals which are no longer serving the purpose for which they were originally built. One example of the latter is a large maternity hospital which is currently running at 40 per cent occupancy in an area with low birth rates where two other maternity hospitals are competing for deliveries. An associated cost study has highlighted the marked difference in cost implications of admitting patients to specialist versus general units and to teaching versus non-teaching hospitals.

These two studies in particular have highlighted the unequal distribution of hospital services in Sydney and have accurately pinpointed the extent of the leakage rates from one region to the other. These leakages are especially important in relation to the speciality hospitals, namely paediatric and maternity hospitals. The studies also highlight the lack of provision for the elderly, and the previous lack of concern for special groups, such as migrants.

One of the interesting findings of the Inner Metropolitan Study has been the demonstration of a very high propensity for populations living near to large hospitals to use not only general medical and surgical services but the super-speciality services. We are at present trying to explain this, and whether it is a feature of the poorer health status of citizens living in the centre of large cities, or whether it is yet another example of that law which states that if a service is provided then it will be used and the people who are closest to the service will be the ones that use it, we are not sure.

What we are sure of is that the cost of providing super-speciality services is very high indeed and with the over-all escalation in hospital

costs it is imperative that some rationalisation of the high-cost areas
be undertaken immediately. We already have far too many renal
units in Sydney and the same could possibly be said for other speciality
areas such as haematology, cardiothoracic surgery, radiotherapy, etc.
We are convinced that we cannot hope to make each of our four regions
self-sufficient in all specialist areas. This conflicts to some extent with
the aspirations of individual hospitals and particularly those teaching
hospitals associated with university medical schools. However, we
have been much heartened by the response of the clinicians and medical
academic staff of the universities, when presenting the findings of our
studies, to note that they are accepting the fact that a certain amount
of rationalisation will have to occur forthwith if only to enable at
least some hospitals to upgrade their physical facilities. There can be
no doubt that the pressures of cost will force even the most independent of hospitals to agree to co-operate in forward planning exercises
and we must be thankful to some extent that the situation in most
Australian cities is that the government pays for most of the hospital
services. In fact in Sydney, the public hospitals are entirely paid for by
government, and there is also some over-all cost exercised by
government over the size and distribution of the private hospitals.

The Health Commission has placed a great emphasis on the development of a forward programme for hospital construction, refurbishing
or modification. Each regional administration has been requested to
list, in terms of its priorities, construction and refurbishing work for
a period of ten to fifteen years so that new building jobs can be taken
in logical sequence on the basis of need as determined from regional
planning studies or regional estimates using less refined techniques such
as bed to population ratios. The first five years of the hospital building
programme is reviewed regularly to ensure that priorities are being met
or that changing needs of individual regional populations do not
warrant a change in direction as regards hospital bed provision. The
costs of the building programme are based on projected rather than
current costs so that a more realistic estimate of total expenditure
can be made. Regionalisation has certainly facilitated this process
although it is always necessary for the central administration to order
the final programme and to arbitrate on the inevitable inter-regional
rivalry that occurs. One additional advantage of having a ten-year plan
for the construction of new hospital beds is that it enables a health
authority to plan well in advance regarding staffing. A survey of future
nursing needs in one region has permitted the early recruitment of
nurses into a training programme sufficiently well in advance of the

opening of several new hospitals, including one of 800 beds, to
guarantee adequate nursing staff for these hospitals.

When one looks at regionalisation in terms of community health
services and ambulatory care there are undoubtedly certain associated
advantages. We have been able to document the extent of primary
care provision in most of the local government areas in Sydney and
have been able to identify populations with low general practitioner
ratios. Furthermore, we have developed a framework for ascertaining
the needs of local populations for community health services and
in these regions we have, for example, deliberately set about to support
the general practitioners by providing support centres or services staffed
largely by community nurses and other ancillary health personnel. The
community nurses have been trained in traditional public health nursing
but many have had previous experience in district nursing, geriatric
nursing, psychiatric nursing and so on. In particular in the Western
Metropolitan Region, which initially had the lowest general practitioner
to population ratios, the concept was initially developed to the extent
of providing two nurses for approximately every 6,000 population,
and these nurses were attached to the local primary schools. The nurses
were responsible for well-baby clinics, school-child screening, and other
related services. The nurses have close liaison with the local general
practitioners, and receive back-up services from what have been called
area health centres, which are staffed by social workers, psychologists,
child health experts, mental health experts and others.

Recently concern has been expressed for the lack of primary care at
night and at weekends, and a detailed study of emergency care departments in two regions of Sydney has highlighted the large load of fairly
non-urgent cases which descend on the emergency departments of
hospitals during these times. We have been liaising with the privately
run general practitioner deputising services to see if a combined effort
cannot be made to close the gaps in out-of-hours services for primary
care. The emergency care studies to which I have referred were done
in an attempt to rationalise casualty departments throughout the city
and to have them categorised region by region according to a three-
level scale. Major accident centres could then be established throughout
the city with a second-tier level of services provided at more peripheral
hospitals which would be staffed and equipped to handle less serious
trauma. Further studies of this nature are planned for the rationalisation
of other important hospital-based services.

We have concentrated on developing detailed projections of
populations of local government areas throughout the city for the next

twenty years. These projections will give us valuable denominator populations for many of our ongoing data collections and *ad hoc* studies. As an example of the former we have just instituted a hospital morbidity statistics programme which is to cover both the private and public hospitals in Sydney and will record details of all discharges from hospital according to local government area of origin of the patient, age, sex, reason for admission, complications of admission, final diagnosis and disposal and length of stay. Thus for the Sydney regions for the first time we shall have detailed information on the rates of admission for all types of illness and also rates concerning surgical procedures. More importantly in the first instance, perhaps, we will have information on the length of stay of all patients in hospitals, and we have adapted the approach developed in Ontario, Canada, of producing relative stay indices which will enable the regional health administrators to investigate those hospitals which are retaining patients with certain categories of illness longer than the state average for that size of hospital. We are hopeful that the use of this approach will not only reduce the length of hospital stay for many patients but will also lead to a critical look at the reasons for admission and the reasons for some surgical operations, particularly those of an elective nature. This we hope will lead both to a reduction in cost and an improvement in the quality of patient care in the near future. We see this too, as a basis of any form of hospital audit and accreditation programme.

The development of detailed population projections also enables us to undertake specific studies into the epidemiology of certain conditions — e.g. childhood accidents, cancer, coronary heart disease, stroke, etc. — and to evaluate the effect of any intervention programme at a regional or subregional level in reducing the incidence of any of these conditions. We are also working towards the detailed projection of need for manpower for our health services on a regional basis. The use of registration data for doctors, dentists, nurses, physiotherapists and others can be correlated with defined population groups in such a way as to identify present and future needs for various categories of health manpower.

One of the problems of all major cities is that certain groups in the population can be lost sight of and only come to notice when a real disaster occurs or when the numbers become so great as to make them patently obvious. In Sydney, as in most other cities in Australia, the proportion of the community who are over the age of 60 is growing year by year and we have recently been made aware of the fact that we have already more beds caring for the aged than we have for any other category of patient. We have something like 24,000 nursing home beds in the state of New South Wales (most of which is concentrated in three regions of Sydney) which approximates the number of acute hospital beds, many of which of course are also taken up by elderly people. A recent survey of all patients in nursing homes has highlighted the very critical situation facing us in Sydney and has indicated that not only are the nursing homes full, but that most of the aged inmates expect to be there for the rest of their lives. Thus we are confronted with a situation where to persist with the existing methods of providing care to the elderly means that we would have to construct several thousand more nursing home beds in the very near future. This is obviously an undesirable answer to the problem and one of the advantages of regionalisation is that one region can be used as an experimental area to see if alternatives to hospital or nursing home care cannot be developed. Any successful experiment or trial of this nature can then be extrapolated to the rest of the city and important innovations made in this way. Regionalisation, therefore, has the advantage of permitting experimentation of any sort to occur within a large city, in a controlled way, and this does not have to be confined to hospital care, but can be applied to community health services, ambulance services, home nursing services, etc.

Regionalisation, too, has given the local population some chance or some expectation of being able to participate in deciding what sorts of services should be provided at the local level, and this has undoubtedly been one of its major advantages. Of course, mistakes have been made and enthusiastic uninformed citizens can always, without proper guidance, push for the development of programmes which are not entirely appropriate and could indeed be wasteful of money and resources. But over all there can be no doubt that a greater understanding of people's needs can be achieved through community participation in the planning of health services at the local level.

From the Health Commission's viewpoint it must be admitted that in establishing regional organisation structures, health service administrators — formerly concentrated in a central office — have been divided among four regional offices and initially this has led to the spreading of talented staff too thinly and the possibly excessive growth of less qualified staff to support them. Some increase in administrative staff does seem to be an inevitable consequence of regionalisation and many express the feeling that a concentration of good people in one place would more than compensate for some of the inefficiencies and bureaucratic delays experienced from time to time in large decentralised organisations. Individual hospitals express this opinion frequently but in time the quality of regional office staff will surely improve and hospitals will benefit from being able to deal with administrators who are more knowledgeable on local matters.

There is no doubt then that regionalisation in large cities has certain advantages. In particular it facilitates the identification of gaps in the provision of services at the local level, and enables the planning of new services to be directed to meet the needs of important sub-groups, whether they be geographic or ethnic. However, cities function as a total organism and, particularly in relation to super-specialist requirements, the city must be viewed as one entity if duplication of services is to be avoided. If cities do regionalise their health services, they must retain a strong central co-ordinating body to ensure that money is spent wisely, to ensure that regions do not attempt to develop self-sufficiency in services which are not appropriate, and to ensure that the quality of care is maintained at all levels. In other words, central monitoring of the distribution and quality of the city's health services is essential, and this means that appropriate data collections and evaluation studies must be developed and maintained centrally.

While budgets may be allocated on a global basis to the regions, the central authority must retain the right and ability to have the final say if expenditure within one region seems unwarranted in relation to the requirements of the rest of the city. What this means is that a city must develop a total plan for its future services on a broad canvas. It must develop firm policies and programmes for the health services of its people and must set standards by which the quality and acceptability of these services is to be measured.

However, once these broad guidelines are set within a city-wide plan, then the regions can develop their own sub-plans which will best be organised to meet the needs of their particular populations. In this way innovative experimentation can take place at the subregional level and this mechanism for testing innovatory health programmes — preventive, curative or rehabilitative — can prove vitally important to the whole of the city's health services. There is nothing more disheartening than to witness the adoption of a solid, monolithic approach for providing health services which becomes encased in bureaucracy or tradition and has no ability to experiment or change itself. We should almost urge change for change's sake and insist on continued experimentation in this age of rapid change in health care technology and health care needs.

The allocation of funds in an equitable manner is something that all health administrators strive for and — except in very ordered societies — too rarely achieve. In large cities where historically the provision of services, particularly hospital services, has been uneven, it is far too simplistic to allocate funds to regions purely on a *per capita* basis. Account must be taken of the cost of those services which serve the city as a whole, the extent of movement of patients resident in one region to hospitals in another, and many other factors. We are working slowly towards developing a financial formula which will take into account these multiple factors and one can only say at this juncture that regionalisation, and the introduction of hospital morbidity data collection systems that document the extent of 'leakage' from one region to another for all types of service on a continuous basis, facilitate this task greatly.

15 PROCEDURES FOR MONITORING HEALTH CARE

R. Alan Hay

Canada is a land of some 23 million people, most of whom live in the southern part of the country within 100 miles, or 150 kilometres, of the border with the United States of America. Ontario is the second largest of the ten provinces and is the most heavily populated of them all. Metropolitan Toronto, with 2.1 million people, is by far the largest population centre in Ontario, and it was upon Metropolitan Toronto that the Ontario Hospital Association (OHA) focused its study for the IHF's 'Health Care in Big Cities' project. The city's downtown district contains a concentration of hospital facilities with all but one of the area's eleven teaching hospitals gathered within a radius of less than two miles (3.2 kilometres).

The OHA is a non-government association, to which all the hospitals of the province voluntarily belong. From its headquarters in the Toronto suburb of Don Mills, a study of health care in Metropolitan Toronto was conducted in 1976. It was in the course of this study (see Chapter 5) that the growing significance of various programmes designed to aid hospitals, physicians and government in monitoring services, and of the evident need for others became apparent. This chapter therefore takes a closer look at what was being done at different levels to monitor health care in the province of Ontario, and how these activities are affecting the delivery of health care.

Not surprisingly, we found a somewhat uneven pattern of monitoring programmes. Voluntary peer review and government-legislated mechanisms are mixed together. Some programmes are province-wide in their scope, while others are confined to individual hospitals or groups. For the purpose of this presentation, I intend to refer first to programmes for monitoring care in hospitals and other settings, and then to services given by physicians. By monitoring, I mean an ongoing data-collection system, which is complemented by an analysis of the data collected.

Monitoring Care Given in Hospitals and Other Settings

Monitoring at the institutional level is carried out in a variety of ways.

302

One of the best known in North America is through the process of
hospital accreditation developed by hospital people and physicians
working together. The programme originated in the United States, and,
since 1959, we in Canada, have been served by the Canadian Council
on Hospital Accreditation. Council provides survey teams to visit
hospitals requesting accreditation. They report upon many aspects of
the care being given, including how it compares with Council's
published standards of acceptability. Approximately 85 per cent
of the beds in the province are in accredited hospitals, which are
re-surveyed periodically.

For hospitals, especially small ones, desiring to know how closely
they meet the standards of the national programme, the OHA, with
the Ontario Medical Association, offers a pre-accreditation service to
tell them how they might fare in a survey. There is also the Joint
Hospital Assessment Programme, conducted as a co-operative effort by
the OHA and the College of Physicians and Surgeons of Ontario.
Unlike accreditation, it issues no certificates. The purpose of this
voluntary programme is to provide hospital boards, which may or may
not have plans to apply for an accreditation survey, with a review, by
outsiders, of many medical and administrative practices, some of which
are not covered by accreditation surveys. Frank discussion of problems
is encouraged. Assessment teams, composed of highly experienced
physicians and hospital administrators, travel to hospitals to look at
patient care, including the important working relationships between
board, medical staff and administration, and the way in which a
hospital and its physicians are complying with provincial laws and
regulations, and the hospital's own by-laws. It is interesting to note
that these three programmes — accreditation, pre-accreditation and
assessment — were developed by non-government associations, which
set their own standards of evaluation, and as a result, both hospital
care and management have approved.

A major problem confronting hospital administrators in Ontario
is that of maintaining financial control. Government provides funds
on the basis of prospective budget approvals. In order to assist them
in monitoring what happens as the year unfolds, the Ontario
Hospital Association has actively supported the Hospital Information
System (HIS), developed in 1968 by the Canadian Hospital Association in conjunction with the federal government. The idea and proposal
came from the Hospital Association. The federal government
provided its computer hardware. The system has just undergone its
second detailed revision in nine years. To participate — and 85 per cent

do in Ontario — hospitals voluntarily report details of their operating results every three months. Government computers process the information and return to each hospital the results of one quarter before the end of the next.

The association receives from Ottawa, each quarter, a record of data produced from the returns made by all its participating members. OHA reprocesses this and provides consolidated reports of 300 statistical indicators with the values of each hospital identified with its name. These reports are supplemented by booklets put out by the association. They are designed to help hospitals use the information By this process, they are assisted in monitoring their operating expenses and experience, and in establishing criteria for future budgets.

This programme is an example of team work between the national and provincial hospital associations, participating hospitals and the federal government, to produce a common and timely data base for evaluating hospital performance. Its full potential has yet to be realised, but it has provided provincial paying agencies and individual hospitals with common means through which to examine management.

Other examples of team work in monitoring are the bed utilisation programmes developed voluntarily by individual hospitals. I wish to refer to one in use at a 600-bed general hospital in Ontario. Using data collected about the medical care provided, and the way it compares with the institution's own previous experience, some interesting trends are revealed. Table 15.1 shows that the average length of stay in medical, surgical, OBS, paediatric and newborn beds in this hospital in 1969 was 8.5 days, decreasing to 6.8 days by 1975, and 6.6 days in 1976, achieved by setting discharge dates on the day of a patient's admission, and by using a computer to monitor length of stay by hospital service, and by individual physician. It shows clearly what happens in a hospital where effective co-operation between board administration and the medical staff leads to critical monitoring of the hospital's care.

The table also indicates that as a result of this shortened stay, there has been a significant increase in the number of admissions. In 1969, the average number per month was 1,676. By 1975 it had increased to 1,897 and in 1976 it went up to 1,924. By this more efficient utilisation, the hospital has been able to avoid opening more beds despite the pressures of a growing catchment area population.

Crucial to good patient care in and out of hospital is accurate laboratory tests. This is the concern of what is known as the Laboratory Proficiency Testing Program, developed by the Ontario Medical

Table 15.1: A 600-Bed General Hospital

Year	Average length of stay (days)	Patient admissions per month
1969	8.5	1,676
1975	6.8	1,897
1976	6.6	1,924

Association and now financed by government. Samples are sent to all
laboratories for testing. Their reports are compared with the known
values by staff of the Ontario Medical Association with the object of
differentiating between laboratories with acceptable performance and
the others that may need technological upgrading, or the services of a
regional facility.

Yet another government monitoring project is concerned with the
province-wide ambulance service. A computer is used to record the
movement of every one of the 512 ambulances, as well as the details
of casualty care provided by ambulance personnel with the aim of
improving utilisation and economy.

Finally, good institutionalised health care depends upon having the
right patient in the right bed at the right time, and for the right length
of time, but it is a great deal easier said than done. Action to achieve
this, however, is not yet being undertaken on a provincial basis, but
some individual hospitals, and groups of hospitals, are working on it.
Probably the best-known to people outside Ontario is the Assessment
and Placement Service (APS), established by the Hospital Council in
the City of Hamilton, some 35 miles west of Toronto. It was discussed
in detail by its Director, Dr Ronald Bayne, at the 1973 IHF Congress
in Montreal, and it is still actively monitoring the progress of bed
patients through the health care facilities of a city of about 300,000
people.

Monitoring Services Given by Physicians

One of the major aids to peer review of physicians' services in
Ontario is a computerised programme conducted by the Hospital
Medical Records Institute (HMRI), located in the OHA Centre. It is
not dissimilar to the American Professional Activities Study (PAS).
The Canadian programme was set up jointly, some ten years ago, by
three non-governmental associations in Ontario representing hospitals,
physicians and medical record librarians, to provide hospitals with a

monthly statistical audit of their clinical activities. HMRI has had its problems in attempting to match ambitions with resources. New objectives, new managers, and an infusion of government funds and technological assistance have recently brought about significant improvements. Participation by hospitals is mandatory.

When a patient leaves hospital and the physician signs off the chart, the medical record librarian abstracts specific information from it for entry on a specially designed abstract form. The completed forms are mailed in batches to the Hospital Medical Records Institute. Over 1.5 million abstracts are processed yearly. The form provides for identification, by number, of the doctors involved in giving care. The key to the numbers is kept confidential by the hospital. The International Classification of Diseases, Adapted, Eighth Revision, or ICDA-8, is used to code the diagnoses and procedures. The form allows additional optional coding for research projects initiated by the hospital. The input flexibility assists medical audit and utilisation review, and thereby serves to upgrade hospital medical practice. This flexibility will be further improved by the introduction of a new redesigned form in 1978.

HMRI provides each hospital with twelve standard reports consisting of indices and analyses for the review of cases discharged, to assist in monitoring quality of patient care, and the use of the hospital's facilities. The details of the care of each case are arranged in columns for easy review. A comparison is also made between a hospital's length of stay figures and those of the Professional Activities Study Canadian data base. Hospitals receive reports within a turn-around time of three to four weeks, but their value is not fully captured without an effective medical staff peer review programme.

HMRI is an example of monitoring in-hospital medical care. There are, however, programmes for the routine scrutiny of physicians' patterns of practice carried out by government through examination of the bills they submit for their services

Hospital and medical care services in Ontario are provided to the public on a prepayment basis through the government's Ontario Health Insurance Plan. Both hospitals and physicians function as private entities, but whereas hospitals are subject to rigid budget controls, physicians operate, for the most part, on a fee-for-service basis, with the payment schedule negotiated between the medical association and the government. While the fee-for-service policy is accepted and supported by the government, its open-ended character is a source of some political uneasiness. To alleviate public concern that the system might give physicians too free an access to the public purse, the Ministry of Health has set up a computer programme, under its Professional Services Monitoring Branch, to scrutinise the volume of services provided to patients by each doctor, and the consequent billings each makes to the Health Insurance Plan.

It examines the profiles of all physicians with particular emphasis on those who appear to have unusual patterns of practice. The profiles are actually statistical analyses of claims submitted for services to patients, and 12,000 physicians in Ontario submit about 4.5 million each month. The pattern of a physicians' practice is compared with that of his peers on the basis of criteria established for the government by the medical profession's licensing body, the College of Physicians and Surgeons of Ontario. The comparison covers, for example, the number of patient contacts in the office, the home, or the hospital. It includes referrals made or received, and the number of specific procedures performed in a month, and their dollar cost. The results of this check are compared in three ways, with the averages recorded by other similarly qualified physicians: first, with those near where he lives, second, with those in his country, and third, in the province generally.

Though it is a department of the government that carries out the initial monitoring and identification of significant variations from the norm, it passes no judgement of its own. Instead, it sends the evidence to the College of Physicians and Surgeons of Ontario, the statutory licensing body of all doctors of the province, which refers it to its Medical Review Committee. This committee consists of 6 physicians and 2 lay people, and must investigate every case referred to it. When its work is complete, the committee makes recommendations to government on the action to be taken, to pay none, part, or all of the physician's billings. Deliberate fraud would generate legal action; suspected misconduct would be referred to the Disciplines Committee of the College for further investigation. The Medical Review Committee is created by legislation, and functions like a peer review committee. It is intended to have the capability of understanding the physician's viewpoint and his explanation of the matters which are under investigation. By its mix of physicians and lay members, it is also expected to have the capacity of understanding the public point of view.

In the course of its investigations, the committee may seek detailed information from the physician himself, or about him, from other sources. This is accomplished, in part, by an inspector appointed by the College, a physician himself, who examines records and documents wherever they are situated.

Summary

This chapter has investigated some of the procedures for collecting, processing and analysing data created by the delivery of health care in Ontario. The intent of them is to reveal a picture about the cost and quality of the services being rendered, and the way in which they are being used, but the picture is incomplete. There are problems in capturing accurate information created by the health care system: one has been the absence of a unique identifier for each member of the population; another is the size and expense of the job. With 4.5 million claims for payment from physicians each month, and 1.5 million patients discharged annually from 250 hospitals, information retrieval is expensive and growing more so every year. It seems obvious that in Toronto, or elsewhere, all the resources cannot be found by non-government agencies alone. The solution to some problems requires a partnership of investigators, both inside and outside the government, working co-operatively together.

With vast and growing expenditures on health, it is inevitable that governments, both to satisfy themselves and the electorate, will seek justification for their outlay. It may have been noticed that the majority of the cost and quality monitoring programmes referred to originated outside of government with associations and groups, who established the criteria and the way they should be used, and they have operated with tacit government approval. Monitoring is not the prerogative of governments alone. Hospital people and physicians, exhibiting necessary concern for patient care and for the efficiency and effectiveness of the publicly financed and privately administered health care system, are well able to design and operate monitoring programmes themselves.

16 HEALTH POLICY AND PLANNING IN BOGOTÁ

Jaime Arias

The aim of this chapter is, first, to present the general methodology
used by the Department of Health of Bogotá, DE (DHB) to plan services
in both the short and long term, and, second, to describe a body of
policy and strategies for the provision of health care in the next 25
years. From 1977, the DHB is due to develop and present a programmed
plan annually, a strategic plan every five years and projections of needs
and resources for the following 25 years. Planning is based on policy
documents which in turn are revised each year in accordance with
national health policies and the relevant policies of the local government
of Bogotá.

Bogotá, DE, is the capital city of Colombia with a population of
about 4 million and a large number of social and economic problems,
particularly in the health field, where more than two million people
depend upon government provision of as yet very limited resources.
The health status of the city is no better than that of European cities
at the beginning of this century and the needs for services grow at a
higher rate than their supply.

Although the DHB has the authority to co-ordinate and control all
types of health organisations, its effectiveness to date is very limited.
There are three independent main health care systems in the city and a
number of small subsystems: the public services, provided directly or
indirectly by the DHB, which represent about 50 per cent of the
population and 30 per cent of the expenditure; the social security
system, which covers about 10 per cent of the population (workers)
and shares 50 per cent of the health money; and finally, the private
system, which accounts for 20 per cent of the population and also
represents 20 per cent of the expenditure. There is 20 per cent of the
population with no coverage whatsoever (see Chapter 6 for details).

Under these circumstances, and as part of the national health system
policies, the DHB has developed the first health plan which is mandatory
for its own programmes, and serves as a guide for the other services
subsystems. It is expected that the plan and regulations will facilitate
the co-ordination of the three subsystems and hence will increase the
output of the services rendered. The process of intervening in the
private and social security systems will be increased very slowly as these

309

systems respond to the present plan and regulations.

Health planning in Bogotá is based on the following principles:

(1)   In order to increase effectiveness, efficiency and quality of health services, it is necessary to plan them on short-, intermediate- and long-term bases.

(2)   The planning process should be based on specific health policies and strategies and should include both general and specific health programmes.

(3)   All interested components of the health system (government agencies, private sector, etc.) should participate actively, at least in the development of guidelines of planning, and each subsystem must carry out the programme plan, including specific activities.

(4)   Health planning should incorporate complete and permanent systems evaluation that makes it possible to provide for ongoing change and adjustments in the programmes.

(5)   It is important that all organisations and individuals engaged in the execution of programmes have adequate access to the planners; among these organisations, consumers play a very important role.

(6)   The metropolitan city should have a central plan (mainly at the level of strategies) and regional, local and even single-institution (hospital-health centre) plans.

(7)   The health plan requires publicity – that is, it should be explained to providers, consumers and others.

The planning process is illustrated in Figure 16.1. In the case of Bogotá, DE, the health plan begins at the level of individual institutions (hospitals, health centre, laboratories, etc.), continues at the level of four regions into which the city is divided (each containing about one million people) and ends at the level of the whole city.

There are three main areas of health planning: medical care, environmental programmes, and services infrastructure. The process of planning is simple and has the following phases: needs and demand analysis; amount, quality and cost of resources; design of programmes and activities; information, evaluation and control.

A. Policies and Strategies for the Next 25 Years

The following list of policies and strategies has served as the base for the development of the annual health plan for the city:

(1)   Organisation, management and control of health services

Figure 16.1: Health Planning Process in the City of Bogotá, DE

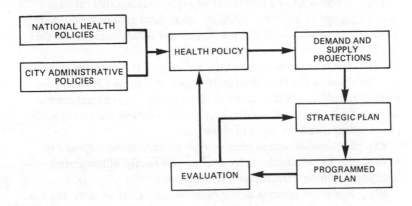

requires the implementation of annual programme planning and long-term guide plans (five or ten year plans) covering programming, monitoring and evaluation of services. For a city of nearly five million people, planning should be developed using available techniques, and should include clear statements of policies and objectives, and descriptions and qualifications of problems and resources and the strategies to tackle with the former.

(2)   A comprehensive evaluation system is necessary to enable policy-makers to change policies, goals or strategies. This evaluation system should include not only programmes but also professional practices and specific procedures which require experimental trials in order to determine output, costs and quality.

(3)   Financial aspects of health services should be treated separately, and some agencies should focus mainly or exclusively on these aspects. For instance, the city's health department (DHB) should develop itself to become an agency engaged in regulation, financing, control and evaluation of the entire health system, handing over direct services to other specialised agencies.

(4)   Regionalisation of the city should follow the population profile and should be based on community needs, rather than the location of existing services or the convenience of providers, as is done now.

(5)   New experimental models should be tried in order to increase the utilisation of human resources, particularly basic and paramedical resources. It is necessary to improve the co-ordination of the DHB and educational institutions so that training of new personnel becomes

relevant to planning.

(6)   It appears to be important to organise integrated medical practice groups to augment specialist work; these groups should have direct access to additional diagnostic aids and common resources that would decrease the costs of the services they provide.

(7)   The projections on costing, not only of the sectional services, but also those of the individual institutions, should be based on complete actuarial-type studies in which are included the characteristics of the population, the disease risk of that population, the use it makes of the services, and the costs of these.

(8)   Systems of comprehensive-type package services should be worked out that assure the individual and his family of integrated, timely, continuing, effective and low-cost care.

(9)   For easier running of the organisation of the services, the use of automated data systems should be promoted, not only for epidemiological information but also for administration at the sectional and individual institution levels. In closed institutions, it is convenient to use computerised record systems for clinical histories.

(10)   As the system grows more complex, simple and universal statistical information systems should be developed.

(11)   It is important to rationalise medical and dental consultations through improved use of filtering at the primary level (health centres and local community hospitals). In a city that spreads over a wide area, the so-called home visit should be avoided.

(12)   It is important to carry out studies on economics and administration that will enable big cities to define what is the ideal size for the different types of hospitals, so that clear policies can be adopted on the building or remodelling of hospitals.

(13)   In the large cities in Colombia, as in other countries where funds are limited, there is a large population of old people and the mentally sick for whom there is no provision of care even at the minimal level within the health systems. In future it is necessary to plan medico-social care for this population.

(14)   As the size of the cities and the complexity of the health services increase, it becomes more difficult for the inhabitants to know exactly how the services are organised. It is thus necessary to provide the large cities with unified public information centres and centres to co-ordinate information on the availability of beds. Also, it is advisable to have a simple and universal telephone line to deal with all the emergency medical cases and enquiries.

(15)   In view of the large number of hospital and medical activities

operational in large cities, it is advisable to develop systems for quality control analysis, not only for individual hospitals and clinics but also for medical, paramedical and auxiliary staff.

(16) It is important to set up committees to deal with disaster situations, on the lines indicated by experience gained in other cities in the world.

(17) In almost all the big cities of the world there has been an evident change in recent years in the pattern of use of services, with the population making more frequent use of the emergency or urgent services. This change can be turned to positive advantage by health organisations who can use it to create a means of easy access to health services. Any plans or organisation concerned with future services should consider the urgent facilities as having a prime role.

(18) As well as this series of guidelines to the organisation of medical care, it is important to note that in the big cities, policies and plans should be developed to embrace a more effective control of the environment, but treatment of this subject is not appropriate here.

B. Projections for the Next 25 Years: Methodology

This section is not concerned with a health plan for Bogotá for the year 2000, for such an undertaking is impossible, but with a series of projections on future needs and demands, resources and the possible interaction between these concepts. At the same time, a list of possible organisational and functioning strategies for the services of that period is presented.

The SSB intends these projections to serve as a point of reference to indicate goals, objectives, strategies and tactics for the five-year health plans. The methodology employed in the projections involves a series of studies on population, the capacity of the population to seek and pay for services, epidemiological shifts, the potential of the different types of resources, a financial analysis of the institutions providing health and medical care, and a consideration of the physical growth of the city, of transport and infrastructural public services, etc. The components of the preparatory analysis are explained in Figure 16.2. As the figure shows, at least three main categories of preparatory analysis are essential for the formulation of the projections; these also correspond to different policy models. Some of the mentioned components are being tested on mathematical simulation models and it is planned that shortly all the categories of exogenous and endogenous variables will be incorporated into a more general projection model, as a joint SSB and CCRP project.

Figure 16.2: Components of Previous Analysis to Determine Health
Problems and Resources in Bogotá, DE

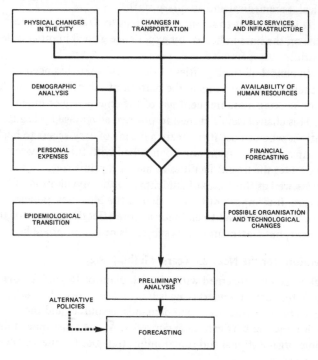

Below, the methodology and sources of information for each
component of the preparatory analysis are explained:

1. (a)   Demographic Analysis

The population census is broken down by sex and five-year age groups,
the net balance of migration is determined, and the births for each
period are aggregated, using the survival data determined for each
period. The three main variables are natality, mortality and migration,
and indirectly the general and total fecundity rates. It is estimated that,
over the twenty-five years, there will be: an increase of 6 years in life
expectancy; a balance of migration at a constant rate of 4 per cent; a
reduction in infant mortality from 45 to 25 per 1,000; a gross birth
rate decreasing from 25 to 14 per cent and a general fecundity rate
falling from 90 to 47 per cent.

1. (b)   Personal Expenditure on Health

This analysis and these projections have been based on the results of Home Enquiries (Encuestas de Hogares) carried out from 1971 to 1973 to investigate the areas of health on which individuals spent their money, how much each type of family spent in relation to income, and what trends in this spending were evident in relation to various factors affecting expenditure.

The foregoing studies were complemented by studies on future changes in personal and family incomes in Bogotá, in which the future increases in the incomes of different groups of individuals are analysed.

1. (c)   Epidemiological Shift

By means of a mathematical simulation model of the health sector of Colombia, using theories of epidemiological shift, it has been possible to project on a long-term basis changes in the incidence of diseases of development, underdevelopment and static conditions, using the experience gained in the country during the last twenty years and that of other countries, and taking into account the changes in a series of indicators of development, such as income and distribution, literacy, spending on infrastructure, electrification, construction of aqueducts, etc.

The changes in the patterns of distribution of diseases taken together with the demographic changes permit the calculation of the potential demand in respect of the different types of diseases.

2. (a)   Availability of Manpower Resources

Our projections are based on some studies by the Ministry of Health of Colombia on the numbers, training, distribution and utilisation of manpower resources, in particular the National Enquiry on Manpower Resources (Encuesta Nacional de Recoursos Humanos) of 1976. In addition, account was taken of present and possible future annual turn-out of professional and other health staff. Each type and sub-type of job has been projected in accordance with the present trend, hypothetical future tendencies. In making the projections, consideration has been given to the 'work functions' of health teams composed of different members, for example, where general doctors can to some extent replace specialists or a certain number of nursing auxiliaries can be interchanged with nurses in some kinds of situations. Finally, the resources that it is possible to offer are compared with the needs determined from demographic, epidemiological, economic and social changes.

2. (b)   Financial Projections for the Institutions

This is one of the most difficult parts of the analysis because any attempt to project the financial positions of individual institutions or of the whole complex of public and private health institutions involves the planner in figures, the reliability of which is very low, due to the large number and unpredictable nature of the variables involved.

In Bogotá, DE, the SSB has carried out studies on the financial performance of the health sector in comparison with other sectors over a period of time and has formulated some projections on the basis of different policies of government spending. These policies may be increases or decreases in spending on health in relation to other sectors, changes in the proportion of public spending, in social security or private insurance, or changes in the investment in the different programmes. In each of the foregoing cases, it is necessary to include possible changes in medical costs.

2. (c)   Possible Organisational and Technological Changes

Up until now, attempts have been made only at the most basic level to treat this important aspect of the preparatory analysis, and this primarily in relation to possible changes in the macro-organisation of services, since the forecasting of technological changes in the field of medicine is more difficult.

In Colombia, an important factor to be taken into consideration is the possible integration of the public assistance and social security systems, which would change the financial and possibly the organisational set-up. As for technology, it seems that in general this is following, with a lag of a few years, the procedures and techniques of the industrialised countries.

3. (a)   Physical Changes in the City

Bogotá is a city that has expanded in all directions at a great pace during the last two decades; it is expected that, though the rate of geographic expansion will not be so high in the next 25 years, nevertheless some of the areas that today are thinly populated will harbour new population groups within the next few years. This physical growth of the city will necessitate changes in the transport system and the building of new health care facilities. Our projections concerning the siting of surgeries, beds and other health facilities have been based on the study 'The Future of Bogotá, Phase II' already mentioned, in which the possible ways in which the physical growth of the city in the next fifteen years will take place are considered (see Figure 16.3).

Figure 16.3: Possible Urban Formations in 1990

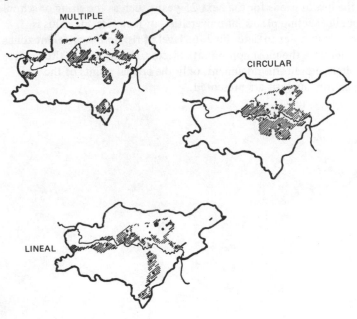

3. (b) Changes in Transport

Another interesting aspect of the preparatory analysis is that of
transport routes, since as far as possible the new facilities should be
built where access to them is easy. In the city of Bogotá, for example,
there are plans to change part of the present system of bus services by
the introduction of a mass-transport system of the metro or underground type. Such a change would force the planners to consider siting
the new facilities near the new lines.

3. (c) Infrastructural Public Services

Knowledge of the expansion of basic services such as water supply,
main drainage, light and telephone services allows limited forecasting
of the social and public health conditions in the different zones of
the city in the next 25 years and thus estimation of the needs for the
different types of medical attention services for each of these zones.
The projections for public services have been described in the study on
'The Future of Bogotá, Phase II'.

There are innumerable factors to be taken into account in forecasting the health needs for the next 25 years, such as the siting of schools, of public meeting places, of universities, of factories, etc. This is necessary in order to determine the level of risk in the different zones and therefore the most appropriate places to build new health centres, hospitals, etc. In this document, only the crucial points of the preparatory analysis are presented.

Bibliography

Financing and deployment of funds of the health system in Colombia: observations on the national home enquiry, CCRP (Heredia, Restrepo and Vivas).

Modelo Seres. Corporacion Centro Regional de Poblacion (CCRP).

Modelo Seres. CCRP and Analisis de los Censos de 1964 y 1973. Edgar Baldion.

Modelo Seres. Salud. CCRP (Arias).

Structural Plan for Bogotá. Study of the urban development of Bogotá. Phase 2. BID. UNDP.

17 MEDICAL ATTENTION FOR IMMIGRANTS COMING TO BIG CITIES

Guillemo Fajardo Ortiz

A. Introduction

Demographic movements are a socio-economic indicator and thus express the type of health services required by towns, cities and nations. Immigration is a demographic movement with characteristics that differ between one country and another, and even within the boundaries of a single country. In this chapter an attempt will be made to analyse the relation between immigration and medical services.

It is surprising that despite the fact that the flow towards the big cities has been the most studied demographic phenomenon, there are hardly any precise statistics on it; another limiting factor which emerged when this present study began was the lack of information on the state of health and the health services in the big urban areas; finally, there is an unfortunate lack of precision in the definition of the term 'big city'.

In spite of these stumbling blocks, we might take the following as our starting points:

(1) It is impossible to separate the health problems of the immigrants from those social, economic, political, educational and industrial circumstances prevailing before and during immigration.

(2) The 'explosive' growth of cities, and especially of the largest among them, has been a phenomenon in all continents for more than twenty years. While the general growth rate of the world population is about 2 per cent per annum, the rate in big cities oscillates between 3.5 and 4.5 per cent. In some extreme cases, it has reached 8 per cent. In Latin America, Sao Paulo, Santiago de Chile, Caracas, Bogotá and Mexico City are particular examples. In the more developed countries, the rate of growth is losing some of its initial impetus.

(3) The definition of the term 'big city' varies widely; in some parts of the world it is based on the size of the locality; in others on the presence or lack of urban characteristics.

At present in Latin America, there are fifteen cities with populations of at least one million. Sao Paulo, Brazil, has more than eight million inhabitants and Buenos Aires, Argentina, more than ten million; there is a similar situation in Mexico City, with thirteen million inhabitants. Indeed, calculations made by the Interamerican Bank of Development, which coincided with United Nations studies, show that in the year 2000 Mexico City will be one of the most populated cities in the world, with some 32 million inhabitants.

The exodus is concentrated, basically, on the outskirts of almost all the cities. Thus in Latin America marginal districts have grown up that in Lima are called 'barriadas' (slums); in Santiago, 'callampas' (mushrooms); in Recife, 'mocambos' (lodges); in Caracas, 'ranchos' (settlements); in Rio, 'favelas' (shanties); in Buenos Aires, 'villas miseria' (misery towns); and in Mexico, 'cinturones de miseria' or 'cuidades perdidas' (misery belts or lost cities).

The uncontrolled growth in extension and density aggravates the health problems of the cities. These are converted into 'metropolitan areas', which later expand to become 'megalopolis' and cosmopolitan cities. Over thousands of square kilometres, the immigrants mix with the city population, sharing nothing other than the communication system, housing, commerce, work, etc. Within this superworld, the health services and other medical organisations cannot find adequate solutions to the resulting 'megalo-sufferings'.

The immigrants have no understanding of the tensions that overwhelm the city-dweller. The inhabitants of a big city face a multitude of problems: the 'city syndrome' involves public administration, health, finance, transport, traffic and environmental contamination. Granted that the big cities provide the opportunities, or at least the possibilities, for cultural, health, work, sporting, scientific and social activities that are not to be found in smaller cities, nevertheless these activities are generally orientated towards productive ends and social service or utility. With regard to these activities, the common man finds himself a mere spectator or compelled to take certain roles because access to such opportunities is limited to a minority.

B. Causes of Immigration

In Latin America, the study of migratory movements and their consequences is of fundamental importance for the solution of health problems. The lack of progress, or its limited extent, towards improvements in living conditions influence the continued displacement and indeed seem to make it irreversible. The immigrant population moves to the big cities. The immigration brings people and it brings their problems, all of which worsen the conditions, already at crisis point, in the metropolis.

One can say that in the majority of cases, it is the limitation on human and material resources, the lack of communications, the scattered nature of the population, the inadequate housing, the shortage of facilities for education, and unemployment that force the pilgrimage to the cities. There is a patent desire among the immigrants to become part of the economic or social development and not to miss out on health and welfare.

Among the attractions that accelerate the transfer of people from a given locality to the cities one must consider the economic factors connected with work opportunities (the attraction exercised by better working conditions, or the belief that more opportunities exist); better pay and in a more general sense, better legal conditions of work (more convenient hours, greater stability, social security, a wider variety of activities and the existence of labour exchanges). Family factors are also important, such as the presence of a relative in the city who can help the immigrant to adapt, parents moving their home, and marriage.

It is also worth taking note of the attraction exercised by ethnic factors, such as the presence of a homogeneous group to which the person belongs. Note must also be taken of 'magical' attractions (myths of the big city) and the cultural attractions (means of acquiring education and culture: schools, colleges, universities). Such psychological motivations would also include an aversion to life in a closed community, dissatisfaction with work, and the desire to reach a certain level in one's calling (desire for social mobility).

C. Immigrants

The differences within an immigrant population are established by the state of health; whether the population is indigent or working; known or unknown; supervised or not; given assistance, permitted or illegal; invasive; permanent or temporary (seasonal); international, internal or interregional.

In general, immigration brings along young people, who for the most part have broken free from the care or the coercion of the family or the group and are therefore at the mercy of a poorly developed stationary environment and exposed to the seduction of the hitherto unknown temptations to be found in the big cities.

Clear evidence of the magnitude of such migratory movements is given by the tendency to urbanisation, the growth rates of the important urban nuclei and the exceedingly high proportion of persons who live in a place other than that in which they were born. The internal migratory movements of the last decades represent one of the most striking characteristics of demography and have the greatest significance for the economic and social changes in Latin America.

The general condition of the immigrants and their state of health are in many ways linked to environmental contamination and the quality of the water; as far as the first is concerned, there is generally a degradation of the atmosphere by the smoke and gases produced by the city industries and by the combustion products of motor vehicles; the indiscriminate discharge into sluices, rivers, lakes and seas of the waste products of industries and factories, etc. reduces the quality of the water; and at the same time, the supplying of drinking water to the urban centres causes water shortages in the rural areas.

D. Health Problems Deriving from Immigration

The fundamental problem of the immigrant concerns both the general quality of life and his precarious personal state of health on account of his lack of adaptation to the city. His lack of experience of city life and even language difficulties make his incorporation into the new habitat even more difficult.

All the studies on health indicate that the health problems of the immigrants are concerned, to a greater or lesser extent, with: malnutrition, dental decay, digestive upsets, respiratory diseases (especially tuberculosis), accidents or injuries at work, inadequate prenatal care and psychiatric disturbances. These last apparently occur more frequently among the immigrants than among the city population, probably on account of the tensions and frustrations involved in the need to adapt to an ecology with new food, weather, cost of living, social habits, type of work and living conditions.

Within industry, the immigrants are faced with working conditions different from those they are used to. They resent the changes in work shifts, the type of machinery and the working procedures; this gives rise to an inability to adapt, expressed as absenteeism and more frequent and more serious illnesses or accidents at work.

The immigrant workers, for the most part males, have left behind their family and friends; they feel that the loneliness is something beyond their control and in addition they have a particular worry about their family that is often disregarded, but which is very real to the immigrants: whether or not their children benefit from the money sent by the father, they suffer from the emigration of the breadwinner, and the mother or grandmother under whose care they are left complains of the difficulties of bringing them up once the parental authority has been removed.

E. Possible Solutions

The health services at the disposal of the immigrant population are diverse as\far as their administrative basis, type of service, financing, etc. are concerned. They can be government-run or private; preventive or curative; free or paying; compulsory, periodic or sporadic.

If in theory the immigrant population possesses the same rights as the inhabitants of the big city, in practice it only makes use of them as a last resort, and for the most part makes no use of them, either through ignorance of them, difficulties in adapting, or because it has only a poor idea of the cultural and economic values that circulate in the big city.

As a general rule, all the established health services of a city should be available to all the inhabitants. In only a few places are there hospitals devoted exclusively to the care of immigrants and their relatives; in others there are small sections that deal with severe emergencies or provide preventive medical care. These centres may have been set up by the government, as a result of private initiative, or by the industry that employs the immigrants.

In the case of immigrant workers, there are some countries whose health authorities carry out very detailed medical examinations usually repeated at frequent intervals; simultaneously information is supplied on customs, food, clothing, climate, housing and working methods. In this last case, a start is made with simple tasks such as instructing them on the prevention of accidents. This is just one way to help the immigrant to adapt to new working conditions.

To deal with the complex health problems peculiar to the immigrant in the big city a wide variety of organisations and specialists is required. For medical care and public health measures, it is most important to determine the type of immigration: whether it is permanent or temporary; whether it involves only men or all the family; if it was produced by the urge to seek new outlets or as a result of rural wretchedness, etc.

Planning and urbanisation studies dealing with waves of immigration must determine the land available, the building of new factories and industries, the availability of energy supplies, transport facilities, etc. On the basis of these facts, the type of medical services required can be determined.

Success depends on a multidisciplinary and global focusing of attention on the problem; each nation and each community should study in detail the tendencies and characteristics of its migratory flow. In all cases it is necessary to extend the cover provided by the health services to the immigrant population which more often than not lives on the edges of the big cities, without access to even the basic health services. Priority must be given to socio-economic aspects, the control of transmissible diseases, mental health, mother-and-child care, poor nutrition and the improvement of the environment.

The extension of the cover implies not only an increase in activity and resources with the aim of achieving a rapid and definable change in the situation, but also requires the prior defining of health policies in such a way as to make clear and explicit the concept of the cover, the strategies for attaining it and, thereby, the human, social, technical and administrative solutions. Each country will need to work out specifications to ensure that the cover satisfies the needs of the immigrant population within its own socio-economic context and that it is in line with the magnitude and true nature of the problems.

With the health problems of immigrants it is not possible to set out a predetermined system or method, with only one category of staff, a fixed demarcation of functions and a single organisation. The appropriate solution will vary with the city concerned, the type of government, and the needs of the city. It is not a universal solution that has to be sought, but integral planning and the rationalisation of the individual migratory movement.

It would be erroneous to consider that immigrations are always detrimental. In many cases they are movements of value because the intake of men who have already been 'shaped' helps the sector that receives them. Demographic strategies are based on social aspects. The same is true of the management of health resources for the immigrants.

In Mexico we have come to the conclusion that the demographic problem has two particular sides to it: the high birth rate and the movement of migrants, the latter being basically of country people moving to towns. For Mexico as a whole, the poles of migratory attraction are, principally, Mexico City, Guadalajara and some towns along the northern frontier zone, e.g. Mexicali, a town which quadrupled its population in only ten years from 174,000 to nearly 700,000, so that the various social services, among them the health services, became inadequate. As the health problems presented were for the most part soluble ones, like diarrhoea, gastro-enteritis and intestinal parasitosis, we attacked them by improving the sanitary infrastructure, carrying out schemes which included supply of drinking water, drainage, pumping plants and storage tanks. A similar solution has been used in other parts of the country, particularly in the outskirts of the capital city.

With our scarce resources, we are trying to provide equal services for all the population, whether migrants or not, by co-ordinating medical services of every kind. If immigrants have a permanent or prospective job, they are immediately covered by social security health services; if not, they can receive assistance from government services, which, as well as providing medical attention, run campaigns to promote health and prevent disease.

We are conscious that in many areas with similar movements of population, plans to discourage immigration have been useless. Education is seen as the long-term solution, so that, without abandoning these methods, we are proceeding with planning the following: programmes for community development, location of schools and industries outside towns, and arrangements seeking to achieve a rational distribution of population, without violating human freedom.

In summary, in Mexico solutions are aimed at the root of the problem, at rationalising immigration and providing services which promote health. Attempts are being made to ensure that immigrants are provided with similar services to those for the rest of the community, while at the same time, their particular needs are attended to.

Bibliography

Fisek, N.H. (1973). 'Turkey: workers' migrations [?and] health. The
    Immigrants in Europe', *World Health* (October), pp. 18-25.
    Geneva: WHO.
Fuentes, J.A. (1974). 'The Need for Effective and Comprehensive
    Planning for Migrant Workers', *American Journal of World Health*,
    vol. 64, no. 1 (January), pp. 2-10. Washington, DC.
Gould, D. (1973). 'British paradoxes. The immigrants in Europe',
    World Health (October), pp. 12-17. Geneva: WHO.
Loskant, H. (1973). 'A Spaniard outside Spain. The immigrants in
    Europe', *World Health* (October), pp. 26-9. Geneva: WHO.
Panamerican Health Organization (1975). 'Demographic Data on the
    Americas', *Bulletin of the Panamerican Health Organization*, vol.
    LXXVIII, no. 5 (May), pp. 460-7. Washington, DC.
World Health Organization (1976). 'Problems of hygiene at work and
    means to resolve them', *WHO Chronicle*, 30, pp. 344-51. Geneva.
Valenzuela, J. and Vernez, G. (1974). 'Popular building and structures
    of the housing market: the case of Bogotá', *Revista Interamericana
    de Planificacion*, vol. VIII, no. 31 (September). Bogota, Colombia.

18 DETERMINING HOSPITAL NEEDS

Odair P. Pedroso and Associates

In the past, the operation of Brazilian hospitals was technically oriented by the findings of experts from more developed countries. However, during these last thirty years, Brazilian hospital experts have become, in a more objective way, aware of the problems of our country and since then foreign data have been used more critically, even though we continue to look for modern patterns from abroad in order to develop our own technology. A new awareness of ecological conditions influencing the diverse regions of our country, of the degree of cultural development, of the existing patterns of communications and, lately, of our specific social and economic problems have permitted us to look at our own situation in a realistic manner.

There is no doubt that the large centres of population and technology are poles of attraction in many contexts, including the search for better health facilities, and no one doubts that the number of beds per 1,000 inhabitants of these centres should be higher than the provision in smaller or less developed areas. The same point was made by Mountin, Pennel and Hoge, of the Public Health Service of the United States, in a paper published in 1945, in which the rates of 4.5 to 5.5 beds per 1,000 inhabitants were accepted as values situated between the 'theoretical and practical' ideal ones. Before reaching this conclusion the authors made a careful study of the bed/population ratios and according to them the figure of 4.5 beds per 1,000 inhabitants is reasonable, if the following conditions are observed:

(1) 'These beds should accommodate all those needing hospitalization, except tuberculosis or mentally ill patients;'
(2) 'the factors that make hospitalization difficult, such as: distance, insufficient accommodation, financial incapacity, unwillingness of the patients to be admitted, should be avoided or reduced to a minimum;'
(3) 'the hospitals should be used, at least, to 80% of their capacity.'

The authors find the utilisation of 4.5 to 5.5 beds per 1,000 population justifiable rates, although below the theoretical idea, based on the facts that:

(a)   'A coordinated scheme of administration of any programme of hospital development should present large fluctuations in the utilization of the existing hospitals;'
(b)   'The harmonic increase of the bed rates in all the areas, at a reasonable level, could avoid excess of constructions.'

According to the standards followed by this study, cities with 250 or more hospital beds would be considered main centres, and those with 100 to 249 secondary centres. Areas with 50 to 99 beds would be called potentially secondary centres and those with less than 50 beds would be denominated isolated districts. The grouping of these different types of areas and cities would form regions and districts, in which a chain of hospitals would function in a hierarchically co-ordinated manner.

The authors proposed 6.5 beds per 1,000 inhabitants for the main centre; 5.0 for the secondary centre; 4.0 for the potentially secondary centre; and 2.5 for the isolated district. The variation in the rate is fully justified, since larger centres (principal and secondary ones) ought to receive a higher number of patients, due to their provision of highly specialised practices.

We do not know how the authors established the 4.5 beds per 1,000 inhabitants rate, but their study is one of great value, since it gives precise indications of how we might proceed in the distribution of beds. We must remember, however, that we cannot suppose that all the cities or counties in the same region or in one state should have the same bed rate. Undoubtedly the larger and wealthier centres attract a larger number of physicians and create a tendency to specialise. As a result, sick people from other localities head in that direction, seeking this type of medical care. This factor, therefore, should be considered in the determination of the hospital bed rate for such communities.

In 1946, the Hill-Burton law was approved by the United States government. According to this law, the American government should help the states in their hospitals construction, providing the bed rate did not exceed 4.5 beds per 1,000 population, this rate referring to general hospitalisation. For chronic diseases, the government set a limit of 2 beds per 1,000 inhabitants.

Also in 1946, a book entitled *Hospital Resources and Needs*, a report of the Michigan Hospital Survey, a W.K. Kellogg foundation publication, similar rates were obtained, following, however, different criteria. A formula is presented, but textually it is said that the study does not presume to supply a complete answer to the problem of calculating hospital bed needs, since a careful and detailed search of the multiple local factors should be considered. However, it does give a more reasonable basis in order to evaluate bed needs than the former methods that utilised arbitrary indices.

The report goes on to suggest that the needs of general hospital beds, in a given area, depend on the actual and future volume of diseases the treatment of which requires hospitalisation. However, a complete analysis of morbidity is rarely possible, since a survey of diseases is very expensive and it is difficult to show a definite relationship between the morbidity data and the hospital bed needs. Thus, another solution must be found.

It was demonstrated that vital and hospital statistics show that in the USA, as a whole, people utilised around 250 days (total of patient-days divided by the number of deaths in a given period) of general hospital assistance for every death and its correlated diseases. This ratio can be expressed in terms of occupied beds per death, dividing 250 (hospital days) by 365 (days of the year) which would give us, roughly, a rate of 0.7. In other words, for each hospital death, 7/10 of a bed was used per year. The practical value of this rate is that it can be used in the prediction of how many additional beds would be necessary, if more deaths (and correlated diseases) took place in the hospital.

The validity of utilising the bed/death rate as an estimating factor is based on the fact that such a rate varies little from state to state and thus can be used to determine the needs of occupied beds in specific communities and local areas. The bed/death rate could be modified from time to time, but its fluctuation would not be evident in short intervals. Its utilisation is simple, since the number of occupied beds necessary is the product of the bed/death rate and the percentage of deaths that one would expect of the hospitalised patients. However, even though we know the number of deaths, the determination of those that we would expect to happen in the hospital is a question of subjective judgement.

In 1936, 33.2 per cent of all the deaths in Michigan occurred in general hospitals. In 1944, the percentage rose to 37.8 per cent and in 1946 reached almost 50 per cent in some states. The Michigan Hospital Survey Committee proposed that, for this state as a whole, at least 50 per cent of the deaths should occur in general hospitals. So, if the mean death rate in Michigan between 1942 and 1944 was around 10.1, the general hospital rate would be 5.05.

The number of occupied beds 'necessary' for 1,000 inhabitants in the state is therefore 0.7 (bed/death rate) × 5.05 = 3.54 (occupied beds). As the occupation of the hospital beds was 75 per cent, the number of beds necessary for 1,000 inhabitants would be 4.72 (3.54 divided by 75 multiplied by 100).

The same experts add that this process could be used to determine the beds necessary in sectors of a state, even for small communities, but it is important to apply it carefully, since it refers only to the residents of the community, and therefore various other factors should be considered when attempting to determine the number of hospital beds needed. It is better to apply, for small communities, the general rate obtained for the state, correcting it for obvious local factors.

Similar results were obtained by the Commission on Hospital Care for the country as a whole (USA) applying the method used in Michigan. In fact, this Commission was the same as that which made the study in the state already referred to.

In 1948, we applied the technique just mentioned in an inland county of the state of Sao Paulo and an increase in the number of hospital beds was proposed as a result. The rate worked out at that time was 4.8 beds per 1,000 inhabitants. The county population was 33,843, the average number of patient-days being 14,077 and the number of hospital deaths 51. The annual number of deaths in the county was 500 on average. Only 10 per cent of that total were hospital ones. So, if the number of hospital deaths happened to go up from 10 per cent to 30 per cent of the county's general mortality, we would need some 4.8 beds per 1,000 population at a 68 per cent bed occupancy.

In 1975 we went over the calculations again, to re-establish the county's bed needs and the following results were obtained:

(a)   the county population went up from 33,843 to 43,911 inhabitants;

(b)   the number of general deaths in the county went down to 491, and the general mortality rate went down from 14.8 to 11.18.

The hospital bed needs were in fact overestimated, due to the average covering only about 90 per cent of our population.

On the other hand, according to the growth of the county's population (which was not properly followed due to suspect local statistical data) the number of hospital beds would grow at the same rate, since it was planned under a pavilion system of construction. In fact in December 1975, the actual number of beds per 1,000 population in this inland county was 4.94 compared to the figure of 4.8 estimated in 1948 for 1975.

These data warn us to be very cautious when studying bed needs for a determined population, since several unpredictable factors may interfere with the calculations, especially if these are being projected on a medium- or long-term basis.

As we can see in the tables presented in Chapter 8, the county of Sao Paulo, in 1975, had 22,959 general hospital beds in 127 hospitals. The total of patient-days was 6,214,723 and there were 764,835 discharges and 31,949 deaths. The total number of deaths in the county in 1975 was 64,253 and the death rate per 1,000 was 8.69.

Applying the formula, we find the following:

$$\frac{\text{Total patient-days}}{\text{Total deaths}} = \frac{6,214,723}{31,949} = 194.5 \ .$$

This means that the people of the county of Sao Paulo utilised 194.5 days of general hospital care for each death and correlated diseases. This ratio expressed in terms of occupied beds per death gives the rate of:

$$\frac{194.5 \text{ hospital days}}{365 \text{ days of the year}} = 0.53 \ .$$

This value 0.53 is the bed/death rate, meaning that for each hospital death, 0.53 of a bed was used per year.

The data show that 64,253 deaths occurred in the county of Sao Paulo during 1975 and, the total deaths occurring in general hospitals during the same year being 31,949, it is evident that around 50 per cent of the deaths of the county occurred in hospitals.

We know that in some hospitals, mainly the non-profit ones, there is a refusal list for admissions (for example for the Santa Casa de Misericordia with 1,000 beds, the rate is two refusals for one admission; at the Hospital das Clinicas with more than 1,500 beds, 3 patients are refused for every patient admitted). Besides this, the length of stay of the patients in the county of Sao Paulo is very low — 8.3 days — if compared with the length of stay in the United States. However, we should not expect that our county could have a hospital length of stay as low as in the US, knowing that the standards of living of our people are far lower than the people of that country; we still live in an era of communicable diseases, an era now past in other countries.

With the data we obtained a bed/death coefficient of 0.53 — yet we would like to have 70 per cent of the deaths occurring in our hospitals. Therefore, applying the formula already presented we have:

Bed/death coefficient of desired deaths in hospitals = 3.13.

However, as only 80 per cent of the beds are occupied, the corrected coefficient of beds per 1,000 inhabitants would be 3.91. This means that, at that time (end of 1975), Sao Paulo was in need of 7,000 more beds. Using the same rate, 3.91 per 1,000 inhabitants, projected requirements are shown in Table 18.1.

Table 18.1: Projection of Bed Requirement to the Year 2000

	Population estimate	Beds required
1980	9,027,605	35,297
1985	11,301,425	44,188
1990	14,147,960	55,318
1995	17,711,465	69,251
2000	22,172,523	86,694

This means that for the year 2000, more than 80,000 beds should be planned. The only way in which this demand could be mitigated would be through some strategy of population control or some health programme that could cut the ratio of beds per 1,000 inhabitants from 3.91 to a more reasonable rate.

19 THE AUXILIARY MEDICAL SERVICE OF HONG KONG

George K.C. Tong

In Hong Kong there is at present a population of 4.5 million people residing over a total territorial area of 400 square miles (see Chapter 9). Hong Kong is particularly prone to disasters in view of its geographical location and topography. Such disasters, which occur especially during the summer months, include typhoons (sometimes called cyclones), rainstorms, flooding and landslides. The house collapses which often follow as the direct result of these happenings involve considerable loss of life and property.

In order to minimise the effects of these natural disasters, the government of Hong Kong formulated emergency plans as early as 1950. The formation of auxiliary units to assist the regular forces is just one of the precautionary implementations.

Formation

In 1950 it was intended that one of the auxiliary units would be a corps of professional doctors and nurses together with trained auxiliary members who would perform tasks to augment the regular medical and health services in times of need. The Auxiliary Medical Service was therefore inaugurated with a membership of some 2,000 volunteers.

Organisation

Despite its meagre membership in 1950, the Auxiliary Medical Service (AMS) has grown from strength to strength with a current membership of nearly 6,000 volunteers, most of whom are aged between 20 and 30 years. These members come from all walks of life, and there are about 4,000 such youngsters in this segment. The other 1,600 or so professionals comprise doctors and nurses working either with the government or in private practice, plus pharmacists, dispensers, radiographers and paramedical personnel who are also willing to render services in times of need. It could be said that it is through the AMS link that many professionals manage to maintain association with the government authorities year after year.

By law the Director of Medical and Health Services of Hong Kong is the Unit Controller of the AMS. This enables the Director to exercise powers to mobilise personnel of the auxiliary unit under his command for reinforcing existing facilities, whether in peacetime or in overcoming a crisis in an emergency. The availability of auxiliary resources whether in terms of manpower or equipment is never far away.

Broadly speaking, the organisation of the AMS could be outlined as follows:

(a)   the hospital section;
(b)   the ambulance section;
(c)   the administration sub-units (which include: transport and general supplies section; food and fuel section; and pay and records section).

Obviously the majority of AMS members are allocated to either the hospital section or the ambulance section for operational purposes. Members of the administrative sub-units comprise only a minority.

Roles and Functions

The roles and functions of the AMS could be described as follows:

(1)   With its corps of professionals and trained auxiliaries, to augment the medical and health services in the event of emergencies.
(2)   In the event of a major disaster requiring the mobilisation of the AMS, then emergency medical facilities would be available from the AMS to treat the injured on the spot, to convey casualties to hospitals, and to care for patients at both acute and convalescent hospitals.
(3)   With its team of uniformed and disciplined members trained in ambulance manning techniques, to reinforce the regular ambulance service of Hong Kong.
(4)   The provision of Mobile First Aid Parties to work in conjunction with rescue forces in the saving of life.

Hospital Section at Work

If and when a major disaster should occur and the AMS were to be mobilised, then the hospital section would be alerted to establish the following:

(1)   Dressing Stations (DSN)

Dressing Stations are housed mainly in government clinics, with some

in private clinics and others in suitable medical institutions. Their
role is twofold:
   (i)   To provide the everyday clinic services as far as possible so
   that the general population can receive treatment for illness or
   injury not necessarily due to the emergency.
   (ii)   To act as a buffer to the casualty clearing hospitals by
   treating the lightly injured and returning the less seriously injured
   for treatment and observation.

(2)   Casualty Clearing Hospital (CCH)

Formulated in the Emergency Hospital Scheme is the list of government and civil hospitals which are earmarked to receive casualties in
the event of major emergencies. When mobilisation orders are issued
each casualty clearing hospital will be reinforced by AMS personnel
and emergency supplies, thereby rendering these hospitals suitable for
accepting casualties from the incident site. In real terms these
hospitals will provide additional acute beds to the extent of several
thousand.

(3)   Convalescent Units (CU)

In a major emergency it is likely that all the beds of the casualty
clearing hospitals will be filled in a very short time. Plans have been
made therefore to create 'relief' hospitals by making use of private
hospitals and major government buildings, such as schools and colleges.
The intention is not to admit cases direct to convalescent units but to
use them for the continuation treatment of those patients who can be
moved from casualty clearing hospitals soon after surgery. This would
ensure that throughout the emergency empty beds are available at
every acute hospital.

(4)   Forward Medical Aid Units (FMAU)

These are mobile units each with an AMS staff of 1 medical officer,
2 auxiliary nurses (female), 8 auxiliary dressers (male) and 1 driver.
Forward medical aid units are based on casualty clearing hospitals and
their function is to render resuscitation and medical aid to casualties
at disaster sites with the minimum of delay.

Organisation of Ambulance Section

The ambulance section of the AMS consists of a few thousand
uniformed and disciplined members who upon mobilisation will be
deployed either to work at disaster sites to save life, or to be affiliated

to the regular ambulance service for casualty evacuation. AMS ambulance depots are organised on the basis of one depot per district, and throughout Hong Kong there are established 36 such depots each with an organisation of two sub-units of 36 officers and members. For ease of control the districts conform to those under police and fire command. Personnel of this section are based at their respective AMS ambulance depots, each of which is under the over-all command of a medical officer. In practice, these members group themselves into either mobile first aid parties (4 members) ready to be deployed for tasks at disaster sites, or into ambulance crews (3 members) to staff and man ambulances.

Briefly the functions of the ambulance section are:

(1)   to treat casualties before transporting them to hospital;
(2)   to hold severely injured casualties for such time as is necessary to ensure safe (medical) evacuation;
(3)   to evacuate casualties to hospitals by all available means.

Duties of the medical officer are:

(1)   to undertake the immediate treatment of severely injured casualties before or after their removal from the scene of the incident;
(2)   to advise members of first aid parties on the application of first aid and handling of casualties;
(3)   to give instructions on the priorities of casualty evacuation.

Training

Except for members of the medical and nursing profession, training is offered to volunteers at weekends and on public holidays. Upon joining the service, every recruit is required to receive an initial 40-hour training period in basic first aid. Thereafter further training related to casualty handling, nursing, the manning of an ambulance and various other practical training at hospital wards and casualty departments is available on an individual basis. Members are also offered training in the field of junior leadership, supervisory techniques and officer training. Throughout the training curricula great emphasis is placed on the inspiration in members of the spirit of service to others of the community.

Emergency Supplies

In order to ensure success of AMS operations, emergency supplies have
been stockpiled at various government clinics and hospitals. All in all,
these supplies are dispersed over some 50 sub-unit stores in both the
urban and rural areas. Essential items range from a simple bandage for
first aid to complex surgical instruments for an operating theatre;
from simple utensils to feed patients to large-scale equipment to
convert a school into a casualty hospital. There are several thousand
blankets and camp beds in stock and millions of bandages and swabs
on the inventory lists. To facilitate control over these items the
equipment has been classified into the following categories:

List A —	*Hardware*	to enable hospital wards to be fully equipped and ancillary services to be maintained
List B —	*Linen material*	these include bed sheets, gowns, and clothing for patients
List C —	*Bandages and dressings*	Also included are cotton wool, gauze, swabs and other items
List D —	*Surgical instruments*	Separate scales are maintained for dressing stations, casualty clearing hospitals and convalescent units
List E —	*Emergency drugs*	these are regularly inspected and replaced by government pharmacy staff
List F —	*Stationery*	these include essential records and stationery required for administrative purposes.

All items of emergency stores are inspected regularly with a view
to ensure the highest degree of serviceability. Where possible, stores
such as linen materials are packed and sealed in 44-gallon drums in
order to prolong the life-span of these materials.

Peacetime Role

Besides being in full readiness to perform emergency roles and
functions all members of the AMS organise themselves in peacetime
in various activities designed to render service to the community.
During weekends and public holidays members work with the regular
staff of the ambulance service in order to learn more and to serve in a
wider field. Many members staff first aid posts at public functions

likely to be attended by large crowds, whilst many more volunteer to act as lifeguards on public beaches and make good use of their knowledge of resuscitation and first aid.

The Auxiliary Medical Service so far has spared no effort in augmenting the regular medical and health services whenever necessary. Members have been mobilised and deployed to assist at mass educational schemes on health and campaigns against epidemics, and on a few occasions have staffed and administered cholera quarantine centres for the Medical and Health Department.

Currently members of the Auxiliary Medical Service are assisting the department in duties at four methadone maintenance centres (daytime); and are themselves staffing and controlling 16 methadone detoxification centres which operate only in the evening (6 pm to 10 pm). All duty members are trained for such procedures as conducting nalline tests and dispensing methadone linctus.

It has been nearly 27 years since the inauguration of the AMS. During its history members have on numerous occasions attended scenes of catastrophe in order to save life. They have been present either as individuals or in groups at scenes of fires, traffic accidents, landslides, floodings, etc., in order to render first aid and to evacuate casualties. Their preparedness to serve in all emergencies has won respect from all segments of the local community. It can be concluded that 'whatever the size of the emergency, the function of the Auxiliary Medical Service is a practical exercise in good citizenship and fellowship'.

20 THE BARANGAY—HEALTH CENTRE LINKAGE IN THE METROPOLITAN MANILA HEALTH CARE DELIVERY SYSTEM*

Gabriel G. Carreon and Associates

Introduction

The Philippines is a Third World developing nation in south-east Asia. It has a population of approximately 44 million and continues to grow at a rate of 2.7 per cent annually. This rapid growth tends to place an increased burden on health services. Health statistics and details of its provision are presented in Chapter 10.

The Department of Health (the national government health agency), in co-operation with the National Economic Development Authority, has formulated a National Health Plan with the goal of raising the level of health of the general population. The rationale behind this plan is that good health services result from the collective effort of various institutions delivering health care. Since the environment and socio-economic forces influence the state of health, the citizenry is also called upon to take an active role in promoting health as a way of life.

The said plan presents the National Health Care Delivery System in terms of three levels of health care: primary, secondary and tertiary. This system involves the government and private sectors and integrates all centres of health care into a comprehensive network of health facilities.

The general and specialised government medical centres, the teaching and university hospitals and the private medical centres provide tertiary health care services. The community, emergency, municipal, city, provincial and regional hospitals provide a broad complex of secondary care facilities. The health centres, rural health units, puericulture centres, clinics in industrial and commercial firms and the clinics of private practitioners form the extensive base of primary health facilities which is the general entry point in health care.

The Department of Health administers the bulk of the government services in the country. They are composed of 894 hospitals with a

* Dr Carreon's associates in the preparation of this chapter are listed in Appendix A at the end of this chapter. Further acknowledgements are included in Appendix B.

total bed capacity of 65,185 and 1,560 primary health care units.
These facilities are dispersed in the twelve regions of the country.
Among these regions is the Metro Manila Area (MMA).

Metropolitan Manila covers about 636 square kilometres of land,
with an estimated population in 1975 of seven million. It is composed
of four cities and thirteen municipalities, within which live around
1,830 barangays, for a description of which see below. For effective
and economical administration, however, these cities and municipalities are grouped into four sectors or districts.

The general health condition of MMA approximates that of the
over-all Philippine setting. To meet the health care needs in the area
there are some 156 hospitals with a total bed capacity of 26,547 and
303 primary health care centres. The over-all health facility to
population ratios in the MMA are as follows:

(a)	hospital to population	1:45,144;
(b)	hospital bed to population	1:265;
(c)	health centre to population	1:23,242.

The Metro Manila Commission governs the area with a fair amount
of autonomy as one of the country's regions. The responsibility for
planning, organising, integrating and developing the MMA's health
and sanitation services is vested in the Action Officer for Health and
Sanitation Services. Final decisions, however, are made by the Governor
of the Commission unless explicitly delegated to the Action Officer.

Following the creation of the Commission's Health and Sanitation
Services in November 1975, the Action Officer established the organisation for these services with the following aims:

(1)   to develop the health and sanitation services (including
structures, methods and facilities) in the MMA;
(2)   to ensure the availability, accessibility, adequacy and continuity of health and sanitation services to the population of the
said area, especially to those who could barely afford the present
health care costs (the so-called 'medically indigent'); and
(3)   to maximise the utilisation of existing health and sanitation
facilities in the area.

Currently, the health and sanitation services in the MMA are
organised in a three-level manner as laid out in the National Health
Plan mentioned earlier. The categories of health services rendered

(primary, secondary and tertiary) are co-ordinated as well as inter-linked with one another and with their clientele through a referral system.

The reasons for this health referral system are as follows:

(1)   each health agency must be interlinked with other health institutions so that the desired total package of services can be delivered to the community;

(2)   within a given locality, there must be systematic co-ordination of all health service outlets in a three-layered concept to avoid overlapping, duplication and fragmentation of services;

(3)   through a hierarchical system of interdependent and inter-related health agencies, maximum utilisation of resources is attained.

In this regard, the Metro Manila health referral system addresses itself to the following objectives:

(1)   to link the consumers of care, particularly the medically indigent patients, with the appropriate health service resources;

(2)   to ensure availability, accessibility and continuity of care to patients; and

(3)   to maximise the utilisation of existing health agencies and facilities within the region.

This referral system defines the catchment area to be served by each of the health facilities and interconnects the facilities with one another operationally and, ultimately, with the recipients of health care in a two-way manner. Thus a tertiary care centre is linked with two or more secondary care hospitals while a secondary care hospital serves several health centres. The health centre, which serves a number of barangays, is the entry point into the health care system.

The Barangay-Health Centre Linkage

Enhancement of the quality of life is a basic desire of every man, community or nation. Good health is a significant component of this goal. This objective can be best achieved by a health agency or a network of health service outlets operating with the enlightened involvement of the individual and the community. Successful health care, therefore, needs the individual and the community as major participating elements while a health agency provides the technology and expertise required in the process. Thus, collaboration is a necessity among the providers of health services and their clientele. In this respect, the critical area of individual and community participation in the Metro Manila health care delivery system is the linkage between a specific barangay and a specific health centre.

The Barangay

A barangay is the smallest unit in the Philippine political structure. It is composed of at least one hundred families residing in a common area and is, therefore, a distinct community by itself. Barangay members face the same environmental forces and try to solve common problems or difficulties. To integrate individual efforts towards the enhancement of the quality of their community life, barangay members (who are at least fifteen years old) elect a barangay council. This council assumes responsibility for the welfare of the whole barangay.

The Health Centre

A health centre is a basic service unit in the Metro Manila health and sanitation structure. A typical health centre is manned by a basic staff of one physician, one dentist, one nurse, one midwife and one lay worker. It performs primary diagnostic and treatment services. Moreover, it provides basic health programmes and facilities such as nutrition, family planning, primary medical care, health education, tuberculosis control, maternal and child health care, immunisation and dental health. It is also responsible for monitoring the general health and sanitation conditions of the community and initiating appropriate measures in the area it is assigned to serve.

In the development of the health and sanitation services at the primary care level in MMA, the barangay councils, as well as the barangay constituents themselves, are encouraged to participate. Linkages between the health centres and the barangays are established in this manner.

The Linkage

The objectives of this barangay-health centre linkage are as follows:

(1) to increase the effectiveness of the health centre by maximising the use of existing health centre resources and developing the capabilities of the health centres;

(2) to ensure the continuity and availability of health services to the barangay;

(3)   to emphasise promotive and preventive health care; and
(4)   to promote active participation of the barangay members in the identification and solution of their community health problems.

Operationally, this linkage takes the following forms:

(1)   assignment of specific barangays to a specific health centre;
(2)   utilisation of the health centre by the members of the barangays it serves;
(3)   regular meetings between the barangay council and the health centre personnel;
(4)   participation of the barangay officials in health and sanitation campaigns of the health centre; and
(5)   establishment and operation of a barangay health post (BHP) in the barangay.

At present, each Metro Manila health centre serves an average of six barangays, or approximately 23,000 people, providing health and sanitation services as required. It therefore helps to improve and maintain the general health and sanitation conditions of a defined area. This catchment allocation also facilitates evaluation of the effectiveness of each health centre.

Usually, a health centre extends services primarily to members of the barangays it serves. Those who belong to other barangays, if they are non-emergency cases, are directed to their respective health centres. This feature 'compels' the recipients of health services to utilise the health centre assigned to them and likewise facilitates orderly keeping and updating of medical records. This procedure also ensures an equitable distribution of patient load among health centres, which helps in the efficient delivery of quality care. Health centres, in this manner, are also compelled to maintain a certain level of competence in terms of expertise and resources as the barangays continuously utilise them.

The Metro Manila health care delivery system encourages the barangays to express their views through the barangay council, which has regular meetings with health centre personnel. These meetings (usually held monthly) provide opportunities to formulate collectively measures or action plans to improve the health and sanitation of the community as well as to develop the responsiveness of the health centre itself. During such occasions, the barangay's problems and the health centre's programmes are discussed and analysed. Difficulties in the

implementation of projects and their corresponding causes are brought
to the attention of everyone concerned. Action plans which are within
the capability of the health centre and the barangay are mapped out.
This system introduces relevant and practical approaches and generates
a situational responsiveness that is well rooted for greater effectiveness.

Other ways by which community participation in the delivery
of health and sanitation services could be realised include the following:

(1)   Attendance by barangay members at training sessions conducted by the health centre. These sessions are designed to
improve the knowledge, skills and attitudes of barangay members
on individual and community health and sanitation practices.

(2)   Dissemination by barangay officials of health and sanitation
information and health centre policies and procedures through
pamphlets, posters or by word of mouth.

(3)   Implementation of health and sanitation measures and
practices in the community.

(4)   Assistance given by barangay officials and members during
immunisation campaigns by giving publicity and information,
identifying the immunisation centres and gathering the patients
accordingly.

The Barangay Health Post: Health Care Delivery at the Grass-Roots Level

Promotive and preventive health care is achieved in the community
where a symbiotic relationship exists between the clientele and the
providers of health services. In the Metro Manila Area, the establishment of the Barangay Health Post (BHP) strengthens collaboration
between the providers (health centres) and the consumers (barangays)
of health care. Manned by auxiliary health workers, the BHP serves
as a sub-station or an extension of the health centre in the barangay.
It broadens the base of primary health care by extending the
accessibility of the health centre to remote barangays. It increases
the capabilities of the health centre in providing information,
education and first aid.

The BHP addresses itself to the following objectives:

(1)   to strengthen and make more effective the current health
care delivery system in Metropolitan Manila by outreach activities;

(2)   to emphasise promotive and preventive health care;

(3)   to encourage the people to become self-directing in the

identification of personal, family and community health problems;
and
(4)   to ensure the continuity and availability of health services at
the barangay level by strengthening the barangay-health centre
linkage.

Given the above-mentioned objectives, the BHP assumes responsibilities for the following:

(1)   promotion of the community's awareness on proper health
and sanitation practices;
(2)   proper information linkage between the community and
the health centre;
(3)   organisation of community health action; and
(4)   provision of the simplest type of emergency care in the
community, such as treatment of wounds.

The BHP updates the barangay members' awareness of proper health
and sanitation practices *vis-à-vis* environmental changes, such as
increased incidence of gastro-enteritis during the summer and of
respiratory ailments during the rainy season. It implements the health
education programmes of the health centre by carrying out health and
sanitation campaigns among the barangay members, distributing
pamphlets and holding informal discussions with barangay members.
The BHP also conducts community surveys from time to time to
provide the bases for defining community health problems, and
designing appropriate programmes or improving existing ones. With
proper guidance and support from the health centre and the barangay
council, the BHP organises the community in the implementation of
specific community health activities such as immunisation and pest
eradication campaigns, deworming programmes and sanitation activities.

Establishing the Barangay Health Post (BHP)
The BHP is established in selected barangays. The required resources
are contributed by the health centre and the barangay. The health
centre provides the appropriate technology and expertise, especially
for training and development. For its part, the barangay provides the
physical structure and the necessary manpower (barangay health
workers — BHW). The BHP is a simple room in a dwelling where small
group meetings and emergency care can take place. Bigger group
meetings and health education sessions can take place in the barangay

hall or in the health centre, which are government-owned but serve as extensions of barangay activities. The local government can extend assistance through the provision of simple facilities (first-aid medicines, health education material, etc.) at the BHP or barangay hall and possibly even stipends or honoraria for the BHWs.

The following conditions in a barangay are necessary for the establishment and maintenance of a BHP:

(1)   the health centre is not easily accessible to the members of the barangay being served;
(2)   there are significant health needs in the barangay to be met due to overpopulation, poor sanitation, economic depression, etc.;
(3)   the idea of establishing and maintaining a BHP is acceptable to the community, its barangay council and the health centre personnel; the people involved are committed to implement and provide the requisite resources to the BHP.

The process of establishing a BHP includes the following activities:

(1)   selection of the barangay;
(2)   recruitment and training of barangay health workers;
(3)   implementation and evaluation.

The establishment of the BHP strengthens the proprietary attitude towards health programmes and the initiative to keep healthy at all times.

The Barangay Health Worker

Health service, in general, is expected to be rendered on a person-to-person basis. With the demands of a growing population and limited personnel and facility resources, there is a need to develop innovative responsiveness. Such responsiveness should be reasonably available and accessible and could be directed at various levels of service. On the basis of the country's major health problems, there is much to be gained by adequate information and education activities in the promotion of health and the prevention of disease. These activities do not necessarily require the full expertise of a physician or nurse. They can be implemented by a less qualified type of health practitioner, such as an auxiliary health worker.

In the Metro Manila area, there is a strong movement in community-orientedness where the young are especially involved. There is a growing desire of young barangay members to commit themselves to community welfare and development. This participation has been significantly evident during natural disasters such as floods and earthquakes and daily occurrences like traffic congestion. With the realisation of the possibility of using barangay members for health and sanitation activities, the concept of the barangay health worker has evolved and is progressively being developed in the Metro Manila Area.

The BHWs assume the role of community health workers, manning the health post and providing the dynamic element in the barangay-health centre linkage. Through continued monitoring of the community's health conditions they contribute vital information to both the barangay and the health centre for collaborative action. They are usually volunteers coming from the barangay itself. The BHW renders health services within his capabilities, disseminates health and sanitation information, reports on community health conditions and initiates and implements organised community health action in his barangay. His specific functions are listed below.

(a)   When he is in the BHP or in the field he:

(1)   participates in community health surveys and submits regular reports on the community health condition to the health centre;
(2)   reports cases of communicable diseases to the health centre immediately;
(3)   informs the barangay members about the services offered by the health centre, and performs information activities like issuing pamphlets, putting up posters and conducting discussions with barangay members, especially in nutrition and sanitation;
(4)   motivates couples in family planning, refers them to the health centres, seeks 'drop-outs', and issues supplies to recipients;
(5)   assists in immunisation campaigns and implements sanitation programmes;
(6)   provides advice on problems like fever, headache, diarrhoea, abdominal pain, constipation, colds and coughs, and simple skin conditions;
(7)   gives first-aid measures within his capabilities as a lay person in emergency cases such as febrile convulsions, vomiting, bleeding, injuries, burns, drowning, poisoning and dog bites;
(8)   refers patients to the health centre or hospital when necessary and if possible makes a follow-up on his referrals; and
(9)   advises patients on the use of common drugs.

(b)   When assigned to a health centre, he:

(1)   assists the physician in the treatment of emergencies such as wounds;
(2)   takes the temperature, pulse rate, respiratory rate, blood pressure and weight of patients;
(3)   assists in obtaining general patient data; and
(4)   performs such tasks as preparing cotton balls and preparing/ sterilising instruments and syringes.

Being a volunteer, the BHW renders services during his free time, which can be scheduled accordingly with his supervisor (the health centre physician or nurse). In view of this, it becomes desirable to develop groups of BHWs so that optimum coverage in time and place may be achieved. This arrangement does not rule out the future possibility of full-time BHWs working in the community, manning the BHPs and receiving stipends or honoraria from the local governments.

The BHW is recruited on the basis of his energy, inclination, potential and capabilities to perform his expected functions appropriately. More specifically, the minimum requirements for recruitment are:

(1)   he should be at least eighteen years of age;
(2)   he should have a minimum educational attainment of two years in the secondary or high school level;
(3)   he should show active interest and commitment in community welfare and development activities; and
(4)   he should be acceptable to and respected by the barangay members.

The BHW lives with the people he serves. This should enhance his commitment, acceptability and effectiveness.

The BHW Training Program seeks to contribute to the proper and speedy development of a system of health care delivery in Metro Manila through the training and development of barangay health workers prior to their actual work. It aims to achieve the following objectives:

(a)   to develop the necessary knowledge, skills and attitudes among BHWs to enable them to participate effectively as primary health service extension workers in the Metro Manila health care delivery system; and

(b)   to develop BHWs as links or intermediaries between the barangays and health centre serving them.

The programme contents include the following:

(1)   Public health: the health care delivery system in the country, particularly in Metro Manila area; proper referral of patients to health centres and hospitals; the team approach; integration of efforts; comprehensiveness in concept; the over-all picture of health and the programmes; statistics and reporting.

(2)   Family planning: BHWs are trained to become motivators for family planning recipients and 'drop-outs'. Subjects covered are population dynamics (growth, resource depletion, pollution), socio-cultural factors, types and methods of family planning, and motivating principles. The BHW learns how to refer recipients to the health centre or the family planning clinics.

(3)   On first aid and emergency care, the BHWs are taught the proper skills to render immediate assistance until the victim is referred to a centre, clinic or hospital. Specific situations are wounds, injuries, bleeding, burns, febrile convulsions, animal bites, artificial respiration and natural calamities.

(4)   Maternal and child health care: this contains lectures and discussions on health services for mothers and children, such as prenatal care, domiciliary obstetrical care, the lying-in clinic, the well-baby clinics, immunisation and early identification of abnormal pregnancies and infant/child development.

(5)   Community development: topics are observations and surveys to be made; how problems are identified in individuals, families and in the community and analysed accordingly; extensive discussions to be held with the barangays after which appropriate action is taken to arrive at solutions; how strong effort is made to involve private and civic organisations. Linkage with the health team is always kept in mind.

(6)   Prevention and control of communicable diseases: the BHWs are acquainted with the seasonal incidence of diseases; how to identify communicable diseases and the need to report them at once to the health centre; preventive and control measures; and immunisation.

(7)   Nutrition: based on identifying causes and features, the proper selection of food is emphasised.

(8)   Drug addiction: the social causes are elaborated upon. The

BHWs are briefed on how to identify prohibited drug users and the procedure of referring them for treatment.

(9)   Environmental sanitation: this is related to the prevention of contagious diseases and to health education. Topics include: proper food and water handling, laws related to environmental sanitation, insect and vermin control, personal hygiene, proper utilisation of sanitary facilities and proper garbage disposal.

The lectures, discussions, demonstrations and workshops take up a five-week period. A six-month field experience is advised under supervision of the health physician. During the formal training period, the health centre nurses act as preceptors. Resource speakers include the health centre physicians, invited experts and health educators from various health agencies and schools in the Metro Manila area. After the formal training period, the BHW works in his barangay and meets his supervisor at the health centre every week for consultation. Apart from this, the BHW is supervised from time to time in the field whenever he requests direct guidance and support, or when his supervisor deems it necessary. Evaluation and retraining periodically go on.

Summary

The involvement of the barangay health workers in community health and the introduction of the barangay health post suggest the possibility of strengthening the health care system at the grass roots. In a modified concept of the three levels of health care, the BHP may, therefore, serve as a first-level care centre emphasising preventive and promotive health measures, health education, information and sanitation. The health centres may thus partake of the role of second-level care units while the hospitals as a group serve as the third-level care units.

Thus the active participation of the recipients of health care is being utilised both in the delivery of health care as well as in the development of the programmes any system of care. In this way, the aspirations of both providers and recipients are closely co-ordinated and translated into practice. Such interaction motivates all people who are involved to improve their own health, and therefore leads to the promotion of a better quality of life.

Appendix A

Those who were associated with Dr Carreon in the production of this chapter were:

Ramon L. Arcadio, MD, Chairman, Department of Family Medicine, UP-PGH Medical Center, and Executive Officer, Metro Manila Health and Sanitation Services.
Alfredo T. Traballo, Jr, Research Associate, UP-PGH Medical Center.
Renato A. Atienza, Senior Research Assistant, UP-PGH Medical Center.
Thelma M. Reyes, MD, Medical Consultant in Family Medicine, UP-PGH Medical Center.

Appendix B: Acknowledgements

We, the authors, hereby extend our deep gratitude to the authorities and members of the Tondo Foreshore Development Project of the National Housing Authority for sharing their experience on the establishment of a Barangay Health Post in Dagat-Dagatan, Tondo, Manila. We also feel deeply indebted to the contributions and assistance of the following: the Metro Manila Health and Sanitation Services Committee on the Barangay Health Post Concept, composed of Dr Teodora V. Tiglao of the UP Institute of Public Health as Consultant, and Professor Minda Luz Quesada of the UP Institute of Public Health, Dr Mona Lisa Hitalia of UP-CCHP and Dr Rafael P. Bantayan, Jr, of the UP-PGH Department of Family Medicine as members; the group of Dr Fe Villanueva-Fernandez who shared some materials on their barangay health workers' training at Tatalon, Quezon City; the Pasay City Health Department, and the Manila Health Department. Finally, we would like to acknowledge the efforts of those who helped us in the preparation of our manuscript.

21 EMERGENCY MEDICAL SERVICES IN TOKYO

Katsumi Takahashi

Tokyo is a megalopolis with an area of 2,045.38 square kilometres and a population of 11,693,560. Regarding the establishment of effective emergency medical care, few problems are encountered in cities with a population of up to two or three hundred thousand. In a city with six to eight hundred thousand people, difficulties become apparent and it would seem that a population of one million is the limit for satisfactory planning of emergency services, because at this threshold mutual co-operation between hospitals becomes strained.

First, I would like to present an analysis of emergency patients entering the Musashino Red Cross Hospital (500 beds), one of the main hospitals on the outskirts of Tokyo proper, in comparison with those of the Santama region, and Tokyo as a whole. Table 21.1 indicates the approximate number of emergency cases in each section; while details of acute medical cases are shown in Table 21.2. The emergency cases hospitalised in the Red Cross Hospital in the past two months are listed in Table 21.3.

As can be seen, about 60 per cent of the emergency patients in Tokyo are medical cases, especially paediatric cases; traffic accident patients make up approximately 15 per cent. About fifteen years ago the number of traffic accidents increased markedly, in particular whiplash injury cases. At the same time there were insufficient emergency medical services and a shortage of neurosurgeons in Japan was first noted. Official and civil efforts in traffic safety have brought down the number of traffic accidents. For example, grade school pupils walk to school in groups, street bridges are provided for pedestrians, safety belts for car drivers and protective helmets for cyclists, etc., are required by law. Deaths due to traffic accidents have gradually decreased from the 1970 peak figure of 16,765 throughout all of Japan.

Since 1970, acute medical diseases have replaced traffic accidents as the principal call for the emergency ambulance services located in fire stations. In 1975 these acute medical emergency calls accounted for 55.8 per cent of all emergency calls received. Among the acute medical emergencies, cerebrovascular disease is the major killer in

354

Table 21.1: Number of Emergency Patients, Musashino Red Cross
Hospital, 1975

			Per cent
Total	7,050	Medical and paediatric	65.5
		Gynaecology and obstetrics	8.0
		Surgical	27.5
		Santama region	
Total	49,831	Medical and paediatric	57.0
		Traffic accidents	16.0
		Civil accidents	15.9
		Other	11.1
		Tokyo as a whole	
Total	247,559	Medical and paediatric	56.4
		Traffic accidents	14.8
		Civil accidents	15.8
		Other	13.0

Table 21.2: Details of Acute Medical Cases, 1974

			Per cent
Total	130,886	Cerebrovascular disease	11.4
		Cardiac disease	7.5
		Nervous system	6.8
		Respiratory system	11.9
		Digestive system	10.7
		Uncertain	41.8
		Other	9.9

Table 21.3: Two Months' Emergency Admissions, Musashino Red
Cross Hospital

	Number	Per cent
Medical	93	39
Paediatric	55	23
Surgical	37	15
Trauma	37	15
Gynaecology and obstetrics	18	8
Total	240	100

Table 21.4: Causes of Death

Rank	First	Second	Third	Fourth	Fifth
Year					
1930	Gastro-enteritis	Pneumonia	TB	CVD	Senility
1940	TB	Pneumonia	CVD	CD	Neoplasma
1950	TB	CVD	Pneumonia	CD	TB
1955	CVD	Neoplasma	Senility	CD	Pneumonia
1960	CVD	Neoplasma	CD	Senility	Accident
1965	CVD	Neoplasma	CD	Senility	Accident
1970	CVD	Neoplasma	CD	Accident	Senility
1975	CVD	Neoplasma	CD	Accident	Senility

CVD = Cerebrovascular disease
CD   = Cardiac disease

Japan, and therefore is one of the main causes of calls, along with cardiac disease, for emergency medical care. Table 21.4 shows the changes in the cause of death among Japanese people over a forty-five year period.

According to the statistics of the World Health Organization, the total of hospital beds available in Japan is almost equal to the number available in the USA and England. However, private hospitals and clinics make up 76.1 per cent of the hospital count and about 56.0 per cent of the total beds available.

The history of the public hospital in Japan is brief. Before the Meiji Restoration (1868) the Tokugawa government had established only one public hospital in Yedo (Tokyo). The Nagasaki hospital founded by the Dutch surgeon, Pompe, is also famous as a pioneer public hospital in Japan. During the years since the Meiji Restoration many public hospitals have been founded, including Red Cross hospitals such as the one at Musashino.

It must be added that any medical institution with more than twenty beds is called a hospital in Japan. Therefore there are a great number of small (mostly private) hospitals.

In Tokyo there are 501 registered hospitals caring for emergency cases (384 hospitals and 117 clinics) of which 466 are private and 35 public. There are 25 hospitals with more than 500 beds which provide emergency services, most of which are public (see Chapter 11 for further details).

The actual status of doctors and nurses on night duty in the hospitals is as follows: one specialist in internal medicine and paediatrics and, except at weekends, always one paediatric specialist; one surgeon who is either a neurosurgeon, urologist, or orthopaedic surgeon; and one gynaecologist-obstetrician. This staff is on duty each night for the care both of patients in the hospital and of emergency out-patients. In other words, the emergency unit of the hospital is not divorced from regular ward care as far as the doctors are concerned. As for nursing, there are three nurses on duty every night for the care of emergency patients. Most other hospitals have about the same number of medical personnel on night duty. Hospitals with radio-logical and laboratory technicians on night duty are quite exceptional. It is also to be noted that young doctors are not adequately trained in the care of emergency cases and trade union contracts in the hospitals make this problem more difficult. In view of these facts one can easily appreciate the importance of the central control facility which directs emergency cases to the hospitals and clinics.

Tokyo is divided into eight large divisions, somewhat parallel to the administrative divisions of the city, for referrals from the emergency ambulance services provided through local fire stations. These divisions are further divided into 146 subdivisions, each equipped with one ambulance. Each divisional centre is fully staffed and equipped and the central control regulates the divisional centres through the use of a computer and television network to which 470 of the 501 hospitals and clinics are connected. These 470 hospitals and clinics are classified in Table 21.5 according to bed count. Thus, although there is an adequate number of emergency medical institutions, 72 per cent of these are small hospitals and clinics with less than 100 beds and only one or a few doctors.

The authorities have undertaken the classification of these hospitals and clinics by the criteria of bed count and the number of specialists since the beginning of the emergency medical programme: that is, primary, secondary and tertiary hospitals. In other words, the primary institution is a small clinic or hospital with one or two doctors; the secondary is a middle-sized hospital with more than ten doctors, that is, a general hospital capable of special services; and the tertiary is the highly specialised centre prepared for the purpose of emergency medical care.

Under these circumstances, the role of the central control is very important. The rescue personnel in the ambulance arriving at the scene of the emergency should be able to diagnose the medical need and which class of hospital can give the needed care; then communicate this

Table 21.5: Classification of Hospitals and Clinics (by bed count)

Number of beds	Number of hospitals/clinics	Per cent
20	110	23
50	120	26
100	110	23
300	85	19
500	20	4
over 500	25	5
Total	470	100

Table 21.6: Distribution of Hospitals and Clinics among the Divisions and Subdivisions of Tokyo

Division number	1	2	3	4	5	6	7	8	Total
Number of subdivisions	14	12	14	17	22	13	18	36	146
Hospitals	40	62	39	58	92	48	41	90	470
(clinics)	(4)	(3)	(4)	(4)	(5)	(1)	(2)	(2)	(25)
Population				8,653,000			3,040,000		11,693,000

information to the divisional centre for confirmation and direction to the proper institution. Sometimes it is necessary to communicate with primary, secondary and even tertiary emergency centres to receive the proper care. This communication and co-operation between the secondary and tertiary hospitals is crucial. However, such ideals are not always practical, and co-operation is not always satisfactory. In most cases, it is possible within seconds or minutes to direct the emergency to a properly equipped hospital for treatment. However, we also find from time to time an unfortunate case, such as an ambulance with a patient having a severe head injury, wandering for more than an hour seeking a suitable hospital. This happens occasionally during the small hours of the night and on holidays.

One additional remark needs to be added. We do not yet have an ambulance service staffed by doctors, and helicopter rescue is exceptional even in Tokyo. There is an Association of Emergency Medical Institutions which was established in 1965 and an Annual Congress of the Japanese Association for Acute Medicine which has met since

1973. The journal of this Congress has already gone into Volume III.

Finally I would like to point out two urgent problems for the improvement of emergency medical service in Japan. The first is to emphasise the role which needs to be taken by the large public hospitals. We need to be more adequately equipped to deal with acute cases such as traumatic shock and infectious disease which are among the more urgent needs of the population. These needs cannot be too strongly exaggerated for a megalopolis like Tokyo.

The second problem is to establish a good training course for primary care during the post-graduate period of all newly qualified doctors. This must be obligatory to all graduates who aim to be a physician or surgeon, because I believe that emergency medical care is the most needed among the many varieties of medical service.

NOTES ON CONTRIBUTORS

[as at May 1977]

Dr Anthony I. Adams is Director of the Division of Health Services Research, Health Commission of New South Wales, Sydney, Australia.

Mr George B. Allen is President of the Hospital Association of New York State (HANYS). He joined the association in 1962, has served as chief executive officer since 1971 and was appointed President in 1974.

Dr Jaime Arias is at present Secretary of Health for Bogotá and a Visiting Assistant Professor at Mount Sinai Medical Center in New York.

Dr Robert F. Bridgman (formerly Inspector-General of Social Affairs, Paris; and formerly Chief Medical Officer, Organisation of Medical Care, WHO, Geneva).

Dr Gabriel G. Carreon is Director of the Philippine General Hospital and Action Officer for Health and Sanitation Services, Metropolitan Manila Commission. He is also currently Professor of Medicine at the University of the Philippines.

Mme Eve Errahmani is Director of Studies at the Regional Health Observatory, Prefecture of the Ile-de-France Region of France.

Mr Miles Hardie became Deputy Director of the King's Fund Hospital Centre when it opened in 1963 and was Director from 1966 until 1975 when he took up his present post as Director-General of the IHF.

Mr R. Alan Hay has been Executive Director of the Ontario Hospital Association since 1966. He is a past President of the Canadian Hospital Association and was also delegate for Canada in the House of Delegates of the American Hospital Association for five years from 1968.

Professor Kenzo Kiikuni joined the newly created National Institute of Hospital Administration, Government of Japan, in 1961 and worked as a senior researcher until his appointment as a Professor of Social Medicine at the Institute of Community Medicine of the University of Tsukuba in 1977.

Mrs Edith Morgan is Deputy Director of MIND (the National Association for Mental Health). She initially worked in the Clinical and Social Services Department, but in 1960 was invited to set up a new section of MIND to guide the development of voluntary community mental health groups (local associations).

Dr Guillermo Fajardo Ortiz is President of the Mexican Hospital Association and Executive Director of the Latin American Hospital Federation. He is also a former member of the IHF Council of Management.

Dr Odaïr P. Pedroso has been Professor of Hospital Administration and Dean of the School of Public Health of the University of Sao Paulo since 1951. He is also President of the Brazilian Hospital Association.

Dr S. David Pomrinse is currently Executive Vice-President of both the Mount Sinai Medical Center and the Mount Sinai Hospital, as well as being Edmond A. Guggenheim Professor and Chairman of Administrative Medicine, Mount Sinai School of Medicine of the City University of New York.

Dr John C. Rossman has been Director of Health Economics at the Hospital Association of New York State since 1970, and before this was a consultant for the Hospital and Educational Research Fund of the Association.

M Jean-Marc Simon is a former legal adviser to the Minister of Health, and in 1976 became Director of Planning, Assistance Publique, Paris, and lecturer in Health Economics at the National School of Public Administration.

Mr Arthur E. Starling served on the Commissioning Unit of the Queen Elizabeth Hospital of Hong Kong which was opened in 1963. He has also been secretary to a number of other major government hospitals in Hong Kong and in 1969 was appointed Chief Hospital Secretary. He is also a part-time lecturer in hospital administration at the Extra

Mural Department of Hong Kong University.

Dr Katsumi Takahashi is currently chief surgeon to Musashino Red Cross Hospital, lecturer at Tokyo Medical-Dental University, a Councillor of the Japanese Society of Clinical Surgery, and a Member of the Board of Directors of the Japanese Association for Acute Medicine.

Mr George K.C. Tong served for many years as a volunteer member of the Hong Kong civil defence organisation – the Civil Aid Services, which he eventually joined as a Training Officer. In 1966 he transferred to the Auxiliary Medical Service, and is currently Medical Defence Staff Officer of that service.

Editor

Mr Lesie H.W. Paine is currently House Governor and Secretary of the Bethlem Royal Hospital and the Maudsley Hospital in London and Editor of the IHF quarterly journal, *World Hospitals.*

INDEX

Australia, *see* Sydney; health
  services, regionalisation of
Auxiliary Medical Service, Hong Kong:
  ambulances 336-7; casualty
  clearing hospital 336; convalescent
  units 336; dressing stations 335;
  formation 334; Forward Medical
  Aid Units 336; methadone centres
  339; organisation 334-5;
  peacetime role 338-9; role and
  function 335; supplies in
  emergency 338; training 337

Barangay–Health Centre Linkage:
  Barangay Health Post 345-7;
  centre itself 342-5; health
  workers 347-50; Metropolitan
  Manila Commission 341-2;
  National Economic Development
  Authority 340; programme
  contents 350-1; summary 351
Bogotá: access to services,
  improving 174; availability 170-1;
  beds, utilisation of 166; changes
  planned 174-7; demography 161-2;
  development 169; doctor per
  capita ratio 165; doctors, numbers
  of 171; economic distribution
  162; elderly, care of 178;
  environment programme 171-2, 177;
  expenditure, table of 166;
  experiments 178; finance 170;
  geographical distribution 162;
  Health Authority control diagram
  167; health centre availability 170;
  Health Service control diagram 167;
  health status 162-7; hospital
  admissions 171, availability of 170;
  incapacitating diseases 163;
  malnutrition 163; mental health
  172, 178; morbidity 162, 165;
  mortality 162, 164; mother/child
  programme 172; national health
  system 168-9; nurses, numbers of
  171; organisation 168; peripheral
  services 177; planning 169;
  policies 169; population 162, 164;
  problems 172-4; quality control

Bogotá–*cont.*
  of services 176-7; regionalisation
  168; rehabilitation 172; resources
  170-1; special group risks 175-6;
  staff, use of auxiliary 178;
  students, numbers of 171; studies
  178; support services 171;
  TRIAGE system 178; tuberculosis
  172; vaccination 172; venereal
  disease 172; vital statistics 164;
  see also planning health policy

Canada, *see* health care, monitoring
  procedures for; Toronto
community involvement, *see* mental
  health, community involvement
  in
contributors, notes on 360-2

emergency medical services, Tokyo:
  acute care cases 354-6, 358;
  admissions, causes of 354,
  numbers of 355; ambulance
  crews, medical duties of 357-8;
  Association of Emergency Institutions 358; beds, table of 358;
  death, causes of 356; divisional
  structure 357; hospitals 356;
  night duties 356-7; number of
  patients 355; problems 359;
  see also Auxiliary Medical
  Service, Hong Kong; Tokyo

financial crisis, *see* health care in
  financial crisis

health matters: care: monitoring
  procedures for: admissions 304,
  ambulance service 305, Assessment and Placement Service 305,
  bed utilisation 304, 305, by
  physicians 305-8, College of
  Physicians 307-8, fees, patients'
  306-7, financial control 303-4,
  Health Insurance Programme
  306, Hospital Accreditation
  Scheme 303, Hospital Information
  System 303-4, ICDA-8 codings